Surgical Management of Infectious Pleuropulmonary Diseases

Guest Editor

GAETANO ROCCO, MD, FRCSEd

THORACIC SURGERY CLINICS

www.thoracic.theclinics.com

Consulting Editor
MARK K. FERGUSON, MD

August 2012 • Volume 22 • Number 3

SAUNDERS an imprint of ELSEVIER, Inc.

W.B. SAUNDERS COMPANY
A Division of Elsevier Inc.

1600 John F. Kennedy Boulevard • Suite 1800 • Philadelphia, Pennsylvania 19103-2899

http://www.theclinics.com

THORACIC SURGERY CLINICS Volume 22, Number 3
August 2012 ISSN 1547-4127, ISBN-13: 978-1-4557-4895-2

Editor: Barbara Cohen-Kligerman
Developmental Editor: Teia Stone

Thoracic Surgery Clinics (ISSN 1547-4127) is published quarterly by Elsevier Inc., 360 Park Avenue South, New York, NY 10010-1710. Months of publication are February, May, August, and November. Business and editorial offices: 1600 John F. Kennedy Boulevard, Suite 1800, Philadelphia, PA 19103-2899. Periodicals postage paid at New York, NY, and additional mailing offices. Subscription prices are $322.00 per year (US individuals), $416.00 per year (US institutions), $154.00 per year (US Students), $400.00 per year (Canadian individuals), $526.00 per year (Canadian institutions), $209.00 per year (Canadian and foreign students), $426.00 per year (foreign individuals), and $526.00 per year (foreign institutions). Foreign air speed delivery is included in all Clinics' subscription prices. All prices are subject to change without notice. **POSTMASTER:** Send address changes to Thoracic Surgery Clinics, Elsevier Health Sciences Division, Subscription Customer Service, 3251 Riverport Lane, Maryland Heights, MO 63043. **Customer Service (orders, claims, online, change of address): Telephone: 1-800-654-2452 (U.S. and Canada); 314-447-8871 (outside U.S. and Canada). Fax: 314-447-8029. Email: journalscustomerservice-usa@elsevier.com (for print support); journalsonlinesupport-usa@elsevier.com (for online support).**

Reprints. For copies of 100 or more, of articles in this publication, please contact Commercial Rights Department, Elsevier Inc., 360 Park Avenue South, New York, NY 10010-1710. Tel: (212) 633-3812; Fax: (212) 462-1935; E-mail: reprints@elsevier.com.

Thoracic Surgery Clinics is covered in *MEDLINE/PubMed (Index Medicus)* and *EMBASE/Excerpta Medica.*

Printed and bound by CPI Group (UK) Ltd, Croydon, CR0 4YY

Transferred to Digital Print 2012

Contributors

CONSULTING EDITOR

MARK K. FERGUSON, MD
Professor of Surgery, Section of Cardiac and
Thoracic Surgery, The University of Chicago
Medical Center, Chicago, Illinois

GUEST EDITOR

GAETANO ROCCO, MD, FRCSEd
Director and Chief, Department of Thoracic
Surgery and Oncology, Division of Thoracic
Surgery, National Cancer Institute, Pascale
Foundation, Naples, Italy

AUTHORS

THIRUGNANAM AGASTHIAN, MBBS
Department of Cardiothoracic Surgery,
National University Hospital, Singapore

MARCO ALIFANO, MD, PhD
Professor, Department of Thoracic Surgery,
Hôtel-Dieu Hospital, Paris Descartes
University, Paris, France

JURY BRANDOLINI, MD
Department of Thoracic Surgery, Hôtel-Dieu
Hospital, Paris Descartes University, Paris,
France

DIANE DAMOTTE, MD, PhD
Professor, Department of Pathology,
Hôtel-Dieu Hospital, Paris Descartes
University, Paris, France

ANGELA DE PALMA, MD, PhD
Department of Thoracic Surgery, University
of Bari "Aldo Moro", Bari, Italy

CLAUDIO DELLA PONA, MD
Division of Thoracic Surgery, E. Morelli
Hospital, Sondalo, Italy

**PIERRE-EMMANUEL FALCOZ, MD,
PhD, FETS**
Service de Chirurgie Thoracique, Hôpitaux
Universitaires de Strasbourg, Strasbourg,
France

SONIA GAUCHER, MD, PhD
Associate Professor, Department of Plastic
Surgery, Hôtel-Dieu Hospital, Paris Descartes
University, Paris, France

CLAUDE GUINET, MD, PhD
Department of Pathology, Hôtel-Dieu Hospital,
Paris Descartes University, Paris, France

RAMSEY R. HACHEM, MD
Associate Professor, Department of Internal
Medicine, Washington University School of
Medicine in St Louis, St Louis, Missouri

SEMIH HALEZEROGLU, MD, FETCS
Professor of Thoracic Surgery and Chair,
Thoracic Surgery Department, Faculty of
Medicine, Acibadem University, Acibadem
Maslak Hospital, Istanbul, Turkey

DAWN E. JAROSZEWSKI, MD, MBA, FACS
Associate Professor of Surgery, Mayo Clinic
College of Medicine; Consultant, Department
of Surgery, Division of Cardiothoracic Surgery,
Mayo Clinic Arizona, Phoenix, Arizona

BENJAMIN D. KOZOWER, MD, MPH
Associate Professor of Surgery and Public
Health Sciences, Department of Surgery,
University of Virginia, Charlottesville, Virginia

RICHARD S. LAZZARO, MD
Chief, Division General Thoracic Surgery, New
York Methodist Hospital, Brooklyn, New York

KEVIN O. LESLIE, MD
Professor of Pathology, Mayo Clinic College of
Medicine; Consultant, Department of
Laboratory Medicine and Pathology, Mayo
Clinic Arizona, Phoenix, Arizona

JOSEPH LOCICERO III, MD
Professor of Surgery Emeritus, Department of
Surgery, SUNY Downstate, Mobile, Alabama

DOMENICO LOIZZI, MD
Department of Thoracic Surgery, University of
Foggia, Foggia, Italy

MICHELE LOIZZI, MD
Department of Thoracic Surgery, University of
Bari "Aldo Moro", Bari, Italy

GILBERT MASSARD, MD, PhD, FETS
Service de Chirurgie Thoracique, Hôpitaux
Universitaires de Strasbourg, Strasbourg, France

FABIO MASSERA, MD
Division of Thoracic Surgery, Maggiore della
Carità Hospital, Novara, Italy

ROBERT E. MERRITT, MD
Division of Thoracic Surgery, Department of
Cardiothoracic Surgery, Stanford University
School of Medicine, Stanford, California

BRYAN F. MEYERS, MD, MPH
Professor, Department of Surgery, Washington
University School of Medicine in St Louis,
St Louis, Missouri

JOHN D. MITCHELL, MD
Chief, Section of General Thoracic Surgery,
Division of Cardiothoracic Surgery,
Department of Surgery, University of Colorado
School of Medicine, Aurora; National Jewish
Health, Denver, Colorado

JOHN A. ODELL, MB ChB, FRCSEd, FACS
Cardiothoracic Surgeon, Mayo Clinic Florida;
Professor of Surgery, Mayo College of
Medicine, Jacksonville, Florida

ERDAL OKUR, MD
Associate Professor of Thoracic Surgery,
Thoracic Surgery Department; Faculty of
Medicine, Acibadem University, Acibadem
Bakirkoy Hospital, Istanbul, Turkey

ANNE OLLAND, MD, MSc
Service de Chirurgie Thoracique, Hôpitaux
Universitaires de Strasbourg, Strasbourg,
France

VINCENZO PAGLIARULO, MD
Department of Thoracic Surgery, University of
Bari "Aldo Moro", Bari, Italy

ELISEO PASSERA, MD
Division of Thoracic Surgery, Humanitas
Gavazzeni Hospital, Bergamo, Italy

ANTOINE RABBAT, MD
Department of Pneumology and Intensive
Care, Hôtel-Dieu Hospital, Paris Descartes
University, Paris, France

JEAN-FRANÇOIS REGNARD, MD
Professor, Department of Thoracic Surgery,
Hôtel-Dieu Hospital, Paris Descartes
University, Paris, France

ADRIANO RIZZI, MD
Division of Thoracic Surgery, Humanitas
Gavazzeni Hospital, Bergamo, Italy

MARIO ROBUSTELLINI, MD
Division of Thoracic Surgery, E. Morelli
Hospital, Sondalo, Italy

GAETANO ROCCO, MD, FRCSEd
Director and Chief, Department of Thoracic
Surgery and Oncology, Division of Thoracic
Surgery, National Cancer Institute, Pascale
Foundation, Naples, Italy

GEROLAMO ROSSI, MD
Division of Thoracic Surgery, Valduce Hospital,
Como, Italy

NICOLA SANTELMO, MD, FETS
Service de Chirurgie Thoracique, Hôpitaux
Universitaires de Strasbourg, Strasbourg,
France

JASON P. SHAW, MD
Attending Surgeon, Division General Thoracic Surgery, Maimonides Medical Center, Brooklyn, New York

JOSEPH B. SHRAGER, MD
Division of Thoracic Surgery, Department of Cardiothoracic Surgery, Stanford University School of Medicine, Stanford; Division of Thoracic Surgery, VA Palo Alto Health Care System, Palo Alto, California

FRANCESCO SOLLITTO, MD
Department of Thoracic Surgery, University of Foggia, Foggia, Italy

MATTHEW D. TAYLOR, MD
Surgical Resident, Joint General Surgery/General Thoracic Track, Department of Surgery, University of Virginia, Charlottesville, Virginia

M. OZAN TANYÜ, MD
Specialist in Radiology, Radiology Department, Acik MR Radiology Center, Nisantasi, Istanbul, Turkey

BRANDON J. WEBB, MD
Clinical Instructor, Department of Internal Medicine, Mayo Clinic Arizona, Phoenix, Arizona

MICHAEL J. WEYANT, MD
Associate Professor of Surgery, Section of General Thoracic Surgery, Division of Cardiothoracic Surgery, Department of Surgery, University of Colorado School of Medicine, Aurora, Colorado

CHAD A. WITT, MD
Assistant Professor, Department of Internal Medicine, Washington University School of Medicine in St Louis, St Louis, Missouri

JESSICA A. YU, MD
Section of General Thoracic Surgery, Division of Cardiothoracic Surgery, University of Colorado School of Medicine, Aurora, Colorado

Contents

diagnostic yield in pulmonary infection include bronchoscopy, ultrasound- and electromagnetic-guided endoscopy, transthoracic needle biopsy, and samples obtained with thoracoscopy. The spectrum of bacterial, mycobacterial, fungal, and viral pathogens implicated in pulmonary disease is discussed. Treatment strategies and guideline recommendations for antimicrobial selection are described for community-acquired, health care–associated, hospital-acquired, and ventilator-associated pneumonia, and for the most common fungal, mycobacterial, and viral infections. The state-of-the art in topical and aerosolized anti-infective therapy and an algorithm for managing hemoptysis are also presented.

Nowadays, antibiotic and antifungal therapy is effective in treating some of the infections that can involve the lung parenchyma in a localized manner, such as bacterial abscess and infection with nonresistant tuberculosis strains. However, other localized pulmonary infections, for example aspergilloma and mucormycosis, are highly resistant to nonsurgical therapy, and in these diseases there are no generally successful options that do not include surgical resection. This article reviews the indications for surgical intervention in the treatment of common infections involving the lung, and also focuses on the general approaches to their management.

Bronchiectasis and lung abscess are generally treated medically, reserving surgery for when medical treatment has failed. Current goals of surgical therapy for bronchiectasis are to offer possible cure and better quality of life after medical treatment has failed and to resolve and prevent complications, such as empyema, severe hemoptysis, and lung abscess. Whenever possible, complete resections of localized disease should be done, reserving palliative resections to selected diffuse bronchiectasis with localized severe disease. Most lung abscesses can be successfully treated medically provided early diagnosis and prompt treatment are instituted.

Aspergillomas are fungal balls within lung cavities. The natural history is variable. Hemoptysis is a dangerous sequela. Medical therapy is ineffective because of the lack of a lesion blood supply. Randomized trials are lacking. Surgery should be the treatment of choice in cases of hemoptysis, and even in asymptomatic patients, if lung function is not severely compromised. Cavernostomy and cavernoplasty may be options for high-risk patients. Percutaneous therapy should be reserved for patients who are not fit for surgery. Bronchial artery embolization is appropriate for symptomatic patients not suitable for surgery. Embolization could be considered a preoperative and temporary strategy.

Surgical participation in the management of fungal infections has changed since the advent of effective antimicrobials. Even so, a surgeon may be called on for a variety of reasons, depending on the specific fungal infection and the evolution of thoracic disease. Specific fungal infections are enumerated. Each organism, its clinical picture, and method of diagnosis are briefly described and the medical and surgical management of thoracic disease are discussed.

Hydatid disease is caused by the parasite *Echinococcus granulosus*. The liver and the lungs are common sites. When a cystic lesion is seen on CT scan, diagnosis is made based on the patient having lived in an endemic area. Serologic tests are used for differential diagnosis. Medical treatment is centered on albendazole. Surgery is recommended either by open or endoscopic technique depending on the characteristics of the cysts and the patient. Complications of surgery are rare except for prolonged air leaks. Mortality occurs when the cyst is located in the central nervous system or occludes major vessels.

Thoracic surgeons often treat children with infections: pneumonia with abscess and/or empyema, multiresistant or complicated tuberculosis, or parasitic and fungal infections. The pediatric patient with serious infection presents anatomic and metabolic-functional frailty. Anesthesiologists and surgeons must consider this aspect to reduce surgical impairment and improve outcome. This article reviews the causes, pathophysiology, clinical aspects, diagnosis, and management of pleuropulmonary infections of surgical interest in childhood.

Infectious complications are a major cause of morbidity and mortality in solid organ transplant recipients. Infections with viruses, bacteria, and fungi have all been associated with the development of bronchiolitis obliterans syndrome (chronic allograft rejection) in lung transplant recipients. Lung transplant recipients have a higher risk of infectious complications than recipients of other solid organs because of the intensity of immunosuppression, blunted cough mechanism, and constant exposure to the environment. This review provides a broad overview of the infectious complications encountered in caring for patients who have undergone lung transplantation.

Surgical treatment of lung diseases is based on removal of the affected lung tissue, achieved by atypical or anatomic lung resection. Infectious lung diseases are generally treated by medical therapy, including medications, chest physiotherapy, bronchoscopic toilet, and respiratory rehabilitation. Surgical management of infectious disease of the lung is integrated in the multispecialty care. This article focuses exclusively on nonresectional surgery and other alternatives to lung resection and addresses bacterial infection and fungal disease of the lung.

> Empyema remains a major source of morbidity and health care expenditure in the thoracic surgery community. Early intervention in pleural space infections is key to prevention of chronic empyemas and the need for surgical intervention. The advent of video-assisted thoracoscopic surgery has made it possible to treat stage I and stage II empyemas with significantly less morbidity. Although management of chronic empyema remains a significant challenge, surgical intervention is usually successful in cleaning up the pleural space.

THORACIC SURGERY CLINICS

DOWNLOAD Free App!

Review Articles
THE CLINICS

NOW AVAILABLE FOR YOUR iPhone and iPad

Preface

Surgery for Thoracic Infections—The Mother of All Surgeries

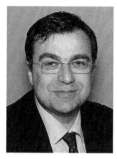

Gaetano Rocco, MD, FRCSEd
Guest Editor

In daily thoracic surgical practice characterized by "oncogenic addiction," the extent and importance of infections of surgical interest are underestimated. However, vast geographic areas of our planet are still plagued by thoracic infections.

In the Western world, reduced exposure to pleuropulmonary infections has rendered surgical training somewhat incomplete. In our current state of knowledge, surgery for infectious disease is misinterpreted as the surgical management of infectious complications. In contrast, the history of thoracic surgery has been marked by surgeons contributing with their skills to the anatomic and biological eradication of pleuropulmonary infections. Experienced surgeons will likely agree that surgery for thoracic infections is the *mother of all surgeries*, decisively contributing to the birth of modern cardiothoracic surgery.

A number of images remain carved in stone in the memories of trainees and thoracic surgeons: severely depleted and emaciated patients, dissection of complex mycetomas growing into the apex, the threat of postoperative bleeding despite extremely cautious hemostasis, and the unrelenting purulent discharge from a Petzer drain of chronic patients on the ward. These images define where we come from and where we belong.

This issue of the *Thoracic Surgery Clinics* is dedicated to the surgical management of these conditions, which require a mix of expertise, experience, and, at times, a lot of courage. I believe that all of these surgical qualities are outlined well in the articles. My appreciation goes to Mark Ferguson—Consulting Editor of the *Thoracic Surgery Clinics*—and to the contributors to this issue for their help in focusing the readers' attention once again on the challenging clinical scenarios often witnessed in desperate patients for whom we can provide the prospect of possible cure.

Gaetano Rocco, MD, FRCSEd
Division of Thoracic Surgery
Department of Thoracic Surgery and Oncology
National Cancer Institute, Pascale Foundation
Via Semmola 81, 80131
Naples, Italy

E-mail address:
Gaetano.Rocco@btopenworld.com

Thorac Surg Clin 22 (2012) xiii
doi:10.1016/j.thorsurg.2012.05.007

The History of Surgery for Pulmonary Tuberculosis

John A. Odell, MB ChB, FRCSEd

KEYWORDS

- Thoracic surgery • Pulmonary tuberculosis • Sanatorium therapy • Collapse therapy

KEY POINTS

- Thoracic surgical procedures evolved from surgical management of tuberculosis; lung resections, muscle flaps, and thoracoscopy all began with efforts to control the disease.
- The discovery of antituberculosis drugs in 1944 to 1946 made sanatorium therapy and collapse therapy in all its forms obsolete and changed thoracic surgery dramatically.
- Currently, management of tuberculosis is primarily medical, and surgery has a minimal role.
- Today surgery is usually only performed in patients with tuberculosis when the diagnosis is necessary, who have complications or sequelae of the disease, or who have active disease resistant to therapy.

Surgery of the twentieth century can boast no more important advance than that now being made in the operative treatment of pulmonary tuberculosis.
—First sentence of John Alexander's book, The Surgery of Pulmonary Tuberculosis.[1]

Collapse therapy, the only important addition to the treatment of pulmonary tuberculosis since the sanatorium was introduced more than fifty years ago, has revolutionized the management of phthisis.
—First sentence of John Alexander's second book, The Collapse Therapy of Pulmonary Tuberculosis.[2]

INTRODUCTION

Pulmonary tuberculosis was the disease that spawned thoracic surgery (including thoracoscopy) and pulmonology. During the eighteenth and nineteenth centuries, the population shift to cities and the ensuing overcrowding contributed to tuberculosis being the most common cause of death.

It was apparent to many that tuberculosis was a communicable disease. When Chopin wished to return to France from the island of Majorca, where it was hoped that the climate would lead to a cure, no cab or carriage would carry him to the boat; the weakened Chopin was finally transported in a wheelbarrow. Similarly, in Rome, no servant could be found who was willing to care for Keats.

Although laymen suspected that the disease was communicable, medical proof had to await Koch's presentation, entitled "Die Tuberculose" (On Tuberculosis), to the Berlin Physiologic Society on March 24, 1882. The electrifying atmosphere that developed at the presentation is vividly described in the book *The Forgotten Plague* by Frank Ryan.[3] Present in the crowded room were Virchow, Loeffler, and Ehrlich, who described "that evening to be the most important experience of my scientific life."[3] Three weeks after the presentation, the lecture was published[4]; 12 days later an English summary was published in the *London Times*, and a few weeks later, on May 3, it was published in *The New York Times*. The rapidity of the spread of the news and its publication in the lay press testify to how pervasive and threatening tuberculosis was at the time. Here at last was an enemy (the tubercle bacillus) to which attention could be directed.

Mayo College of Medicine, Mayo Clinic Florida, 4500 San Pablo Road, Jacksonville, FL 32224, USA
E-mail address: odell.john@mayo.edu

Thorac Surg Clin 22 (2012) 257–269
doi:10.1016/j.thorsurg.2012.05.003
1547-4127/12/$ – see front matter © 2012 Elsevier Inc. All rights reserved.

Folk Remedies

Many folk remedies existed for treatment of the disease. Society attempted to reduce communicability of the disease (**Fig. 1**). One of the most popular myths was of a change in climate and diet. It was well recognized that individuals in rural communities were less likely to get the disease and, if affected, to live longer than those in urban communities, but this was more likely a reflection of overcrowding. Ultraviolet light kills acid-fast bacilli in the laboratory, and therefore patients were encouraged to spend time exposed to sunlight (**Fig. 2**). Physical activity in children supposedly conferred resistance; in adults, rest was advocated following the suggestion of Hippocrates that horizontal rest was good for leg ulcers. When Laennec discovered he had the disease, he returned to his childhood home in Brittany to breathe the fresh air and drink goat's milk.

Sanatoria

The first sanatorium specific for tuberculosis was established by Brehmer, who was supposedly cured of his cavitating tuberculosis when he traveled to the Himalayas. At Gobersdorf, Germany, where the sanatorium was situated, high altitude, bed rest, exposure to the environment, and good nutrition were pursued as therapeutic options. Other famous sanatoriums included the Trudeau sanatorium in the Adirondacks. The most famous was in Davos, Switzerland, the highest town in Europe, where Robert Louis Stevenson was treated. This sanatorium was the setting for Thomas Mann's novel *The Magic Mountain*.[5] Davos is now better known for the World Economic Summit and winter sports than tuberculosis. The sanatoria have been turned into hotels; the rooms once occupied by patients now accommodate politicians and economists, and the spittoons lining

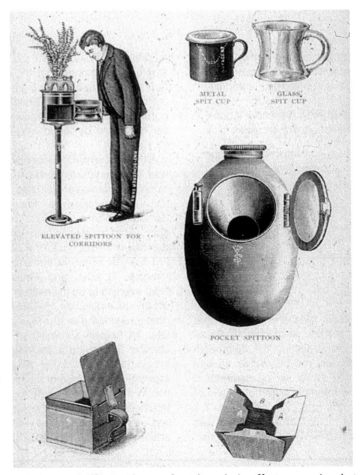

Fig. 1. Before the development of effective therapy for tuberculosis, efforts were aimed at reducing spread of the disease. Spitting in public was abhorrent and could engender a fine. Illustrated is a catalog page offering spittoons for sale. (Available at: http://www.flickr.com/photos/94515086@N00/1601158457/.)

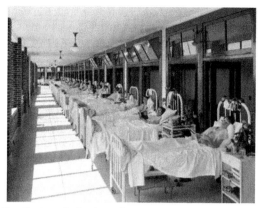

Fig. 2. A typical tuberculosis ward. Patients were expected to lie in bed most of the day exposed to the elements. (*Courtesy of* University of Louisville Photographic Archives, ULPA CS 076031; with permission.)

the hallways have been replaced with flowerpots. The sanatorium in Battle Creek, Michigan was associated with Dr William Kellogg, who developed the breakfast cereals associated with his name. One of his patients was C.W. Post, who developed his own breakfast cereal, Post Toasties.

Despite the hundreds of tuberculosis sanatoria built around the world, no scientific proof exists that sanatorium therapy had any influence on the disease. Sanatorium therapy did, however, concentrate patients with the disease in one place, which contributed to better understanding of the disease. Many of the physicians treating these patients saw their practice disappear after the discovery of drugs to treat the disease; they branched into a new field of medicine, pulmonology, using many of the skills acquired in managing lung disease and interpreting chest radiographs.

SURGICAL APPROACHES TO TUBERCULOSIS
Drainage Therapy

The adult form of pulmonary tuberculosis is characterized by cavities predominantly affecting the apex of the upper and lower lobes. Abscess cavities elsewhere in the body are managed with simple drainage, and therefore it is not difficult to imagine that drainage of these tuberculous cavities would be the first surgical procedures pursued in an attempt to control the disease. Isolated reports of this surgical approach can be found[6,7]; some are from before the discovery of radiography by Roentgen in 1885, testifying to the clinical skills of the physicians involved. Until Monaldi[8] published a series of cases in 1939, drainage was uncommonly performed; thereafter it had a temporary period of enthusiasm, which waned after the realization that improvement was usually temporary.

The Barrier to Chest Surgery, and Early Resection Procedures

One of the barriers to surgical procedures on the lung in the late nineteenth and early twentieth century was that the lung collapsed whenever the chest was opened. Sauerbruch was one of thoracic surgery's great pioneers. Von Mikulicz in Breslau, Sauerbruch's mentor, stated to him while he was working as a voluntary assistant, "Hundreds of thousands of people are succumbing to tuberculosis, because as yet no one has been able to operate within the thorax."[9] This statement had two implications: it indicated that surgical resection was being considered to deal with the disease, and it stimulated Sauerbruch to find a solution. His solution of a negative pressure chamber, which worked to some degree, was unfortunately cumbersome. The chamber was soon replaced by a simpler method of positive pressure ventilation, initially through a chamber around the head, then a mask, and later an endotracheal tube. Sauerbruch's efforts to solve the problem, and his surgical ability and forceful personality, made him famous throughout Europe. Sauerbruch anesthetized Mikulicz during his laparotomy, during which widespread metastatic gastric cancer was found, unfortunately.

Adhesions at the apex are commonly found in patients with tuberculosis, and surgeons used this knowledge, before the previously mentioned techniques had gained favor, to their benefit. Sarfert[10] of Berlin stated that "by excising the second rib from its sternal end to the axilla one can shell out the whole of the apex of the lung, delimit the cavities by palpation, and incise and tampon them extrapleurally, without fear of invading the pleural cavity."

The first attempt to resect a portion of tuberculous lung occurred in 1883 when Block operated on his own cousin, who was thought to have apical tuberculosis.[11] Block resected apices of both lungs, but his cousin died. At postmortem no evidence of tuberculosis was found. The distraught Block shot himself. Other early attempts at resection were made, with similar poor patient results. Tuffier[12] in 1891 and Doyen[13] in 1895 reported single successes with wedge excision of apical lesions, but most were unsuccessful.

In 1907 Gluck[14] performed a lobectomy on a 5-year-old with success. The first lobectomy for tuberculosis in the United States was performed by Babcock[15] in 1908. The right lower lobe was delivered through the chest wall and clamped sequentially and oversewn. The patient died, and at postmortem the remaining lobes were atelectatic and had tuberculosis. A hiatus of 27 years followed before the next reported lobectomy in the United States.[16] During the next several years, resections were performed sporadically and in small numbers. At the meeting of the American Association of Thoracic Surgery in 1938, 18 cases were reported; at the 1940 meeting, 50 cases were reported, with 16 deaths.[11] In discussion, resection was suggested to be better after thoracoplasty to diminish the dead space and possibility of infection; others emphasized that resection was dangerous.[11] Resection was not actively pursued as a means of managing the disease, because collapse therapy (the advance mentioned by Alexander at the beginning of the article) and its variations were the preferred treatment options. In fact Alexander, in the chapter on the Evolution of Surgical Therapy in his book devoted to collapse therapy, places the description of pulmonary resection into the section "proposed operations which have not been generally adopted."[2] Surgical resection was performed in patients in whom collapse therapy had failed, the cavities had not collapsed, who had a stenotic bronchus, and who experienced recurrent hemoptysis—all patients who would be expected to have a high mortality.

In 1943, Churchill and Klopstock[17] challenged the prevailing view of resection after collapse therapy and once all other options had failed. They published a small series in which patients with lobar involvement underwent lobectomy using the individual vessel ligation technique rather than thoracoplasty. They believed that lobectomy was more conservative of pulmonary function than a seven-rib thoracoplasty. After this report, the surgical attitude swung to some degree against collapse therapy and toward surgical resection primarily.[11] However, mortality was still high in the pre-streptomycin era; in 1946 Overholt and colleagues[18] had 200 cases with a mortality of 25%.

Four years later, after several years of streptomycin use, the picture was different; surgical procedures performed for tuberculosis and surgical complications and mortality had decreased dramatically. Chamberlain[19] of New York proposed segmental resection to control the disease. He noted that the disease was commonly localized to three segments: the apical and posterior segments of the upper lobe and the superior segment of the lower lobe. By 1953 he had performed 300 cases with a low mortality of 3%.

Unusual Operations

Some of the procedures undertaken to treat tuberculosis were bizarre in nature. What was the thinking and logic behind these procedures? They were performed in a similar vein to other therapeutic approaches—some previously discussed with respect to sanatorium treatment and others involving many different bizarre medications—

with a sense of frustration and desperation in treating an extremely common lethal disease. Instead of being critical, one must be aware of the clinical circumstances of the time.

In 1858 Freund, as reported by others[20,21] (no original report can be found), based on necroscopy observations, concluded that active apical tuberculosis was more common in patients whose first rib was shorter or whose first cartilage was stiffer than normal. He also noted evidence of healed tuberculosis in cadavers in which spontaneous rupture of the first costal cartilage and false-joint formation had occurred. The absence of apical tuberculosis in children was explained by the apex of the lung being inferior to the first rib, and therefore uninfluenced by abnormalities of the first rib. He advocated subchondral resection of approximately 0.5 cm of the first rib cartilage and interposition of a portion of pectoralis major. This bizarre operation with illogical basis was popular for some time, and represented the first attempt at managing pulmonary tuberculosis using a surgical procedure on the chest wall.

Scaleniotomy and scalenectomy, the division or excision of the scalene muscles in the neck, was advocated to lessen respiratory movements of the upper lung.[22,23] It was usually performed in association with a collapse procedure, or to assist the resection of the anterior portion of the first rib at a subsequent thoracoplasty.

In 1913 Alvarez[24] operated on four patients with advanced tuberculosis. He stretched the second, third, and fourth intercostal nerves "to paralyze by excess of stimulation via the rami communicantes, the vasoconstrictor fibers supplying the lung." He hoped that congestion of the lung would be produced and that the hyperemia would influence the disease. The dyspnea and dullness that lasted 3 to 6 days was attributed to encroachment on the alveolar spaces by the dilated blood vessels, rather than the likely pneumothorax or hemothorax. Three of the four patients soon died. He later reported on a further 12 patients, who were improved but not cured, because they did not complete the sanatorium treatment.[25]

In 1921 Sayago[26,27] proposed placement of a bone graft removed from the tibia and placed in a subpleural position between the first and forth ribs. The presence of the graft was to excite a reaction in the lung, increasing blood supply and causing growth of fibrous tissue, which would encapsulate the tuberculous lesions. Three patients underwent the procedure; "one died, one improved," and one later underwent a thoracoplasty.[28]

Ligation of the pulmonary artery was initially reported by Sauerbruch[21] and later by Schlaepfer,[29,30] who also performed animal experiments to assess effectiveness. The lungs shrunk to approximately half their normal size; collateral bronchial arteries enlarged and the alveolar walls became thickened. Based on his experiments, Schlaepfer[30] recommended ligation of the lobar branches of affected lung in conjunction with phrenic paralysis, in preference to collapse therapy using pneumothorax or thoracoplasty. Baumgartner and also Eloesser, reported by Alexander,[2] proposed ligation of the pulmonary artery and veins in patients with severe hemoptysis. Blood supply from pleural adhesions was expected to keep the lung viable. Others proposed simply ligating the pulmonary veins to the affected lobe.[31] Significant pleural adhesions made the surgical intent difficult; only small series of patients were reported.

The vascular approach to tuberculous surgical treatment gets even more unbelievable. In 1929 Babcock[32] divided the common carotid artery and jugular vein on the side of the tuberculous lung and anastomosed their proximal ends. His theory was that diversion of blood would decrease the rate and amplitude of respiratory movements and produce a hyperemia around the tubercles. At 17 days he reported that the respiratory rate in the 28-year-old patient had been reduced such that 11,500 respiratory cycles per day had been saved the patient, who was discharged with a less productive cough.

Adams[33,34] suggested induced bronchial stenosis. In experimental animals he had induced bronchial stenosis by applying 35% silver nitrate through a bronchoscope. He had noted after injecting tubercle bacilli into the blood stream that induced bilateral pulmonary lesions healed quicker in the atelectatic lobes.[33] Of the five patients on whom he reported, only one experienced questionable benefit.[34]

Collapse Therapy

Terms used within this section are summarized in **Box 1**. James Carson[35] of Liverpool proposed compressive therapy, largely through creating a pneumothorax, to treat a lung abscess or tuberculosis. He wrote that "the diseased part would be placed in a quiescent state and not be disturbed by the movements of respiration, and the divided surfaces (the cavity walls) would be brought into close contact by the same resilient power (air) which before had kept them asunder." Carson[35] apparently experimented on animals, and even persuaded a surgeon to attempt the procedure on two patients, but, because of extensive adhesions, no free space could be found. He thought that disease in both lungs could be managed by alternating the pneumothorax.

John Alexander, the seventeenth president of the American Association for Thoracic Surgeon, wrote two books on the surgical treatment of

Box 1 Explanation of terms	
Thoracoplasty	The resection of ribs with the intention of decreasing the size of the chest cavity
Scaleniotomy and scalenectomy	The division or excision of the scalene muscles in the neck
Pneumolysis	The division of adhesions within the chest to improve an induced pneumothorax
Apicolysis	Freeing the apex of the lung in the extrapleural plane
Plombage	Filling of the extrapleural space by artificial material or tissue

tuberculosis, while himself bedbound with the disease and recovering from his own thoracoplasty.[1,2] He expanded on the rationale for bedrest and collapse therapy. The rationale is somewhat difficult to understand given current thinking, but an attempt to do so is made using Alexander's own words. He stressed that tuberculosis heals through fibrous encapsulation.

Individual resistance to the disease, which could be influenced by environmental factors or tuberculin therapy, was likely the most important factor for healing. The next most important factor—the most important one capable of control—is functional rest of the diseased part. Rest is the keystone of successful treatment of tuberculosis of any organ and the more completely it can be achieved the better is the result. Compression therapy, whether by artificial pneumothorax or by thoracoplasty or other surgical method causes partial or complete rest of the more diseased lung. Thereby the most important condition for the repair of the tuberculous lesion is accomplished.[1]

He elaborated that with rest, lymph flow, carrying toxins to the general circulation, ceases. The temperature of the patient decreases and coughing and spread of infected secretions to other healthy areas of the lung diminishes. "Next to rest probably the most important clinical effect of compression therapy is the lessening in size of the cavities, ulcers and other tuberculous lesions and of the alveoli and smaller bronchi." He likened the compressed lung being emptied of its waste products being "like a pressed sponge." He reported that "cavities whose walls are not very stiff are obliterated to mere clefts by thoracoplasty; mechanical compression accomplishes part of this and secondary fibrous shrinkage the rest. The clefts then fill with granulation tissue rich in blood vessels and become obliterated, or a smooth clean mucous membrane replaces the previous dirty lining." These selected passages do not encompass, nor do justice, to the concept that Alexander elaborated on in his two books, one of which was 700 pages devoted to collapse therapy.[1,2]

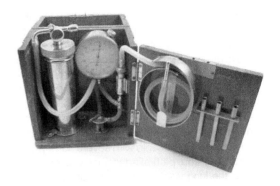

Fig. 3. Apparatus used to induce an artificial pneumothorax. (*Image courtesy of* Phisick: Medical Antiquities; with permission. Available at: http://phisick.com/; accessed June 25 2012.)

Induced Pneumothorax

In 1882 Forlannini[36] of Pavia, 60 years after Carson's proposal, published his first article on artificial pneumothorax. He had noted that some patients with tuberculous who developed a pneumothorax seemed to get better. Those who developed a pyopneumothorax obviously worsened. He reasoned that if a pneumothorax is induced and compressed the lung, the procedure could be used therapeutically. Forlannini's initial report was overshadowed by Koch's famous lecture and report of the same year. The technique resurfaced in 1894 when Forlannini's second article was published and the results presented in Rome.[37] He placed small volumes of nitrogen, because it tended to get absorbed slowly, into the chest daily until he believed sufficient volume was present. He recognized that adhesions limited the curative value.

John Murphy, the famous Chicago surgeon, heard of Forlannini's work and sent his assistant, William Lemke,[38] to learn about the procedure. In characteristic fashion, Murphy popularized the procedure,[39] so that in Germany, where it was adopted by Brauer,[40] an internist, it became known as the Murphy operation. Murphy and Lemke proposed instilling large volumes of nitrogen in the early stages of disease, before adhesions had formed, with short treatment duration[41]; Forlannini was less cavalier and believed the pneumothorax needed to be maintained for years.[42] In Europe, pneumothorax became the most popular form of treatment for many years, but was only used more frequently in the United States from the mid 1920s. **Fig. 3** shows an example of apparatus used to regulate the extent of pneumothorax.

A major problem with induced pneumothorax is that adhesions may prevent the establishment of adequate collapse. It was the frequent inability to collapse the lung with an induced pneumothorax that spawned other operations to affect collapse.

Pneumolysis procedures were performed to divide the adhesions so that a pneumothorax would be possible. The open operation was first performed by Friedrich[43] in 1908, but the patient died. Other surgeons also performed the procedure with poor results and a high incidence of complications, and the procedure was basically abandoned. Closed intrapleural pneumolysis refers to attempts to divide the adhesions without thoracotomy. Some of these attempts were made using radiographic fluoroscopic control but were soon abandoned because of poor definition.[44] The procedure that made closed intrapleural pneumolysis possible was thoracoscopy, devised by Jacobeus[45–47] of Stockholm, the forerunner of modern day video-assisted thoracoscopic and laparoscopic surgery. He used a cystoscope-like instrument introduced through one intercostal space, with a cautery instrument introduced through another.

Thoracoplasty

Thoracoplasty had actually been used to manage empyema before being considered for management of pulmonary tuberculosis. de Cerenville[7] of Lausanne was the first to perform the operation for tuberculosis, and reported on four cases with apical cavitary disease. However, he only removed small portions of anterior ribs. Brauer,[48] an internist working in Marburg, recognized that, for thoracoplasty to work, the lung needed to collapse as much as with a pneumothorax. He persuaded Friedrich (see previous paragraph), who had previously been Sauerbruch's chief, to remove the second to ninth ribs. Under local anesthesia, Friedrich resected the ribs, periosteum, intercostal muscle, and nerves. This operation produced considerable paradoxic movement. The first patient remarkably survived and 14 months later was much improved. Of the next six patients, three died. It seems surprising that the mortality was not higher. Over time, Brauer, the internist, and Friedrich, the surgeon, made several modifications to reduce the high mortality of approximately 30%.[49] The team went through phases, including removing 11 ribs in one stage; performing the procedure in two stages; resecting ribs subperiosteally to allow regeneration and stabilization; combining the procedure with pneumothorax and phrenic nerve avulsion; and, lastly, only removing upper ribs.[50]

Meanwhile, Wilms[7,51] of Heidelberg and Sauerbruch, Friedrich's previous pupil now working in Zurich and operating on patients with tuberculosis at the tuberculous sanatorium at Davos, independently developed operations that were a compromise between the earlier limited, low-risk, but less successful procedures of de Cerenville and the extensive, high-risk procedures of Brauer and Friedrich. Their operations were more conservative in that they preferentially resected the posterior portions of the ribs and transverse processes of the thoracic vertebra, an operation that became known as an *extrapleural paravertebral thoracoplasty* (**Fig. 4**). Both surgeons modified their procedures over time. Sauerbruch, in particular, performed hundreds of thoracoplasties. The author's own mentor, Andrew Logan, visited Sauerbruch in Berlin before World War II and described him performing a thoracoplasty in approximately a half hour. Sauerbruch was a tyrant in the operating room; many of the procedures were performed under local anesthesia.[52] Logan described that alongside the patient

was a metal table covered in sterile towels. As each portion of rib was removed, still attached to the rib cutter, Sauerbruch would bang the instrument loudly against the metal table, causing the rib fragment to fly off the instrument around the room. He was too impatient to remove the rib fragment in any other way. Rib fragments were flying around the room at roughly 1-minute intervals.

Sauerbruch was a pioneer in thoracic surgery. In 1911 he performed the first thymectomy for myasthenia gravis using the transcervical approach.[53] In 1913 he described phrenicotomy for the treatment of pulmonary tuberculosis.[53,54] He performed the first successful pericardiectomy for constrictive pericarditis.[21] His autobiography describes the treatment of Lenin, Rothschild, and King Constantine of Greece, among others.[9] When war broke out in 1914, he volunteered and was appointed surgeon to the German army. He was exposed to the carnage at Ypres. While treating many amputees, he developed a crude artificial hand.

In 1918 he was offered the chair of surgery at Munich by the Bavarian government. He described vividly the revolution, the great influenza epidemic, and severe inflation that nearly crippled Germany.[9] At that stage Nissen was his assistant, as was Lebsche. He met Hitler in 1925 for the first time when Hitler attempted to appoint General Ludendorff, a patient of Sauerbruch's, Field Marshall.

In 1927 Sauerbruch succeeded Bier (who pioneered the Bier's block technique) as the surgical chair of surgery in Berlin. His operating room became a Mecca for thoracic surgeons worldwide. His patients included Röntgen and Hindenburg.

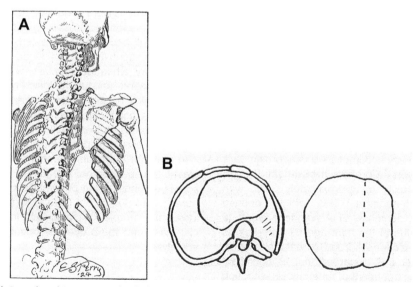

Fig. 4. (*A, B*) Sauerbruch's paravertebral thoracoplasty. The reduction in size of the chest is diagrammatically shown in the axial view. (*From* Alexander J. The collapse therapy of pulmonary tuberculosis. Springfield (IL): Charles C Thomas; 1937.)

In recognition of his treatment of Hindenburg, he was given the honorary title of State Councilor by Goering. In 1933, under the Third Reich, Jews were being persecuted. After a visit to Turkey, he recommended his assistant Nissen, a Jew, for a position there.

In Berlin, Sauerbruch became a member of the Mittwochsgesellschaft, the Wednesday Society, a club founded in the 18th century by Wilhelm von Humboldt, in which a limited membership of 16 eminent people met alternate Wednesdays at one of the member's houses. At these meetings the host gave a talk on a subject of his particular field. Five of these members, who were close friends of Sauerbruch's, were involved in planning the assassination attempt on Hitler and were executed.[55,56] In 1943 Sauerbruch was asked to treat von Stauffenberg, Hitler's would-be assassin, who had been wounded in Africa and had been brought to Berlin. von Stauffenberg did not allow Sauerbruch to remove the bullet that had passed through his eye and had lodged in the occipital bone, nor did he allow construction of a Sauerbruch-arm.[55]

In the purge that followed the failed assassination attempt, in which hundreds were imprisoned, tortured, and executed, Sauerbruch's son Peter was arrested because of correspondence discovered between him and von Stauffenberg. Sauerbruch himself was interrogated, but Gebhardt, a former student of Sauerbruch's working with the SS and as Himmler's doctor, convinced Hitler of Sauerbruch's innocence, and he and his son were released from prison. Gebhardt was hanged later after the Nuremberg trials.[55,56]

To return to the story of thoracoplasty, the operation slowly became refined and more standardized. The surgeon who popularized the procedure in the United States was Alexander.[1,2] The number of ribs resected usually was not more than seven to nine and tended to be of the same extent as the Brauer-Friedrich operation. Portions of the posterior and lateral ribs are removed, but usually no more than two to three ribs at one time, requiring staged procedures (**Fig. 5**). In Alexander's hands, mortality was approximately 10%, with sputum negativity accomplished in approximately 75% of survivors.[2] Compare this with the Brauer-Friedrich mortality of approximately 30%, with 35% sputum-negative. This article opened with the first sentence of Alexander's book to show the status of the fight against tuberculosis up until the discovery of drugs to treat the disease. Thoracoplasty was regarded as a significant advance in the treatment of tuberculosis, although currently it has a reputation for being a painful disfiguring operation, and many surgeons have never seen one performed. However, it does have a small

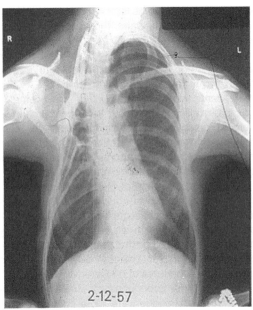

Fig. 5. Chest radiograph of a patient who had a thoracoplasty for treatment of tuberculosis. An eight-rib thoracoplasty, including the first rib, was performed. Note the inevitable scoliosis toward the side of the thoracoplasty. The ribs seem to have been resected subperiosteally as regeneration and formation of a bony carapace has occurred. (*Courtesy of* Mayo Clinic archives; with permission.)

place in the management of postresection residual spaces or a pulmonary cavity.[57]

It is not difficult to imagine why thoracoplasty was popular. The operation involved the chest wall, and efforts were concentrated on keeping extrapleural. Many operations were performed using local anesthesia. Operations for resection within the chest were difficult because of the extensive adhesions generally present. In the first 4 decades of the twentieth century, when thoracoplasty was a predominant operation for tuberculosis, no antibiotics, blood banks, double-lumen endotracheal tubes, or accurate monitoring of oxygen saturation or arterial blood pressure were available. A thoracoplasty was obviously a safer procedure for most surgeons.

In many of the patients undergoing a thoracoplasty, the apex did not adequately collapse, and some surgeons added pneumolysis to the procedure.[58] Carl Semb,[58,59] instead of mobilizing the lung in the intrapleural plane, did it in the extrafascial plane and the procedure became known as apicolysis.

Extrapleural Apical Procedures

The following procedures are included under collapse procedures because they follow the apicolysis procedure popularized by Semb.[58,59] In addition, many of the procedures whose descriptions follow were also performed in combination with thoracoplasty.

In 1891, Tuffier[12] performed an extrapleural dissection before his apical resection. Two years later he performed a similar procedure of extrapleural apical dissection (apicolysis) for severe hemoptysis, which stopped. In 1910 he performed a similar procedure in which he filled the space with body fat, hoping to establish a permanent collapse.[60] Thereafter followed a series of different collapse procedures in which the apex of the lung was freed extrapleurally and the space between the extrapleurally mobilized lung and the unresected chest wall was filled with either air[61,62] (extrapleural pneumothorax), pedicled muscle,[63,64] oil and wax (oleothorax) (**Fig. 6**),[2,65] inflatable rubber bags (the forerunner of tissue expanders),[66] polyethylene sheeting,[67] or hollow spheres of polymethyl methacrylate (perspex) (**Fig. 7**).[68] In 1934 Alexander described the use of pectoralis major and minor muscles with intact neurovascular structures as extrapleural filling—the forerunner to the present-day muscle flap transfer.[69] The rationale for these procedures was that disfigurement and paradoxic movement of the chest wall was avoided. Despite attempts at sterilizing the foreign material that was placed, inevitably, in most patients, infection ensued, with development of chronic sinuses, empyema, and fistula formation. Occasionally patients survived, and decades later the chest radiographs became the subject of interesting historical teaching.[70]

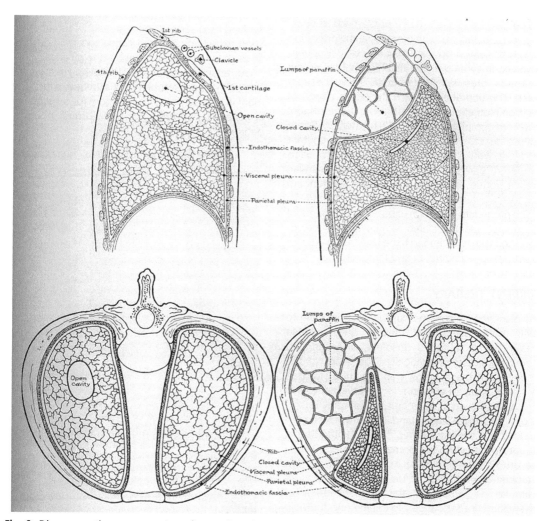

Fig. 6. Diagrammatic representation of extrapleural pneumonolysis with paraffin filling. The warmed lumps of paraffin with a melting point of 51°C are introduced via a small defect created in the chest wall. The goal was to collapse cavities to allow healing. (*From* Alexander J. The collapse therapy of pulmonary tuberculosis. Springfield (IL): Charles C Thomas; 1937.)

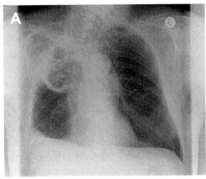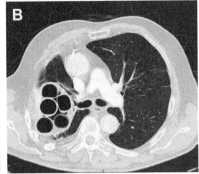

Fig. 7. (*A, B*) Hollow spheres of polymethyl methacrylate (perspex) used as an apical plombage. (*From* Tezel CS, Goldstraw P. Plombage thoracoplasty with Lucite balls. Ann Thorac Surg 2005;79:1063; with permission.)

Induced Diaphragmatic Paralysis

In 1911, Stuertz[71] proposed paralysis of the diaphragm in patients in whom a pneumothorax could not be induced. Sauerbruch[54] performed the operation on five patients with benefit. As the operation was relatively simple it became very popular; however, in some patients diaphragmatic function returned, presumably because of accessory fibers. The operation evolved through a period of avulsion (sometimes associated with hemorrhage) to a more complete procedure in the neck.[72] Some advocated crushing in selected patients so that recovery would occur[73]; later others proposed temporary paralysis as a first step.[74] There was even a vogue of inducing a pneumoperitoneum to cause elevation of the hemidiaphragms (**Fig. 8**).

The procedure, although used as an independent procedure, was associated with lower-lobe atelectasis, and with time tended to be used as an adjunct to induced pneumothorax and thoracoplasty.

CURRENT THERAPY

The discovery of antituberculosis drugs in 1944 to 1946 made sanatorium therapy and collapse therapy in all its forms obsolete, and changed thoracic surgery dramatically. The story of the discovery of these drugs was beautifully written by Frank Ryan.[3] Lehmann[75,76] in Sweden (para-aminosalicylic acid), Domagk in Germany (isoniazid), and Waksman and his researchers[77] working with the Mayo Clinic[78] in the United States (streptomycin) were the prime discoverers. When the drug treatments were made known, a more dramatic event could not be imagined; it was as dramatic as would be the announcement of a genuine cure for cancer. Medicine and thoracic surgery were changed forever. The era that saw the birth of thoracic surgery[79] has passed, and requests for a Tuffier retractor, a Lilienthal guillotine, a Doyen raspatory, or a Sauerbruch rib holding forceps have been replaced by requests for sternal saws, Favaloro retractors, oxygenators, microvascular instruments, and loupes. The history of thoracic surgical procedures shows that they evolved from surgical management of tuberculosis. Lung resections, muscle flaps, and thoracoscopy all began with efforts to control the disease.

Currently surgery has a minimal role in the treatment of pulmonary tuberculosis, because management is primarily medical. Surgery for tuberculosis is generally performed for three broad groups of patients:

- Those in whom surgery is necessary to make the diagnosis

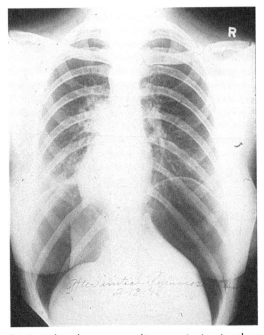

Fig. 8. Induced pneumoperitoneum to treat pulmonary tuberculosis. The disease involves the superior segment of the left lower lobe. (*Courtesy of* Mayo Clinic Archives; with permission.)

- Those with complications or sequelae of the disease
- Those who have active disease resistant to therapy, in whom surgery is performed with the goal of disease control (resectional).

Collapse therapy, previously so popular in tuberculosis disease management, has fallen by the wayside.

REFERENCES

1. Alexander J. The surgery of pulmonary tuberculosis. Philadelphia; New York: Lea and Febiger; 1925. p. 17.
2. Alexander J. The collapse therapy of pulmonary tuberculosis. Springfield (IL): Charles C Thomas; 1937. p. 3.
3. Ryan F. The forgotten plague. How the battle against tuberculosis was won and lost. Boston: Little, Brown and Company; 1992.
4. Koch R. Die aetioloie der tuberculose. Berliner Klinische Wochenschrift 1882;19:221–30 [in German].
5. Carter R. The mask of Thomas Mann (1875-1955): medical insights and last illness. Ann Thorac Surg 1998;65:578–85.
6. Fenger C, Hollister FH. Opening and draining cavities in the lungs. Am J Med Sci 1881;82(164): 370–92.
7. de Cerenville EB. De l'intervention operatoire dans les maladies du poumon. Rev Med Suisse Romande 1885;441–67 [in French].
8. Monaldi V. A propos du procede d'aspiration intracavitaire des cavernes. Rev Tuberc 1939;5:848–56 [in French].
9. Sauerbruch F. Ferdinand Sauerbruch, a surgeon' life. London: Andre Deutsch Limited; 1953.
10. Sarfert H. The operative treatment of phthisis pulmonalis. Ann Surg 1902;35:540–1.
11. Meade RH. Surgery for pulmonary tuberculosis. A history of thoracic surgery. Springfield (IL): Charles C Thomas; 1961. 98–161.
12. Tuffier T. De la resection du sommet du poumon. Semin Med Paris 1891;2:202 [in French].
13. Doyen. Chirugie du poumon. Cong Fran Chir 1895; 104 [in French].
14. Gluck T. Die entwicklung der lungenchirurgie. Arch klin Chir 1907;83:581–601 [in German].
15. Babcock WW. The operative treatment of pulmonary tuberculosis. Report of an excision of over one-half of the right lung. JAMA 1908;50:1263–5.
16. Freedlander SO. Lobectomy in pulmonary tuberculosis. J Thorac Surg 1935;5:132–42.
17. Churchill ED, Klopstock R. Lobectomy for pulmonary tuberculosis. Ann Surg 1943;117:641–69.
18. Overholt RH, Langer L, Szypulski JT, et al. Pulmonary resection in the treatment of tuberculosis. J Thorac Surg 1946;15:384–417.
19. Chamberlain JM. Segmental resection for pulmonary tuberculosis. In: Steele J, editor. Surgical management of pulmonary tuberculosis. Springfield (IL): Charles C Thomas; 1957. p. 52–67.
20. Andrews EW. Chondrectomy or operative treatment of bronchial asthma. JAMA 1914;63(13):1065–9.
21. Sauerbruch F. Die chirurgie der brustorgans. 2nd edition. Berlin: Julius Springer; 1920.
22. Gale JW, Middleton WS. Scaleniotomy in the surgical treatment of pulmonary tuberculosis. Arch Surg 1931;23(1):38–46.
23. Alexander J. Multiple intercostal neurectomy for pulmonary tuberculosis. Am Rev Tuberc 1929;20: 637–84.
24. Álvarez C. Nuevas orientaciones para el tratamiento quirurgico de la tuberculosis pulmonar par la simpatectmia toracica. Sem Med 1920;27:733 [in Spanish].
25. Álvarez C, Terapéutica de la tuberculosis. Ensayos experimentales para el tratamiento quirúrgico de la tuberculosis pulmonar por intervención directa sobre el simpatico torácico. Rev Esp Tuberc 1931; 38(21):323–6 [in Spanish].
26. Sayago GyA JM. Dos intervenciones quirurgicas en tuberulosis pulmonar. Sem Med 1921;28(1):164 [in Spanish].
27. Sayago G. Los metodos ortopedicos en al tratamiento de la tuberculosis pulmonar. Sem Med 1923;30(2):562 [in Spanish].
28. Sayago G. The surgical treatment of pulmonary tuberculosis. Am Rev Tuberc 1927;15:544–63.
29. Schlaepfer K. Ligation of the pulmonary artery combined with resection of the Phrenic nerve in chronic inflammatory conditions, especially tuberculosis of one lung. Am Rev Tuberc 1924;10: 35–66.
30. Schlaepfer K. Ligation of the pulmonary artery of one lung with and without resection of the phrenic nerve. Experimental study. Arch Surg 1924;9: 25–94.
31. Kerschner F. Die ligatur der vena pulmonalis bei lungentuberkulose. Archiv fur klinische Chirurgie 1931; 167:141–2 [in German].
32. Babcock WW. Carotid-jugular anastomosis in the treatment of advanced pulmonary tuberculosis. Surg Clin North Am 1929;9:1043–5.
33. Adams WW. Rapid healing of embolic lung abscess in atelectatic lobes. Proc Soc Exp Biol Med 1932;24: 539.
34. Adams WE. Detailed description of a safe and reliable method for closing large bronchi. J Thorac Surg 1933;3:198–200.
35. Carson J. Essays, physiological and practical. Liverpool (UK): BF Wright; 1822.
36. Forlannini C. A contribuzione della terapia della tisi. Ablazione del polmone? Pneumotrace artificiale? Primo caso di tisi polmonare monolaterale avanzata

curato felicemente col pneumotrace artificiale. Gaz d Osp 1882;68:537–9 [in Italian].

37. Forlannini C. Primi tentativi di pneumotorace artificiale dell tisi polmonare. Gazz med di Torino 1894;45:381–401 [in Italian].

38. Lemke AF. Report of cases of pulmonary tuberculosis, treated with intrapleural injections of nitrogen, with a consideration of the pathology of compression of the tuberculous lung. JAMA 1899;33(16):959–63.

39. Murphy JB. Surgery of the lung. JAMA 1898;31(4):151–65.

40. Brauer L. Die Behandlung der enseltigen Lungenphthisis mit kunstlichen Pneumothorax (nach Murphy). Munch Med Wochenschr 1906;53:338–9 [in German].

41. Murphy JB, Kreuscher PH. Pneumothorax and rest treatment in the management of pulmonary tuberculosis. Interstate Med J 1914;21(3):266–78.

42. Forlannini C. Zur behandlung der lungenschwinsucht durch kuntlich erzeugten pneumothorax. Dtsch Med Wochenschr 1906;32:1401–5 [in German].

43. Friedrich PL. The operative treatment of unilateral lung tuberculosis by total mobilization of the chestwall by means of thoracoplastic pleuropneumolysis. Surg Gynecol Obstet 1908;7:632–8.

44. Herve R. Liberation par etincelages adherences pleurales au cours du traitment par le pneumothorax. Rev Tuberc 1922;3:420 [in French].

45. Jacobeus HC. Endopleurale operationen unter der leitung des thorakoskops. Beitr Klin Tuberk Spezif Tuberkuloseforsch 1915;35:1–35 [in German].

46. Jacobeus HC. The cauterization of adhesions in artificial pneumothorax therapy of pulmonary tuberculosis. Am Rev Tuberc 1922;6:871–97.

47. Jacobeus HC. The practical importance of thoracoscopy in surgery of the chest. Surg Gynecol Obstet 1922;34:289–96.

48. Brauer L. Lungenkollpstherapie unter anwendung einer extrapleuralen thorakoplastik. Munch Med Wochenschr 1909;56:1866 [in German].

49. Friedrich PL. Statisches und prinzipielles zur frage der rippenresektion ausgedehnten oder beschranken umfanges bei kavernoser lungenphtise und bei hamoptoe. Munch Med Wochenschr 1911;58:2041–6 [in German].

50. Brauer L. Die wirkungsweise und die formen der extrapleuren thorakoplastik zur behandlung der einseitigen lungentuberkulose. Dtsch Med Wochenschr 1927;49:2060–2 [in German].

51. Wilms M. Eine neue methode zur verengerung des thorax bei lungentuberkulose. Munch Med Wochenschr 1911;58:777–8 [in German].

52. Odell JA. Dr Andrew Logan: the passing of a pioneer. Ann Thorac Surg 2006;82(4):1567–9.

53. Sauerbruch F. Thymektomie bei einem Fall von Morbus Basedowi mit Myasthenia. Mitteilungen aus den Grenzgebieten der medizin und Chirugie, Jena 1913;25:746–65 [in German].

54. Sauerbruch F. Die beeinflussingvon lungenerkrankungen durch kuntstliche lahmung des zwerchfelles (Phrenikotomie). Munch Med Wochenschr 1913;60:625–6 [in German].

55. Hoffman P. Stauffenberg: a family history, 1905-1944. Cambridge (UK); 2003.

56. Hoffman P. The history of the German Resistance 1933-1945. Cambridge (UK): McGill-Queens Press; 1996.

57. Stefani A, Jouni R, Alifano M, et al. Thoracoplasty in the current practice of thoracic surgery: a single-institution 10-year experience. Ann Thorac Surg 2011;91(1):263–8.

58. Semb C. Thoracoplasty with extrafascial apicolysis. Acta Chir Scand 1935;76:5–85.

59. Semb C. Technique of plastic operation of apicolysis. Acta Chir Scand 1934;74:478.

60. Tuffier T. Decollement pleuroparietal en chirugie pleuro-pulmonaire. Arch med-chir de l'appareil resp 1926;1:28–45 [in French].

61. Roberts JE. Extrapleural pneumothorax. Brit J Tuberc 1938;32:68–73.

62. Churchill ED. Discussion of extrapleural pneumothorax. J Thorac Surg 1938;7:586.

63. Shivers MO. Surgical treatment of pulmonary tuberculosis. Colo Med 1919;16:27–33.

64. Archibald EW. Extrapleural thoracoplasty and a modification of the operation of apicolysis utilizing muscle flaps for compression of lung. Am Rev Tuberc 1921;4:828–41.

65. Eloesser L. Subcostal extrapleural compression of the lung. J Thorac Surg 1932;1:672–7.

66. Haight C, Harvey SC, Oughterson AW. Surgical treatment of peripheral lung abscess. Extrapleural compression with a rubber bag. Yale J Biol Med 1931;3:235–40.

67. Lilienthal H. Tuberculosis of the lungs: apicolysis by two different methods. Surg Clin North Am 1928;8:235–54.

68. Rmada O, O'brien WB, Vindzberg WV, et al. Extraperiosteal plombage thoracoplasty: operative technique and results with 161 cases with unilateral surgical problems. J Thorac Surg 1956;32(6):797–813.

69. Alexander J. Supraperiosteal and subcostal pneumonolysis with filling of pectoral muscles. Arch Surg 1934;28:538–47.

70. Tezel CS, Goldstraw P. Plombage thoracoplasty with Lucite balls. Ann Thorac Surg 2005;79(3):1063.

71. Stuertz. Kunstliche zwerchfellahmung bei schwerern chronschen einseitigen lungenerkrankungen. Dtsch Med Wochenschr 1911;37:2224 [in German].

72. Gotze O. Die radicale phrenikotomie als selbstandiger therapeutischer eingriff bei der chirrugischen lungentuberkulose. Munch Med Wochenschr 1922;69:838 [in German].

73. Friedrich PL. Die operative methodik bei der chirurgischen behandlung der lungentuberkulose durch ribbenabtragung operative phrenicus und

intercostalnervenlahmung. Arch fur klinische Chirurgie 1914;105:429–57 [in German].

74. Alexander J. Temporary phrenic nerve paralysis. Its advantages over permanent paralysis in the treatment of phthisis. JAMA 1934;102:1552–3.

75. Lehmann J. Para-amino salicylic acid in the treatment of tuberculosis. Lancet 1946;1:15–6.

76. Lehmann J. Twenty years afterwards. Historical notes on the discovery of the anti-tuberculous effect of para-amino salicylic acid (PAS) and the first clinical trials. Am Rev Respir Dis 1964;90:953–6.

77. Schatz A, Bugie E, Waksman SA. Streptomycin, a substance exhibiting antibiotic activity against Gram-positive and Gram-negative bacteria. Proc Soc Exp Biol Med 1944;55:66–9.

78. Feldman WH, Hinshaw HC. Effects of streptomycin on experimental tuberculosis in guinea pigs: a preliminary study. Proc Staff Meet Mayo Clin 1944;19:593–9.

79. Naef A. The 1900 tuberculosis epidemic - starting point of modern thoracic surgery. Ann Thorac Surg 1993;55:1375–8.

Multidrug-Resistant Pulmonary Tuberculosis: Surgical Challenges

Michael J. Weyant, MD[a],*, John D. Mitchell, MD[a,b]

KEYWORDS

- Multidrug-resistant tuberculosis • MDR-TB • Extensively drug-resistant tuberculosis
- Parenchymal lung resection

KEY POINTS

- Despite the lack of prospective randomized studies regarding the surgical efficacy, the rising rates of multidrug-resistant tuberculosis (MDR-TB) and extensively drug-resistant tuberculosis necessitate the consideration of surgery and other adjunctive therapies in carefully selected patients.
- The morbidity of surgical resection ranges from 12% to 39%, with the most common complications being bleeding, empyema, wound complications, and bronchopleural fistula. Overall mortality ranges from 1% to 5%, indicating the relative safety of these operations.
- The rationale for surgical resection of lung affected by MDR-TB is to remove a large focal burden of organisms present in destroyed nonviable lung tissue because the destroyed lung parenchyma and associated cavities create an ideal environment for the bacillus.
- Surgical procedures are still required to treat the complications of tuberculosis, which include massive hemoptysis, bronchopleural fistula, empyema, bronchiectasis or destroyed lung, broncholiths, and aspergilloma.

BACKGROUND

Multidrug-resistant tuberculosis (MDR-TB) and, most recently, extensively drug-resistant tuberculosis (XDR-TB) have emerged over the last 20 years.[1] MDR-TB is defined as those strains resistant to at least isoniazid and rifampicin. XDR-TB strains are defined as those resistant to rifampicin, isoniazid, fluoroquinolones, and any of capreomycin, kanamycin, or amikacin.[1] Resistance to these antitubercular drugs is a result of spontaneous mutations in the genome of the *Mycobacterium tuberculosis* organism.[1] These resistant strains then proliferate and become the dominant organism. There are several factors thought to be contributing to the development of these resistant strains but, ultimately, they develop from the inadequate treatment of active pulmonary tuberculosis.[2] Inadequate therapy occurs for many reasons, including poor prescribing practices with insufficient treatment duration and poor drug selection. Societal problems such as inadequate public health support or unpredictable drug supplies also play a role. Irregular medicine intake, which can be due to insufficient patient education or socioeconomic determinants, can contribute to resistance. Finally, MDR-TB can be transmitted to previously uninfected patients merely because they live in an environment with a high prevalence of the disease.[2]

EPIDEMIOLOGY OF MDR-TB

Control of the global spread of MDR-TB will be a significant challenge moving forward. It is estimated that there are 440,000 new MDR-TB cases identified each year worldwide and many of these arise in previously treated patients.[3] Approximately 3% to 4% of all new tuberculosis cases

[a] Section of General Thoracic Surgery, Division of Cardiothoracic Surgery, Department of Surgery, University of Colorado School of Medicine, 12631 East 17th Avenue, MSC310, Aurora, CO 80045, USA; [b] National Jewish Health, 1400 Jackson Street, Denver, CO 80206, USA
* Corresponding author.
E-mail address: Michael.Weyant@ucdenver.edu

Thorac Surg Clin 22 (2012) 271–276
doi:10.1016/j.thorsurg.2012.04.003
1547-4127/12/$ – see front matter © 2012 Published by Elsevier Inc

identified worldwide are either MDR-TB or XDR-TB.[3] Alarmingly, only 7% of new MDR tuberculosis cases are reported to be diagnosed and treated.[4] The disease is not distributed equally worldwide with nearly 50% of cases occurring in India and China.[1] In other countries such as Peru, where drug-sensitive cases are decreasing, MDR-TB cases are on the rise. The ideal way to identify and monitor the disease is by culture and drug-susceptibility testing that allows surveillance and tracking of these cases. Unfortunately only 22% of countries worldwide mandate this type of testing. In high-burden countries, only 1% of new patients undergo drug-susceptibility testing[4] The prognosis of treatment of MDR-TB or XDR-TB is significantly worse than that for drug-susceptible disease.[2] Two recent meta analyses reported that the average proportion of successful treatment outcomes in MDR-TB patients is 62%, whereas in XDR-TB patients it was only 42%.[5,6]

CURRENT TREATMENT OF MDR-TB

The standard treatment of drug-susceptible tuberculosis is well defined and borne out by prospective studies. Conversely, treatment of MDR-TB and XDR-TB is less well defined and is based predominantly on either anecdotal case reports or expert opinion as opposed to randomized clinical trials.[7] The World Health Organization (WHO) has recently updated and put forth recommendations for treating MDR-TB. The summary of recommendations includes[3]

1. Rapid drug-susceptibility testing of isoniazid and rifampicin should be performed at the initial diagnosis of tuberculosis
2. The use of sputum microscopy and culture should be used instead of microscopy alone
3. Later-generation fluoroquinolones, as well as ethionamide, should be used in patients with MDR-TB
4. In the treatment of MDR-TB, regimens should include at least pyrazinamide, a flouroquinolone, a parenteral agent (kanamycin, amikacin, or capreomycin), ethionamide, and either cycloserine or p-aminosalicylic acid
5. An intensive of treatment of at least 8-months duration is recommended.

These recommendations are put in place to attempt to standardize treatment of MDR-TB throughout the world. The success of MDR-TB therapy ranges from 36% to 79% with a mortality rate of 11%.[2] However, it is estimated that less than 10% of people with MDR-TB are receiving appropriate treatment according to international guidelines.[7]

SURGERY TO TREAT TUBERCULOSIS

Surgical therapy for tuberculosis is one of the oldest documented treatments for the disease. After initial attempts at drainage of tuberculosis cavities failed, collapse therapy prevailed until the institution of chemotherapy in 1945.[8] Collapse therapy was thought to be efficacious because it prevents a space by which the M tuberculosis, an obligate aerobic organism, can access oxygen.[9,10] Collapse therapy encompassed many forms, including induced pneumothorax, thoracoplasty, phrenic nerve interruption, pneumoperitoneum, and extrapleural plombage. These procedures were used almost exclusively in patients with unilateral disease.[7] These procedures were significantly complicated by infection, hemorrhage, and erosion of foreign material into the lung and other structures. These therapies, for the most part, were phased out after the introduction of streptomycin in 1943.[7] Historically, surgery was also indicated for the complications of tuberculosis such as hemorrhage, bronchopleural fistula, empyema, bronchiectasis, broncholiths, and the development of aspergilloma.[8] In the modern treatment era, surgery is used as an adjunct to chemotherapy to effect and aid in a cure and consists mainly of parenchymal lung resection.

Indications for Surgical Resection to Aid Cure

The rationale for surgical resection of lung affected by MDR-TB is to remove a large focal burden of organisms present in destroyed nonviable lung tissue.[7,9] The destroyed lung parenchyma and associated cavities are an ideal environment for the bacillus to grow owing to its isolation from blood circulation and, therefore, the host's defenses.[7] Even in patients who are found to be sputum-negative, live bacteria are often found in these destroyed areas of lung tissue.[9] These necrotic "homes" for the bacteria are thought to be a potential cause of drug resistance.

The most common surgical procedure used to effect treatment of MDR-TB is lung resection. The literature guiding these recommendations continues to consist of expert opinion and observational studies instead of prospective randomized data. In 1990, Iseman and colleagues[11] reported selection criteria, based on observation of a large number of cases, which are still used today. Surgery is recommended in MDR-TB patients with extensive drug resistance—those with localized disease amenable to resection and those with high drug activity (**Box 1**).[11] The WHO promotes the same indications but assert that pretreatment is required for at least 2 months before surgery to reduce the bacterial burden,

---

Box 1

Indications for surgery of drug-resistant tuberculosis

- High risk of relapse based on drug-resistance profile
- Persistently positive sputum despite aggressive drug therapy
- Localized lesions
- Complications of disease:
  - Empyema
  - Hemoptysis
  - Aspergilloma
  - Bronchiectasis
- Sufficient drug treatment available

---

followed by 12 to 24 months of treatment after surgery.[12]

Results of Surgical Treatment

Despite the lack of prospective randomized trials regarding the use of adjunctive surgery to treat MDR-TB, it is worthwhile to mention the collective results of the largest series of surgical resections of MDR-TB because it helps illustrate complication rates and safety of surgery[13–18] (**Table 1**). The morbidity of surgical resection ranges from 12% to 39%, with the most common complications being bleeding, empyema, wound complications, and bronchopleural fistula. The overall mortality ranges from 1% to 5% indicate the relative safety of these operations. One measure of success used in evaluation of surgical approaches to MDR-TB is the rate of postoperative negative cultures. In these largest series, the rate of sputum sterilization ranges from 78% to 96%. The rates of culture conversion from positive to negative range from 47% to100% (median 92.5%). The WHO states, however, that sputum conversion should not be considered equivalent to cure because a certain proportion of patients may initially convert and later revert to positive sputum culture. The factors associated with this reconversion and its implications are not currently known.[12]

A patient is considered cured by WHO standards when a defined treatment program has been completed and at least five consecutive negative cultures from samples are collected at least 30 days apart in the final 12 months of treatment. If only one positive culture is reported during that time, and there is no concomitant clinical evidence of deterioration, a patient may still be

considered cured, provided that this positive culture is followed by a minimum of three consecutive negative cultures taken at least 30 days apart.[12] In addition, this definition does not address the outcome after patients have discontinued treatment and the issue of long-term durable sterility of sputum.

Using the WHO definition of cure, Kang and colleagues[18] describe their experience of surgical treatment for MDR-TB and XDR-TB in 72 patients. Preoperative sputum cultures were positive in 81% despite aggressive multidrug therapy. Surgical resection was performed mainly in patients with focal disease. In patients who had bilateral disease, the side with greater number or size of lesions was operated on and the remaining disease left to medical treatment. Using the WHO guidelines for cure, 65% of these patients met the criteria strictly. The investigators mention that only 5.6% of patients failed treatment using the WHO definition of treatment failure (two or more of the five cultures recorded in the final 12 months of therapy are positive or one of the final three cultures is positive).[12,18]

Chan and colleagues,[19] from the United States, describe a cohort of 205 patients treated for MDR-TB from 1984 to 1998. Lung resection was performed in 130 of these patients, including 63 pneumonectomies and 59 lobectomies. The patients were classified into three microbiologic outcomes groups: (1) initial favorable response included patients with at least three consecutive negative sputum cultures over a period of at least 3 months while on treatment, (2) microbiologic failure included patients who failed to achieve three consecutive negative sputum cultures over at least a 3-month period, and (3) indeterminate included patients with insufficient respiratory samples. Surgical resection in this study was associated with a nearly fivefold increase in odds of initial favorable outcome. The investigators also performed a statistical analysis of predictors of microbiologic outcome indicating that surgical resection and flouroquinolone therapy were associated with improved microbiologic and clinical outcomes.[19]

Gegia and colleagues[20] examined a series of 380 patients treated for both MDR-TB and XDR-TB in relation to adverse prognostic factors affecting treatment. Thirty-seven patients underwent lung resection as part of treatment. Factors leading to poorer outcomes included retreatment cases, XDR-TB, bilateral disease, and low body mass index (BMI). Patients who underwent surgical resection were more likely to have a favorable outcome. These data suggest that, in properly selected cases, surgical treatment of

Table 1
Case studies of patients with MDR-TB undergoing surgical resection (n≥60)

Author	Country	Year	n	Age	Preoperative Culture Positive (%)	Postoperative Culture Negative (%)	Morbidity (%)	Mortality (%)
Kir et al,[13] 2006	Turkey	2006	79	38	15	96	39	2.5
Kim et al,[14] 2006	South Korea	2006	79	29	98	72	23	1.2
Somocurcio et al,[15] 2007	Peru	2006	121	27	79	78	23	5
Pomerantz et al,[16] 2001	United States	2001	172	39	50	98	12	3.3
van Leuven et al,[17] 1997	South Africa	1997	62	34	39	89	23	1.6
Kang et al,[18] 2010	South Korea	2010	72	31	81	78	15	1.4

destroyed lung or cavitary disease has an integral role in the treatment of MDR-TB. Given the lack of prospective randomized trials, however, it is unclear whether there is selection bias in surgically treating focal and limited disease, which may have a more favorable outcome on its own. Given the continued presence of MDR-TB throughout the world, the opportunity to study this in prospective fashion will likely present itself.

SURGERY TO TREAT COMPLICATIONS OF MDR-TB

Although the main discussion in this article pertains to lung resection in an attempt to cure patients of tuberculosis, it is important to mention that surgical procedures to treat the complications of tuberculosis are still required and should be discussed. Perelman and Strelzov[8] describe the most common complications of tuberculosis requiring surgical intervention, including:

- Massive hemoptysis
- Bronchopleural fistula
- Empyema
- Bronchiectasis or destroyed lung
- Broncholiths
- Aspergilloma.

Dewan[21] reports a large series over 15 years in the modern era of tuberculosis treatment in India in which 2878 patients had some form of intervention for the treatment of complications of tuberculosis. Procedures included 830 lung resections, 12 primary thoracoplasties, 295 space-reducing thoracoplasties, 158 decortications, 744 open-window thoracoplasties, and 837 tube thoracostomies. Massive recurrent hemoptysis was treated in 645

patients, bronchiectasis in 298, and cavitary disease or destroyed lung in 298. These data illustrate the importance of knowledge of the treatment of the disease and the adjunctive procedures used to manage it.

Preoperative Evaluation

Thoracic surgeons are usually not the entry point of care of most MDR-TB patents and most patients are significantly imaged before visiting the surgeon. CT scan is ubiquitously used to image patients being treated for MDR-TB because it is the most common way of identifying areas of destroyed lung to be targeted by resection.[9] Increasingly, PET is being used to identify areas of active disease.[22] The surgeon's main concern is evaluating patients' baseline physical status to reduce the chances of morbidity after surgery. Routine cardiac and pulmonary function testing is required before any resection. Additionally, because many of these patients have marginal lung function, enhanced pulmonary function testing with technetium 99m perfusion scanning may be useful.

The nutritional status of a patient with MDR-TB is often compromised and a low BMI is associated with poor outcomes after surgical treatment.[2,20] Most patients have had a significant amount of weight loss and adjunctive nutrition support with enteral feeding tubes to improve calorie intake can significantly decrease the chances of surgical morbidity in the postoperative period. Evaluation of laboratory nutritional parameters such as albumin levels may help to optimally time the surgery.

Pain management of the patent with tuberculosis undergoing lung resection is crucial to aiding postoperative pulmonary toilet. Liberal use of epidural catheters can significantly aid pulmonary toilet after these often difficult lung resections.

Surgical Technique

The most common surgical approach used is a posterolateral thoracostomy, although anterior thoracostomies are used by some investigators.[9] Recently, video-assisted thoracoscopic techniques have been used by Kang and colleagues[18] with the caveat that the lesions need to be surrounded by lung parenchyma, not involve the pleurae, and be small and focal.

The most common parenchymal resections that will be performed are lobectomies, followed by pneumonectomies. It is extremely important to consider sparing the latissimus dorsi muscle during the thoracostomy portion of these cases because it may be used as a space filler or to cover the bronchial stump (**Fig. 1**). The infectious process often involves the pleural space and it is useful to perform an extrapleural dissection to minimize contamination or bacterial superinfection of the resection cavity (**Box 2**). There is no clear recommendation regarding when to use tissue transfer, such as muscle flaps or omentum, to cover the bronchial stump although several investigators advocate this in most cases (**Box 3**).[9,18] Pomerantz[9] advocates the use of muscle flaps to cover the bronchus in patients who still have

> **Box 2**
> **Surgical pearls regarding resection of MDR-TB**
>
> Use extrapleural dissection in cases involving the pleura
>
> Cover bronchial stump in those patients with positive sputum smear, history of bronchopleural fistula, or polymicrobial contamination.
>
> Intrapericardial control of pulmonary vessels may be easier
>
> Consider pneumonectomy plus intentional Eloesser in severely contaminated pneumonectomy

positive sputum smear, have had a bronchopleural fistula, or if there is polymicrobial contamination.

Pneumonectomy in patients with MDR-TB presents a few unique challenges. The formation of a bronchopleural fistula after pneumonectomy is a significant complication with a high mortality rate. This has led several investigators to recommend muscle flap coverage of the bronchus in all patients undergoing this procedure. Pomerantz[9] has also gone so far as to suggest leaving an intentional Eloesser flap in extremely contaminated pneumonectomy cases. The space is then closed 4 to 6 weeks later with instillation of modified Claggett solution. Additionally, in the completion pneumonectomy patient, it may be helpful to ligate the pulmonary vessels in the intrapericardial space.

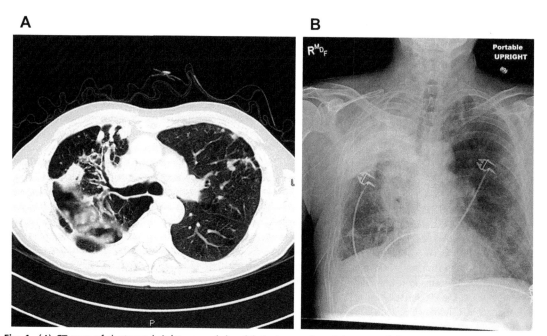

Fig. 1. (*A*) CT scan of destroyed right upper lobe. (*B*) Postoperative right upper lobectomy and use of latissimus dorsi flap to cover bronchial stump and fill resection space.

> **Box 3**
> **Autologous tissue used to fill resection space and cover bronchial stump**
>
> Latissimus dorsi
> Intercostal muscle flap
> Omentum
> Serratus anterior
> Pectoralis major

SUMMARY

This review of the surgical management of MDR-TB demonstrates the potential benefits of surgical resection as a therapy to complement multidrug treatment regimens. Despite the lack of prospective randomized studies regarding the efficacy of surgery, the rising rates of MDR-TB and XDR-TB necessitate the consideration of surgery and other adjunctive therapies in carefully selected patients. The available data demonstrate acceptable morbidity and mortality rates as well as a trend toward improved outcome with the use of surgery as an adjunctive therapy. Collective expert opinion and recommendations from the WHO also support the use of surgery in selected cases to treat MDR-TB. Further study through prospective trials will only help surgery become a more effective adjunctive treatment of MDR-TB.

REFERENCES

1. Gandhi NR, Nunn P, Dheda K, et al. Multidrug-resistant and extensively drug-resistant tuberculosis: a threat to global control of tuberculosis. Lancet 2010;375:1830–43.
2. Johnston JC, Shahidi NC, Sadatsafavi M, et al. Treatment outcomes of multidrug-resistant tuberculosis: a systematic review and meta-analysis. PLoS One 2009;4:e6914.
3. Falzon D, Jaramillo E, Schünemann HJ, et al. WHO guidelines for the programmatic management of drug-resistant tuberculosis: 2011 update. Eur Respir J 2011;38:516–28.
4. Caws M, Ha DT. Scale-up of diagnostics for multidrug resistant tuberculosis. Lancet Infect Dis 2010;10:656–8.
5. Orenstein EW, Basu S, Shah NS, et al. Treatment outcomes among patients with multidrug-resistant tuberculosis: systematic review and meta-analysis. Lancet Infect Dis 2009;9:153–61.
6. Jacobson KR, Tierney DB, Jeon CY, et al. Treatment outcomes among patients with extensively drug-resistant tuberculosis: systematic review and meta-analysis. Clin Infect Dis 2010;51:6–14.
7. Kempker RR, Vashakidze S, Solomonia N, et al. Surgical treatment of drug-resistant tuberculosis. Lancet Infect Dis 2012;12(2):157–66.
8. Perelman MI, Strelzov VP. Surgery for pulmonary tuberculosis. World J Surg 1997;21:457–67.
9. Pomerantz M. Surgery ro the management of mycobacterium tuberculosis and nontuberculous mycobacterial infections of the lung. Shields 6th edition general thoracic surgery. Philadelphia (PA): Lippincott Williams and Wilkins; 2005. p. 1251–61.
10. Koch R. Classics in infectious diseases: the etiology of tuberculosis. Rev Infect Dis 1982;4:1270–4.
11. Iseman MD, Madsen L, Goble M, et al. Surgical intervention in the treatment of pulmonary disease caused by drug-resistant *Mycobacterium tuberculosis*. Am Rev Respir Dis 1990;141:623–5.
12. World Health Organization. Guidelines for the programmatic management of drug resistant tuberculosis. Geneva (Switzerland): World Health Organization; 2008.
13. Kir A, Inci I, Torun T, et al. Adjuvant resectional surgery improves cure rates in multidrug-resistant tuberculosis. J Thorac Cardiovasc Surg 2006;131:693–6.
14. Kim HJ, Kang CH, Kim YT, et al. Prognostic factors for surgical resection in patients with multidrug-resistant tuberculosis. Eur Respir J 2006;28:576–80.
15. Somocurcio JG, Sotomayor A, Shin S, et al. Surgery for patients with drug-resistant tuberculosis: report of 121 cases receiving community-based treatment in Lima, Peru. Thorax 2007;62:416–21.
16. Pomerantz BJ, Cleveland JC Jr, Olson HK, et al. Pulmonary resection for multi-drug resistant tuberculosis. J Thorac Cardiovasc Surg 2001;121:448–53.
17. van Leuven M, De Groot M, Shean KP, et al. Pulmonary resection as an adjunct in the treatment of multiple drug-resistant tuberculosis. Ann Thorac Surg 1997;63:1368–72.
18. Kang MW, Kim HK, Choi YS, et al. Surgical treatment for multidrug-resistant and extensive drug-resistant tuberculosis. Ann Thorac Surg 2010;89:1597–602.
19. Chan ED, Laurel V, Strand MJ, et al. Treatment and outcome analysis of 205 patients with multidrug-resistant tuberculosis. Am J Respir Crit Care Med 2004;169:1103–9.
20. Gegia M, Kalandadze I, Kempker RR, et al. Adjunctive surgery improves treatment outcomes among patients with multidrug-resistant and extensively drug-resistant tuberculosis. Int J Infect Dis 2012;16(5):e391–6.
21. Dewan RK. Surgery for pulmonary tuberculosis— a 15-year experience. Eur J Cardiothorac Surg 2010;37:473–7.
22. Treglia G, Taralli S, Calcagni ML, et al. Is there a role for fluorine 18 fluorodeoxyglucose-positron emission tomography and positron emission tomography/computed tomography in evaluating patients with mycobacteriosis? A systematic review. J Comput Assist Tomogr 2011;35:387–93.

Surgical Treatment of Atypical Mycobacterial Infections

Jessica A. Yu, MD[a], Michael J. Weyant, MD[a],
John D. Mitchell, MD[a,b],*

KEYWORDS

- Nontuberculous mycobacteria • Bronchiectasis • Lobectomy • VATS lobectomy
- Pneumonectomy • Thoracoplasty

KEY POINTS

- Pulmonary NTM infection is the most common manifestation of NTM disease.
- Medical therapy consists of multi-agent antimycobacterial regimens and symptom control.
- Despite optimal medical treatment, relapse/reinfection, or persistent or progressive parenchymal damage may still occur. Resection aims to remove all of the bronchiectasis and damaged lung parenchyma, which might predispose patients to later recurrence of disease.
- Indications for surgery most often include the presence of focal, persistent lung damage (bronchiectasis, cavitation, consolidation, and destroyed lung) amenable to complete anatomic resection after initiation of appropriate antimicrobial therapy.
- Anatomic lung resection for bronchiectasis or cavitary lung disease associated with NTM pulmonary infection provides several technical obstacles when compared with a similar operation for thoracic malignancy (eg, bronchial circulation hypertrophy, adhesions, pleural symphysis).

Nontuberculous mycobacterial (NTM) pulmonary infections represent a complex clinical challenge to pulmonologists and thoracic surgeons. We present a brief background of the definition, epidemiology, and diagnosis of the disease, followed by an in-depth review of the key issues relevant to the modern thoracic surgeon confronting pulmonary NTM disease.

DEFINITION AND EPIDEMIOLOGY

NTM pulmonary disease is characterized most frequently by focal fibronodular bronchiectasis with or without cavitary lung disease. Progressive lung damage extends the spectrum of disease to larger cavities, pleural symphysis/obliteration, and completely destroyed lung.[1] The causative organisms are referred to in the literature as NTM,

"atypical" mycobacteria, "mycobacteria other than tuberculosis" (MOTT), or "environmental mycobacteria" (EM). These organisms are ubiquitous in the soil and water and resistant to chlorination treatment. In contrast to *Mycobacterium tuberculosis*, NTM are not obligate pathogens and do not always cause clinical disease. There is no evidence of human-to-human disease transmission; thus, it is not a reportable infectious disease. Although the true incidence and prevalence is unknown, it is increasingly recognized worldwide with lung disease being the most common manifestation of NTM infection.[2,3] In the United States, the most recent population-based study of pulmonary NTM disease found an overall prevalence of 5.4 per 100,000 people, with a higher burden of disease in women and patients older than 60 years.[3] Patients with preexisting lung damage are

a Section of General Thoracic Surgery, Division of Cardiothoracic Surgery, University of Colorado School of Medicine, 12631 East 17th Avenue, C310, Aurora, CO 80045, USA; b National Jewish Health, 1400 Jackson Street, Denver, CO 80206, USA
* Corresponding author. Division of Cardiothoracic Surgery, University of Colorado School of Medicine, 12631 East 17th Avenue, C310, Aurora, CO 80045.
E-mail address: John.Mitchell@ucdenver.edu

Thorac Surg Clin 22 (2012) 277–285
doi:10.1016/j.thorsurg.2012.05.004

especially at risk. As a result, bronchiectasis is both *a consequence of and a risk factor for* pulmonary NTM infection.[4]

In patients without preexisting lung disease, identification of predisposing features remains elusive. Mutations in the cystic fibrosis transmembrane conductance regulator (CFTR) gene are more prevalent in pulmonary patients with NTM compared with the general population.[5] The distinct female predominant phenotype of Lady Windermere Syndrome, characterized by right middle lobe and lingular bronchiectasis in patients with a lower body mass index and higher incidence of mitral valve prolapse, has prompted the investigation of familial clustering of pulmonary NTM disease.[6,7] Some immune phenotypes have been associated with NTM disease, but no consistent findings have been established.[8] Thus, both immune-compromised and immune-competent individuals remain susceptible.

DIAGNOSIS

Before obtaining a diagnosis of NTM infection, it is not uncommon for patients to have had pulmonary symptoms for months if not years. The most commonly reported pulmonary symptoms are shortness of breath, chronic cough, recurrent upper respiratory infections, and hemoptysis. Systemic symptoms are common, and include fatigue, night sweats, and weight loss.[1] Diagnostic guidelines have been put forth by the American Thoracic Society in conjunction with the Infectious Disease Society of America (ATS/IDSA) (**Box 1**).[2]

NTM species identification requires genotypic techniques,[9,10] and appropriate diagnosis at the species level most often requires the expertise of a laboratory familiar with NTM organisms. Within the subset of NTM organisms that are more frequently encountered in lung disease, there is a distinction between rapid-growers and slow-growers. The most common pulmonary NTM pathogens are listed in **Box 2**.

TREATMENT AND PROGNOSIS
Medical Therapy

Suggested treatment regimens are detailed in the most recent ATS/IDSA guidelines for *Mycobacterium avium* complex disease, and ideally consist of rifampin, ethambutol, and a macrolide. Medical therapy alone has a success rate of approximately 55% to 67%.[2,11,12] For the rapid-grower *Mycobacterium abscessus,* the success rate of medical therapy is half that, at 28%.[13] The difficulties with medical therapy are multifactorial. First, mycobacterial organisms have the propensity to

---

Box 1
Diagnostic guidelines for NTM infection

Clinical

1. Pulmonary symptoms, nodular or cavitary opacities on chest radiograph, or an HRCT scan that shows multifocal bronchiectasis with multiple small nodules.

and

2. Appropriate exclusion of other diagnoses.

Microbiologic

1. Positive culture results from at least two separate expectorated sputum samples. (If the results from the initial sputum samples are nondiagnostic, consider repeat sputum AFB smears and cultures.)

or

2. Positive culture results from at least one bronchial wash or lavage.

or

3. Transbronchial or other lung biopsy with mycobacterial histopathologic features (granulomatous inflammation or AFB) and positive culture for NTM or biopsy showing mycobacterial histopathologic features (granulomatous inflammation or AFB) and one or more sputum or bronchial washings that are culture positive for NTM.

4. Expert consultation should be obtained when NTM are recovered that are either infrequently encountered or that usually represent environmental contamination.

5. Patients who are suspected of having NTM lung disease but who do not meet the diagnostic criteria should be followed until the diagnosis is firmly established or excluded.

6. Making the diagnosis of NTM lung disease does not, *per se*, necessitate the institution of therapy, which is a decision based on potential risks and benefits of therapy for individual patients.

Adapted from Griffith DE, Aksamit T, Brown-Elliott BA, et al. An official ATS/IDSA statement: diagnosis, treatment, and prevention of nontuberculous mycobacterial diseases. Am J Respir Crit Care Med 2007;175:367–416; with permission.

---

develop drug resistance. This necessitates multi-agent therapy, and in severe disease, regular intravenous antibiotics. Second, these multiagent regimens are responsible for high rates of side effects and intolerance requiring antibiotic discontinuation or modification. Antibiotics are stopped because of adverse effects or toxicity in as many as 65% of patients[13]; indeed, antibiotic intolerance

> **Box 2**
> **Common pulmonary NTM pathogens**
>
> *Slow growers*
>
> Mycobacterium intracellulare (MAI) or Mycobacterium avium complex (MAC)
>
> Mycobacterium kansasii
>
> Mycobacterium simiae
>
> *Rapid growers*
>
> Mycobacterium abscessus
>
> Mycobacterium chelonae
>
> Mycobacterium fortuitum

is frequently an indication to consider surgical intervention.[14] The addition of macrolide antibiotics has made some improvements in medical treatment; however, the recurrence rate in the postmacrolide era continues to be high, with 20% to 44% of patients experiencing relapse and or reinfection.[11,12]

Surgical Resection

Parenchymal disease is a major risk factor for recurrent infection, as these permanently damaged areas of lung are poorly penetrated by antibiotics and may serve as a reservoir for organisms. A number of studies have suggested that the use of surgical resection as an adjunct to medical therapy in pulmonary NTM disease may alter the cycle of recurrence and progressive parenchymal tissue damage.[6,13,15–20] A study comparing combined surgical resection and medical management to medical treatment alone in M abscessus pulmonary disease revealed a conversion rate of 28% in the medical group versus 57% in the group receiving surgical management as an adjunct to best medical practice.[13] In the case of M abscessus in particular, surgical resection of localized disease in conjunction with antibiotics is recommended by the ATS/IDSA as providing the best chance for cure.

SURGICAL MANAGEMENT

A multidisciplinary approach is critical to successful treatment of pulmonary NTM disease. At our institution, these patients are managed in collaboration with physicians from a wide array of specialties who have extensive expertise in treating mycobacterial disease. Patients are discussed at a weekly conference attended by pulmonologists, infectious disease specialists, and surgeons.

Computed tomography (CT) confirms the presence of focal parenchymal damage and accompanying cultures obtained from sputum or bronchoscopy confirm the pathogen. Bronchoscopy is not required, but can be used for diagnostic purposes and to eliminate the presence of endobronchial pathology. If hemoptysis is a presenting symptom, bronchoscopy is helpful in localizing the source within the bronchial tree to the segmental or even subsegmental level.

Indications for surgery include the presence of focal, persistent lung damage (bronchiectasis, cavitation, consolidation, and destroyed lung) amenable to complete anatomic resection after initiation of appropriate antimicrobial therapy. Symptoms such as hemoptysis or recurrent pulmonary infections (treatment failure) add additional impetus to consider surgical resection, as do issues such as antibiotic intolerance or significant antibiotic resistance. Consideration of surgical therapy occurs for many patients at the initial consultation, when evidence of irreversible, focal parenchymal injury is noted on the radiologic evaluation. In others, surgery is offered after the lung damage fails to improve or even progresses despite adequate therapy.

When surgical resection is considered, adequate pulmonary reserve should be ensured using standard pulmonary function testing, remembering that the targeted areas for resection usually add little to the patient's pulmonary function. Appropriate cardiac evaluation should also be performed. Nutritional status requires careful attention and nutritional specialist consultation can be obtained as needed. Dietary supplementation with or without nasojejunal or gastrostomy feeding tube placement may be required to ensure adequate intake. This is more of a concern in the patients with destroyed lung and severe pulmonary compromise. We do not consider routine dietary supplementation in patients with a localized disease process. Gastroesophageal reflux is not an uncommon comorbidity associated with NTM pulmonary infection. All patients should be assessed for the presence of significant gastroesophageal reflux and, if present, antireflux surgery can be performed concomitantly, or soon after pulmonary resection.

Targeted antimycobacterial therapy, often including intravenous aminoglycosides, is administered for at least 2 to 3 months before surgical intervention. This duration of preoperative antibiotic therapy aims to reach a nadir in organism counts (bacterial load) before surgery, and in many cases, dictates the timing of surgical resection.

Anatomic lung resection for bronchiectasis or cavitary lung disease associated with NTM pulmonary infection provides several technical obstacles when compared with a similar operation for thoracic malignancy. Pleural adhesions are almost always present in some form, and in some cases can be extensive and vascular in nature. They usually involve the affected areas of lung, but can also be present throughout the hemithorax. In cavitary upper lobe disease, the adhesions to the overlying parietal pleura can be significant. The preoperative CT scan may predict the presence of dense adhesions, but frequently underestimates the amount of pleural symphysis. The adhesions can usually be divided through a minimally invasive approach, often with improved visibility compared with thoracotomy. In this setting, indications to convert to open thoracotomy would include a perceived requirement for extrapleural dissection, or because of concern regarding underlying vital structures.

The bronchial circulation in patients with bronchiectasis or cavitary lung disease is almost always hypertrophied, and in most cases should be directly ligated with clips to minimize bleeding. Considerable lymphadenopathy may be present, and in the setting of chronic pulmonary granulomatous disease can make dissection of the hilar vessels extremely difficult. When developing a fissure with a stapling device, we tend to err toward the uninvolved lobe to ensure complete resection. In addition, the diseased tissue is thickened and tends to compress poorly, thus making it a poor substrate for staple closure.

As mentioned, areas of lung with cavitary disease often have concomitant, adjacent pleural symphysis, and care must be taken during lung mobilization to avoid spillage of infected debris within the pleural space. Following segmentectomy or smaller lobar resections, a significant "residual space" is typically not an issue given the degree of parenchymal collapse or consolidation usually present preoperatively. This should be assessed on a case-by-case basis, for residual ipsilateral lung can be poorly compliant and may contribute to a space problem. In larger resections, or if a significant space is anticipated, use of a transposed muscle flap (typically the latissimus dorsi) may be considered.

We do not routinely buttress the bronchial stump closure with autologous tissue following resection for NTM lung disease. Situations where buttressing of the bronchial stump with transposed muscle or omentum might be considered would be in the presence of a multidrug resistant organism, in the setting of poorly controlled infection before surgery, or in the case of right pneumonectomy.

It is our bias to perform anatomic lung resection in the setting of focal bronchiectasis/cavitary lung disease associated with NTM lung infection, believing this approach removes all of the bronchiectasis and damaged lung parenchyma, which might lead to later recurrence of disease. However, an isolated nodule or small cavity may occasionally be addressed with nonanatomic (wedge) resection in combination with anatomic resection of a more heavily diseased area of lung. In this setting, the target for nonanatomic resection should be small, peripheral, amenable to complete resection, and not associated with visible bronchiectasis on high-resolution CT.

Surgical Technique: Thoracoscopic Approach

Focal fibronodular bronchiectasis and isolated small cavities can usually be treated with a minimally invasive operation (**Figs. 1** and **2**). We have recently reported our experience with thoracoscopic anatomic resection for bronchiectasis, with most of our patients having NTM pulmonary infection.[21] Our results demonstrate the feasibility of a minimally invasive approach in patients with infectious lung disease, with similar outcomes compared with thoracoscopic resection for oncologic purposes.

The thoracoscopic approach to resection in these patients is not routinely accompanied by epidural catheter placement for postoperative pain control, but epidurals are available to all patients. Patients are placed under general anesthesia and intubated using a double-lumen endotracheal tube, or less frequently using a standard lumen endotracheal tube with a bronchial blocker. Video-assisted thoracoscopic lobectomy and segmentectomy are performed using two 10-mm ports and a 4-cm "utility" incision. The trocars are placed first: one in the seventh or eighth intercostal space in the anterior axillary line, the second placed one intercostal space below the tip of the scapula. At this point, inspection of the hemithorax confirms the feasibility of a thoracoscopic approach and the utility incision is made in the anterior axillary line over the anterior hilar structures or major fissure, depending on the planned resection. The latissimus muscle is typically spared. No rib spreading is used, but a small

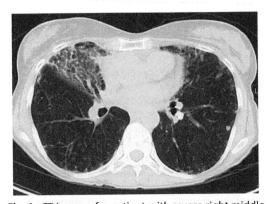

Fig. 1. CT image of a patient with severe right middle lobe and, to a lesser degree, lingular bronchiectasis associated with NTM infection. This is an ideal patient for a thoracoscopic approach.

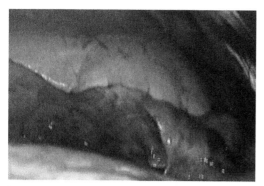

Fig. 2. Same patient as in **Fig. 1**. Intraoperative photo of a consolidated and bronchiectatic right middle lobe.

Alexis Wound Retractor (Applied Medical Co., Rancho Santa Margarita, CA, USA) is used to simultaneously protect the wound from infected tissue, as well as provide some soft tissue retraction. Adhesions are commonly encountered on entering the thorax and are divided with blunt or sharp dissection, or electrocautery. The pulmonary vessels and bronchus are divided using Endo-GIA staplers (Auto Suture Company, United States Surgical Corp., Norwalk, CT, USA), identical to those used in cases of pulmonary malignancy. Not infrequently there is incomplete development of the major fissure secondary to underlying anatomy or significant inflammatory changes. When this is encountered, resection should favor the noninvolved side of the fissure. This is a key technical point that we feel ensures complete excision of diseased lung tissue. An EndoCatch (Auto Suture Company) is used to remove the specimen from the hemithorax, taking care to avoid contamination of the port sites. Cultures should be sent to microbiology laboratories familiar with culture techniques for mycobacterial organisms. Intercostal nerve blocks with 0.25% bupivicaine are placed using a mediastinoscopy aspiration syringe and needle.

Surgical Technique: Open Approach

For more involved lesions, very large cavities, or prohibitive adhesions, an open approach is preferred (**Fig. 3**). We offer epidural catheters to all patients undergoing an open procedure. A lateral thoracotomy incision is adequate for most operations. The serratus muscle is spared. In the reoperative setting, the previous incision is used. When performing lobectomies or segmental resections, the procedure is the same as outlined for a thoracoscopic resection.

For extrapleural or completion pneumonectomies, a posterolateral incision is made. The latissimus dorsi muscle can be harvested for muscle transposition and the serratus anterior is spared. An intercostal muscle, if needed for buttressing of the bronchial stump, is mobilized at this point to avoid pedicle trauma owing to the subsequent placement of the chest spreader. We typically "shingle" the sixth rib posteriorly for planned entry through the fifth intercostal space; for planned extrapleural dissection, the fifth rib is resected. On entering the thoracic cavity, significant inflammatory changes can be encountered in extensive adhesions or erosion into the chest wall, necessitating extrapleural dissection. Extrapleural dissection is completed bluntly, with occasional use of cautery. Great care should be taken in the vicinity of known vascular and neural structures. Once the lung is freed, the planned resection usually can be accomplished without undue difficulty. For completion pneumonectomy, an intrapericardial

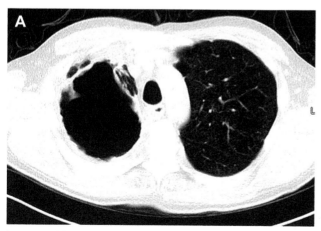
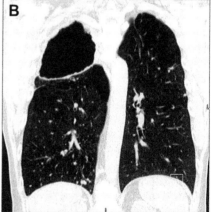

Fig. 3. Axial (*A*) and coronal (*B*) CT images of a patient with cavitary right upper lobe disease associated with *M avium* complex infection. The thin cavity wall and high degree of pleural symphysis suggest the need for an open approach for resection.

Table 1
Summary of outcomes for anatomic resection of pulmonary NTM disease

First Author, Years	Reference No.	No. Patients	Lesion	NTM Pathogen	Procedures (No.)	Mortality, %	% Overall Surgical Morbidity, % Complications (No.)	Preop/Op Culture (+), %	Postop Culture (−), %
Pomerantz, 1983–1996	6	13	Bronchiectasis Destroyed Lung	Mixed NTM	RM Lobectomy (11) Lingulectomy (4)	0%	8% Overall 8% Pneumothorax (1)	NR	85%
Nelson, 1989–1997	17	28	Bronchiectasis Cavity Destroyed Lung	Mixed NTM	Pneumonectomy (8) Lobectomy (20)	7%	32% Overall 17% BPF (1) 11% Prolonged air leak treated with thoracoplasty (3)	54%	93% of survivors
Shiraishi, 1993–2001	18	21	Bronchiectasis Cavity Destroyed Lung	Mixed NTM	Pneumonectomy (3) Lobectomy/ Combination (18)	0%	29% Overall 10% BPF (2) Space issue treated with thoracoplasty (2) 5% Pneumonia (1) Prolonged air leak (1)	62%	95%
Shiraishi, 1983–2002	23	11	Cavity Destroyed Lung	Mixed NTM	Pneumonectomy (11)	18%	36% Overall 27% BPF (3) 9% Empyema (1) Respiratory failure (1)	NR	100%
Watanabe, 1990–2005	19	22	Bronchiectasis Cavity	Mixed NTM	Lobectomy/ Combination (15) Segmentectomy (3) Wedge (4) VATS resection (1)	0%	5% Overall 5% Space issue treated with thoracoplasty (1)	100%	100%
Jarand, 2001–2004	13	24 Surg 46 Med	Bronchiectasis Cavity	Mycobacterium abscessus	Pneumonectomy (6) Lobectomy/ Combination (24)	17% Surg 16% Med	25% Overall 4% Postoperative bleeding (1) BPF (1), Respiratory failure (1) Frozen shoulder (1) Brachial plexus injury (1) Wound infection (1)	64%	57% Surg 28% Med

Study	N	Indication	NTM	Procedure (N)	Complications		
Sherwood, 1994–2003 [14]	26	Cavity Destroyed Lung BPF	Mixed NTM	Pneumonectomy (26) 23%	46% Overall 27% BPF (7) 19% Respiratory failure (5), Pneumonia (5) 12% Arrhythmia (3) 8% ARDS (2), DVT (2), Wound complication (2) 4% Myocardial infarction (1)	65%	NR
Mitchell 1983–2006 [16]	236	Bronchiectasis Cavity Destroyed Lung	Mixed NTM	Pneumonectomy (44) 2.6% Lobectomy/Combination (126) Lingulectomy (46) VATS resection (68)	19% Overall 4% BPF (11) 3% Pneumonia/Respiratory failure (9) 2% Reexplored for bleeding (4) 1% Pneumothorax requiring intervention (3) <1% Wound infection (2) Myocardial infarction (1)	43%	NR
Koh 2002–2007 [24]	23	Bronchiectasis Cavity	Mixed NTM	Pneumonectomy (4) 4.3% Lobectomy/Combination (16) Segmentectomy (3) VATS resection (4)	39% Overall 13% Pneumonia (3) 9% BPF (2) Prolonged air leak (2) 4% Post-pneumonectomy syndrome (1) Wound dehiscence (1)	74%	100% of survivors
Yu 2004–2009 [20]	134	Bronchiectasis Cavity	Mixed NTM	VATS RM Lobectomy/Combination (102) VATS Lingulectomy (70) 0%	7% Overall 4% Prolonged air leak (6) 1% Pneumothorax (2) <1% Atrial fibrillation, (1) Wound infection (1) Pleural effusion (1)	44%	84%

Abbreviations: ARDS, acute respiratory distress syndrome; BPF, bronchopleural fistula; DVT, deep vein thrombosis; NR, not reported; NTM, nontuberculous mycobacteria; Op, operative; Preop, preoperative; RM, right middle; VATS, video-assisted thoracic surgery.

approach may provide the safest technique for vessel division. We typically divide the pulmonary vessels and left mainstem bronchus with the same Endo GIA staplers as described previously. The right mainstem bronchus is typically closed with manual suturing instead of stapling, using a tension-free, interrupted suture technique with 4-0 Vicryl (Ethicon, Inc., Johnson & Johnson, Somerville, NJ, USA). As noted previously, buttressing of the bronchial stump should be considered in the setting of poorly controlled or drug-resistant infection, and in the setting of right pneumonectomy. In the setting of gross contamination of the pleural space after pneumonectomy, an Eloesser procedure (open thoracostomy) may be fashioned at the lower, dependent portion of the thoracotomy wound. Careful planning of the initial thoracotomy incision is helpful if this finding is anticipated preoperatively. In complex pleural space infections without pneumonectomy, myoplasty with or without concomitant thoracoplasty may be used to obliterate the space.[22,23]

When there is gross purulence in the bronchial tree, toilet bronchoscopy should be performed both at the beginning and at the end of the procedure, as secretions from the diseased lung can pool in the dependent, contralateral lung. Patients are extubated in the operating room and transported to the surgical intensive care unit.

Postoperative Care

Routine postoperative care emphasizes pain control, pulmonary toilet, early mobilization, and maintenance of nutrition. Prophylactic low-dose beta-blockade is typically used to reduce the incidence of postoperative atrial fibrillation. Patients are fluid restricted to 1500 mL per day with a goal of maintaining a net negative fluid balance. For patients who present with bilateral focal disease, staged resection of the contralateral diseased lobe or segment can occur 2 to 6 weeks later. Patients with Eloesser flaps have dressings removed on postoperative day 2, with dressing changes every 2 days. We use quarter-strength Dakin solution-soaked Kerlix gauze. Eloesser closure is performed 6 to 8 weeks after discharge depending on the presence of granulation tissue.

Preoperative antimycobacterial antibiotic regimens should be continued throughout the perioperative period. Culture results from tissue obtained at the operation are used to adjust antimicrobial regimens as needed. Typically, antibiotic therapy is continued until culture-negative for at least 12 months.

OUTCOMES

Postoperative outcomes and complications vary by approach and severity of pathology. **Table 1** summarizes rates of major complications and sputum conversion after surgical resection compared with medical treatment alone. Discussion of these outcomes is outlined in more detail in this section.

Outcomes: Thoracoscopic Approach

Indications to convert to open are mostly secondary to adhesions, specifically severe inflammation in the fissure and in the perihilar dissection. In our most recent review of 212 thoracoscopic lobectomies or segmentectomies for predominantly NTM disease, conversion to open occurred in fewer than 5% of cases.[21] Mortality and major complications are negligible. The morbidity in these series is approximately 7% to 8%, consisting of prolonged air leak most frequently, followed by pneumothorax, atrial fibrillation, effusions, and atelectasis.[16,20]

Outcomes: Open Approach

Although the largest series to date demonstrated no intraoperative deaths,[16] mortality following open resection for advanced disease still occurs, resulting from postoperative complications, such as bronchopleural fistula (BPF) and pneumonia leading to respiratory failure. BPF is most frequently a complication after pneumonectomy, particularly right pneumonectomy, and is rarely seen after lobectomies and segmentectomies. In the largest series of pneumonectomies for pulmonary NTM disease, we reported a BPF rate of 20% for patients undergoing pneumonectomy. In the next 2 largest series by Sherwood and colleagues[14] and Shiraishi and colleagues,[23] the BPF rate after completion pneumonectomy for chronic mycobacterial disease, was 27%. Right-sided pneumonectomy and positive preoperative sputum were risk factors for BPF. In the series by Mitchell and colleagues,[16] 50% of patients who had a BPF did not undergo bronchial stump buttressing. No patients who had omentum at the bronchial stump developed a fistula. Shiraishi and colleagues[23] and Sherwood and colleagues[14] specify that 33% and 57% of BPFs respectively occurred within 30 days of the operation.

Despite prolonged preoperative antibiotic therapy, most the patients with advanced disease will still have positive preoperative or intraoperative (tissue) cultures for NTM. More than 80% of patients convert their sputum postoperatively. Importantly, a large percentage of patients with mycobacteria cultured in operative tissue subsequently convert to sputum culture–negative status postoperatively.

The retrospective nature of all of the studies limits the formation of definitive conclusions about conversion rates of pulmonary NTM after medical therapy alone, compared with surgical resection as an adjunct. Microbiologic data are not collected or assessed with standardized techniques or at consistent time points. Without standardization, relapse and or reinfections are also ill-defined. Furthermore, surgical patients have been carefully selected and this may bias the beneficial outcome of the surgical group.

Despite these limitations, anatomic resection of damaged lung parenchyma appears to benefit patients with pulmonary NTM disease when used as part of multimodality therapy with careful attention to patient selection and operative timing. A minimally invasive approach is feasible for focal bronchiectasis and small cavities. Surgical management of more advanced pathology may also benefit select patients and, in severe disease, may be the only option to palliate symptoms and slow the progression of ongoing lung destruction.

REFERENCES

1. Field SK, Cowie RL. Lung disease due to the more common nontuberculous mycobacteria. Chest 2006;129:1653–72.
2. Griffith DE, Aksamit T, Brown-Elliott BA, et al. An official ATS/IDSA statement: diagnosis, treatment, and prevention of nontuberculous mycobacterial diseases. Am J Respir Crit Care Med 2007;175:367–416.
3. Prevots DR, Shaw PA, Strickland D, et al. Nontuberculous mycobacterial lung disease prevalence at four integrated health care delivery systems. Am J Respir Crit Care Med 2010;182(7):970–6.
4. Aksamit T. Mycobacterium avium complex pulmonary disease in patients with pre-existing lung disease. Clin Chest Med 2002;23:643–53.
5. Ziedalski TM, Kao PN, Henig NR, et al. Prospective analysis of cystic fibrosis transmembrane regulator mutations in adults with bronchiectasis or pulmonary nontuberculous mycobacterial infection. Chest 2006;130:995–1002.
6. Pomerantz M, Denton JR, Huitt GA, et al. Resection of the right middle lobe and lingula for mycobacterial infection. Ann Thorac Surg 1996;62:990–3.
7. Colombo RE, Hill SC, Claypool RJ, et al. Familial clustering of pulmonary nontuberculous mycobacterial disease. Chest 2010;137:629–34.
8. Kim RD, Greenberg DE, Ehrmantraut ME, et al. Pulmonary nontuberculous mycobacterial disease: prospective study of a distinct preexisting syndrome. Am J Respir Crit Care Med 2008;178:1066–74.
9. Telenti A, Machesi F, Balz M, et al. Rapid identification of mycobacteria to the species level by polymerase chain reaction and restriction enzyme analysis. J Clin Microbiol 1993;31:175.
10. Woods GL. The mycobacteriology laboratory and new diagnostic techniques. Infect Dis Clin North Am 2002;16:127–44.
11. Field SK, Cowie RL. Treatment of Mycobacterium avium-intracellulare complex lung disease with a macrolide, ethambutol, and clofazimine. Chest 2003;124:1482–6.
12. Tanaka E, Kimoto T, Tsuyuguchi K, et al. Effect of clarithromycin regimen for Mycobacterium avium complex pulmonary disease. Am J Respir Crit Care Med 1999;160:866–72.
13. Jarand JM, Levin A, Zhang L, et al. Clinical and microbiologic outcomes in patients receiving treatment for Mycobacterium abscessus pulmonary disease. Clin Infect Dis 2011;52:565–71.
14. Sherwood JT, Mitchell JD, Pomerantz M. Completion pneumonectomy for chronic mycobacterial disease. J Thorac Cardiovasc Surg 2005;129:1257–64.
15. Pomerantz M, Madsen L, Goble M, et al. Surgical management of resistant mycobacterial tuberculosis and other mycobacterial pulmonary infections. Ann Thorac Surg 1991;52:1108–12.
16. Mitchell JD, Bishop A, Cafaro A, et al. Anatomic lung resection for nontuberculous mycobacterial disease. Ann Thorac Surg 2008;85:1887–93.
17. Nelson KG, Griffith DE, Brown BA, et al. Results of operation in Mycobacterium avium-intracellulare disease. Ann Thorac Surg 1998;66:325–30.
18. Shiraishi Y, Nakajima Y, Takasuna K, et al. Surgery for Mycobacterium avium complex lung disease in the clarithromycin era. Eur J Cardiothorac Surg 2002;21:314–8.
19. Watanabe M, Hasegawa N, Ishizaka A, et al. Early pulmonary resection for Mycobacterium avium complex lung disease treated with macrolides and quinolones. Ann Thorac Surg 2006;81:2006–30.
20. Yu JA, Pomerantz M, Bishop A, et al. Lady Windermere revisited: treatment with thoracoscopic lobectomy/segmentectomy for right middle lobe and lingular bronchiectasis associated with nontuberculous mycobacterial disease. Eur J Cardiothorac Surg 2011;40:671–5.
21. Mitchell JD, Yu JA, Bishop A, et al. Thoracoscopic lobectomy and segmentectomy for infectious lung disease. Ann Thorac Surg 2012;93:1033–40.
22. Stefani A, Jouni R, Alifano M, et al. Thoracoplasty in the current practice of thoracic surgery: a single-institution 10-year experience. Ann Thorac Surg 2011;91:263–9.
23. Shiraishi Y, Nakajima Y, Katsuragi N, et al. Pneumonectomy for nontuberculous mycobacterial infections. Ann Thorac Surg 2004;78:399–403.
24. Koh WJ, Kim YH, Kwon OJ, et al. Surgical treatment of pulmonary diseases due to nontuberculous mycobacteria. J Korean Med Sci 2008;23:397–401.

Surgery for the Sequelae of Postprimary Tuberculosis

Gilbert Massard, MD, PhD, FETS*, Anne Olland, MD, MSc,
Nicola Santelmo, MD, FETS,
Pierre-Emmanuel Falcoz, MD, PhD, FETS

KEYWORDS

- Postprimary tuberculosis • Pneumonectomy • Thoracoplasty • Fibrostenosis

KEY POINTS

- Surgery may be indicated when the sequelae of tuberculosis cause troubling symptoms.
- Intraoperatively, special care should be addressed to a careful step-by-step hemostasis while taking down adhesions and dissecting out hilar structures.
- Because of the increased risk for bronchial fistula, cautious preparation of the bronchial stump and respect of its blood supply is mandatory; the bronchial stump after pneumonectomy should be covered routinely.
- Historic techniques such as thoracoplasty should be available in the surgeon's armamentarium because they may be helpful in particularly difficult situations.
- Preventive surgery is recommended in case of aspergilloma only; in most other categories, observation is legitimate.
- Indications for postoperative antituberculous treatment include the presence of *Mycobacterium tuberculosis* and/or active granulomas, and a history of tuberculosis in a patient who did not receive modern antituberculous multidrug therapy or who did not comply with it.

INTRODUCTION

Tuberculosis remains an endemic disease in most countries, except in western Europe and North America. Surgical concerns are raised when active disease is not controlled by antituberculous chemotherapy, especially in the presence of multiresistant or panresistant *Mycobacterium tuberculosis*, or when sequelae cause annoying symptoms. This review focuses on the latter category.

After healing of active tuberculosis, scarring of bronchi and parenchyma may determine a whole spectrum of elementary lesions, which include bronchiectasis, bronchial fibrostenosis, and lung cavitation; these lesions, isolated or combined in various amounts, may generate destruction of a lobe or even a complete lung. Healing of mediastinal lymphadenitis leads to calcifications, which may subsequently erode into the bronchi and cause broncholithiasis (**Table 1**).

The usual symptoms are:

- Cough
- Dyspnea
- Purulent sputum
- Hemoptysis
- Recurrent pneumonia.

Sequelae of tuberculosis may also lead to catastrophic emergencies such as massive hemoptysis and bronchoesophageal fistula (BEF).

The authors comment briefly on long-term sequelae of historic treatments of tuberculosis, mainly collapse therapy, knowing that these patients have become the exception nowadays.

Service de Chirurgie Thoracique, Hôpitaux Universitaires de Strasbourg, 1, place de l'hôpital, 67091 Strasbourg, France
* Corresponding author.
E-mail address: Gilbert.Massard@chru-strasbourg.fr

Thorac Surg Clin 22 (2012) 287–300
doi:10.1016/j.thorsurg.2012.05.006
1547-4127/12/$ – see front matter © 2012 Elsevier Inc. All rights reserved.

Table 1
Elementary lesions determined by tuberculosis

	Lesion	Complications
Lung	Bronchiectasis	
	Fibrostenosis	
	Cavitation	Aspergilloma
Nodes	Broncholithiasis	Bronchoesophageal fistula

BRONCHIECTASIS

Bronchiectasis may result from numerous other causal factors besides tuberculosis. Congenital varieties of bronchiectasis are usually diffusely distributed and related to hereditary diseases such as cystic fibrosis, ciliary syndromes, immunoglobulin A deficiency, or polycystic lung disease. Acquired bronchiectasis may be due to recurrent infection with or without sinusitis, bronchial obstruction, post-traumatic stenosis and, last but not least, tuberculosis.[1] The 2 histologic variants, acinar and tubular bronchiectasis, differ from a physiopathologic point of view. The usual acinar subtype has virtually no systemic blood supply. By contrast, the tubular subtype presents with a considerable hypertrophy of bronchial vessels. On rare occasions, hypertrophy of bronchial arteries determines a significant left-to-right shunt with hemodynamic alterations adding to the respiratory symptoms; this has been referred to as the acquired patent ductus syndrome.[2] Most available publications on bronchiectasis accumulate cases of various origins and are not specifically dedicated to tuberculosis. With some caution the discussion can be orientated to the following.

Bronchiectasis is the most common elementary lesion observed in patients with history of tuberculosis, occurring in at least 11% of the affected patients.[3,4] The usual mechanism leading to bronchiectasis in tuberculosis patients is either traction on the bronchi due to fibrotic scarring and retraction within the parenchyma, or chronic peripheral infection consecutive to bronchial obstruction attributable to fibrostenosis or broncholithiasis (see later discussion). It develops about 3 months after the initial infection and, by definition, in the same anatomic district.[3,4] There seems to be a female predominance.[5] The left side is more often involved because of anatomic features of the left main bronchus.[6,7]

Diagnostic Workup

A high level of suspicion should be maintained in patients with a history of tuberculosis who complain of chronic cough and sputum; this allows for early diagnosis, which is easily established with high-resolution computed tomography (CT) or spiral CT.[8] Careful analysis with CT does not only confirm diagnosis but is mandatory in planning for a targeted resection. As such, modern imaging is credited with sensitivity and specificity in excess of 95%, and false-negative and false-positive rates of less than 2%.[9,10] Hence, it is not surprising that contemporary CT imaging has been replacing classic bronchography for more than 2 decades. Fiberoptic bronchoscopy completes diagnostic workup: it may identify particular features such as fibrostenosis or broncholithiasis, and allows for the collection of protected samples for microbiology.[11]

Surgical Resection

Surgical resection is recommended in presence of repeated hemoptysis, recurrent infection, or abscess formation. In addition, it should be considered when symptoms are interfering with social and professional life, when medical treatment fails, and when there is lack of compliance with treatment.[1]

Resection should be both complete and economical, and relies on segmental resection techniques. It is well established that staged bilateral operations are safe and do not increase the complication rate.[12] Mini-invasive resection with the use of video-assisted thoracoscopic surgery is increasingly offered as a viable alternative to a classic open thoracotomy approach.[13] Success of operation also depends on adequate preoperative preparation of the patient. Aggressive physiotherapy combined with antibiotics chosen in accordance with microbiologic assessment of sputum samples should aim at bringing the patient to the operating room with a "dry bronchial tree".[14] Postoperative complications are observed in 8.8% to 23% of patients in contemporary publications (**Table 2**).[11,14–17] The relatively diverse rate of complication may depend on the investigators' different definition of complication and patient selection. Pleural adhesions and hypertrophy of bronchial vessels account for perioperative bleeding. Despite optimal physiotherapy, sputum retention is common and may be complicated by atelectasis or even pneumonia. Segmentectomy following the classic peeling technique exposes the patient to prolonged air leak and bronchopleural fistula, which can further lead to residual space and eventually empyema. In extreme cases, when fibrotic changes within the remaining lung oppose to full reexpansion, repeated surgery with thoracoplasty may be required.

Table 2
Operative risk related to resection of bronchiectasis

Authors,[Ref.] Year	No. of Patients	Mortality (%)	Morbidity (%)
Balkanli et al,[15] 2003	238	0	8.8
Kutlay et al,[16] 2002	166	1.7	10.5
Eren et al,[11] 2002	143	1.3	23
Hiramatsu et al,[17] 2012	31	0	18
Prieto et al,[14] 2001	119	0	15

Long-term results are encouraging, with 60% to 75% of the patients becoming symptom-free and another 15% significantly improved (**Table 3**).[11,18] However, logistic regression analysis showed that history of tuberculosis and incomplete resection were independent predictors of postoperative complications and failure to improve at medium term.[11] In other words, the results of surgery for posttuberculous bronchiectasis may actually be less optimistic than those reported in global reviews.

FIBROSTENOSIS

Fibrostenosis results from healing of endobronchial tuberculosis, which is defined as microbiological or histopathologic evidence of tuberculous infection of the tracheobronchial tree.[19] Both a left-sided and female predominance have been reported[20] for an infection that is observed in 10% to 37% of patients.[21] Endobronchial tuberculosis seems to be supported by 2 different pathogenetic mechanisms. In brief, one hypothesis refers to direct implantation of the disease into the bronchial mucosa; the second refers to compression by infected lymph nodes, which may ultimately ulcerate into the bronchial tree. Whatever the mechanism, ultimate fibrostenosis results from scarring with circumferential retraction and submucosal fibrosis. Bronchoscopic findings at initial assessment range from moderate bronchitis to confirmed fibrostenosis, including:

- Nonspecific bronchitis with moderate edema and hyperemia
- Edematous-hyperemic bronchitis
- Actively caseating bronchitis
- Granular bronchitis with a scattered cobblestone aspect
- Ulcerative bronchitis
- Pseudotumoral lesions
- Fibrostenosis.[22]

Multiple aspects may combine in the same patient. The natural history of any stage is progression to fibrostenosis. Fibrostenosis is particularly likely to develop if excessive granulation tissue appears within the lumen. At the end stage, fibrostenosis typically presents as a rigid narrowing of the bronchus lined with normal-looking mucosa.[23,24]

Treatment of endobronchial tuberculosis at the acute initial stage has 2 main goals:

- Eradication of *Mycobacterium tuberculosis*
- Prevention of bronchostenosis.

Despite optimal therapy, the prognosis is uncertain and ranges from complete clearance to severe fibrostenosis; the beneficial effect of corticosteroids remains controversial.[25] In a recently published series reviewing 67 cases, 41.8% of patients developed persisting fibrostenosis. Multivariate analysis identified the following risk factors:

- Age greater than 45 years
- Delay between onset of symptoms and initiation of antituberculous treatment longer than 90 days.

Isolated fibrostenosis or combined with other lesions at initial bronchoscopy was not reversible, whereas other aspects such as caseating, ulcerative, granular, or pseudotumoral bronchitis responded well to treatment.[21]

Clinical presentation of fibrostenosis obviously depends on its location. The most common complaint is dyspnea. When fibrostenosis involves

Table 3
Long-term results after resection of bronchiectasis

Authors,[Ref.] Year	No. of Patients	Cured (%)	Improved (%)	Unchanged (%)
Eren et al,[11] 2007	143	75.9	15.7	8.2
Zhang et al,[18] 2010	790	60.5	14.1	14.8

main stem bronchi or trachea, audible wheezing may be perceived. Peripheral stenoses, located in lobar or segmental bronchi, can be asymptomatic and are obviated by atelectasis at chest radiography. However, long-lasting fibrostenosis may be further complicated by chronic infection determining bronchiectasis or even destruction of the underlying territory; symptoms then include cough, sputum, and infectious exacerbations with fever.

Surgery for Fibrostenosis

The treatment of fibrostenosis usually requires surgery. The operation should be carefully planned. The main issue is to evaluate the underlying lung. In the case of extensive bronchiectasis or even destruction, conservative procedures do not make sense; only resection of the diseased lobe or lung is advisable. CT scanning allows for excellent visualization. Resection is also the only reasonable option when the stenosis involves a lobar or segmental bronchus. On the other hand, stenosis of the central airways with normal underlying lung or only mild bronchiectasis should be managed with parenchyma-saving bronchoplastic procedures. Careful fiberoptic bronchoscopy and virtual bronchoscopy with 3-dimensional CT are helpful tools in evaluating the feasibility by measuring the involved segment of airway. Possible operations include segmental resection of trachea or main bronchus, sleeve upper lobectomy, and even carinal reconstruction. Several series show excellent postoperative and medium-term outcome.[20,26,27]

In complex cases with extended stenotic segments not amenable to resection, invasive bronchoscopy techniques with bougienage or balloon catheter dilatation and insertion of stents may achieve satisfactory results. Low and colleagues[28] reported that the luminal diameter of the trachea increased from 4.5 to 11.9 mm on an average, and the main stem bronchial diameter from 2.6 to 8.3 mm. Stents were used in 52%. Furthermore, 19% of patients required multiple bronchoscopies. At 25 months of follow-up, 52% of patients remained asymptomatic.

Lee and colleagues have undertaken a retrospective study to identify features on CT scan that might predict outcome after reexpansion procedures. Their study analyzed a series of 30 patients: 5 underwent surgical bronchoplasty, 2 exclusive dilatation, and 23 stent placement. Predictors of failure were parenchymal calcifications and bronchiectasis within atelectasis. By contrast, factors such as mucous plugging, extent of stenosis, loss of volume, or active tuberculosis did not affect outcome.[29]

CAVITATION AND ASPERGILLOMA

Saprophytic infection of a lung cavitation with Aspergillus species, leading to the development of a fungus ball or megamycetoma, is probably the most typical long-term complication of tuberculosis. The natural history of the disease starts with healing of cavitary tuberculosis and conversion of sputum. The next step is spontaneous detersion of the cavitation, with progressive elimination of caseous necrosis and lining with bronchial mucosa. Finally, aerosolized Aspergillus may reach the cavitation through the bronchial tree. Local hygrometry and temperature of 37°C are conditions most favorable for fungal growth and development of the megamycetoma. The mycetoma itself may increase the size of the cavitation by secretion of proteolytic enzymes and progressive erosion of the surrounding parenchyma. Sooner or later, the erosive process will ulcerate into blood vessels and cause hemoptysis. Hemoptysis is further favored in the apical area of the upper lobes, where the inflammatory process appeals for systemic neovascularization arising from intercostal arteries. The same inflammatory reaction may determine loss of weight or fatigue. Respiratory function may be altered by the destructive process of previous tuberculosis, or by previous surgical resection.

Depending on various factors, patients may be asymptomatic or present with cough, sputum, and hemoptysis. In the authors' initial report including about 80% of patients with previous tuberculosis, half of the patients were asymptomatic.[30] The most annoying symptom is hemoptysis, which may reach a catastrophic level.

Diagnosis is easy in patients with a known cavitation and who are subjected to a regular follow-up, but is also obvious in patients undergoing incidental chest radiography. The typical presentation is a parenchymal cavitation containing a rounded solid mass, determining the so-called air crescent sign.

Clinical and radiologic presentations led Belcher and Plummer[31] to define 2 opposite categories, called respectively simple and complex aspergilloma. Simple aspergilloma occurs in a thin-walled cavitation embedded into normal-looking parenchyma, without any pleural scar, in asymptomatic patients; in this category, the underlying lesion is bronchiectasis or cystic areas in otherwise normal lungs. Patients with a history of tuberculosis usually belong to the complex aspergilloma type. In the latter, the cavitation is thick-walled and surrounded by fibrotic scarring and/or pleural peel; these patients may be heavily symptomatic, with altered nutritional status or chronic respiratory failure.[31] Besides tuberculosis, other granulomatous diseases such as sarcoidosis or histoplasmosis may host complex aspergilloma.[32,33]

Positive serodiagnosis is a further argument for positive diagnosis. However, radiologic features are usually pathognomonic.

Treatment of Cavitation and Aspergilloma

There are various treatment options.

- The most radical treatment is anatomic resection of the diseased lobe, which eliminates both the mycetoma and the underlying cavitation.
- The most frequent type of resection is lobectomy.
- Segmentectomy or wedge excision is not recommended, because of a significant risk of opening the cavitation and spilling its content into the pleural space.
- Pneumonectomy carries an increased risk of postoperative septic complications, with an empyema rate in excess of 25% (see later discussion on destroyed lung).[1]

When the patient is unfit for anatomic resection, the radical alternative is represented by a direct approach of the cavitation with removal of the fungus ball, combined with immediate thoracoplasty to collapse the cavitation. Both types of treatment may be considered to be radical and provide a permanent cure in the vast majority of patients.[30] In desperately ill patients, cavernostomy may be helpful. Systemic antifungals are ineffective, and intracavitary injections do not guarantee a permanent cure; relapse of aspergilloma is likely to occur if the cavitation is not obliterated or resected.[30] The reverse side of operative management is risk for mortality and complications. Two recent updates of the authors' series showed a progressive decline of postoperative problems:

- Mortality decreased from 5% to zero
- Postoperative bleeding decreased from 44% to 6%
- Pleural space problems decreased from 47% to 12%.

This decrease in complication rate is definitely related to a changing profile of the patients: during the years 1974 to 1991, 80% of patients had complex aspergilloma; this category has decreased to 12% in the most recent period, from 1998 to 2009.[34,35] Obviously this time trend reflects the dramatic decrease of the prevalence of tuberculosis during the past 4 decades in France.

Another issue is treatment strategy. Given the high complication rate reported in historical series, it has been considered that only symptomatic patients should undergo surgery. However, postoperative outcome is improved in asymptomatic patients, even in those with complex aspergilloma and a previous history of tuberculosis.[30] Accordingly, the authors recommend elective surgery in asymptomatic patients mainly to prevent ultimate deterioration. One should be aware that, also in the most contemporary series, the overall complication rate of complex aspergilloma is slightly higher than that of simple aspergilloma.[36,37]

BRONCHOLITHIASIS

Broncholithiasis is defined as a condition in which calcified or ossified material is present within the bronchial lumen. It is most often attributable to progressive erosion of the bronchus by calcified mediastinal nodes in relation to granulomatous infections or inflammation. Tuberculosis is the leading cause in most parts of the world except North America, where the leading cause is fungal infections primarily due to *Histoplasma capsulatum* or *Coccioides immitis*.[38] Other more exceptional conditions are silicosis,[39] aspiration of bone tissue or calcification of aspirated foreign body,[40] or sequestration of ossified bronchial cartilage plates into the bronchus.[38] On rare occasions, calcified endobronchial tumors such as carcinoids and hamartomas may mimic broncholithiasis.[41,42]

There seems to be a mild predominance of female patients; median age is close to 60 years.[43] The most common location of broncholiths is the bronchus intermedius.[44]

Potential anatomic complications of broncholithiasis are obstructive pneumonia with subsequent development of bronchiectasis and/or parenchymal destruction, and acquired benign BEF.

Broncholiths become symptomatic when the calcified node impinges on or erodes into the lumen of the airway. Symptoms include chronic cough, hemoptysis, lithoptysis, recurrent pneumonia, and fistulas between bronchi and mediastinal structures (see later discussion). Cough is the most frequent symptom, closely followed by hemoptysis of varying amount. By contrast, lithoptysis, though pathognomonic, is rare and accounts for less than 10%.[43] Most broncholiths are symptomatic; Cerfolio and colleagues[44] reported on 50 patients with 76% being symptomatic, whereas 44 of 47 patients reported by Potaris and colleagues[43] presented with symptoms.

Radiographic findings of broncholithiasis include visualization of calcified mediastinal nodes occurring together with signs of airway obstruction such as atelectasis, mucoid impaction, bronchiectasis, or expiratory airway trapping.[45] Disappearance or displacement of a previously identified calcified nidus on serial radiographs is very suggestive.[45] CT typically depicts an endobronchial calcified nodule, which may be associated with signs of bronchial obstruction. However, conventional CT may suffer from a volume-averaging artifact of broncholith, bronchus, and peribronchial tissues, and lead to erroneous interpretation. Contemporary helical CT performed with thin collimation and multiplanar reformation is most helpful in distinguishing endobronchial and peribronchial calcifications.[45]

Broncholiths eroding the bronchial wall are easily identified at bronchoscopy, and may present as either mobile or fixed. Mobile broncholiths, also referred to as rockable broncholiths, are either loose in the airway or move when probed with bronchoscopic instruments. Fixed broncholiths or airway stones do not exhibit any movement when probed at bronchoscopy.[44]

Surgery for Broncholithiasis

Active treatment relies on either bronchoscopic removal or open surgery.

Bronchoscopic removal

Cerfolio[46] has succinctly described the technique of endoscopic removal. The procedure is performed under general anesthesia with intubation, with a rigid number-8 bronchoscope and jet ventilation. Once identified, the broncholith is gently probed to check for mobility. If the stone is loose or becomes loose after manipulation, it is removed through a 0° lens straight-A head grasper. Stones that cannot be grasped may be pulled up to the proximal airway with help of an inflated 4- to 8-mm angioplasty balloon catheter. Because bleeding may arise from surrounding granulation tissue, laser or electrocautery must be available during the procedure. Irrigation is performed at the conclusion to check that all fragments have been removed, and the distal airway is inspected to ensure that all subsegments have been recruited. In Cerfolio's experience, 67% of broncholiths were mobile, and all mobile stones could be retrieved endoscopically without significant bleeding.[44] Hence, the classic fear of massive bleeding seems unfounded.[47,48] However, manipulation of a broncholith located contiguous to the pulmonary artery may be dangerous; the amount of broncholith located outside of the airway should always be carefully evaluated on CT. Three patients of 29 reported by Cerfolio and colleagues[44] required subsequent procedures to remove other broncholiths that moved into the airway.

Open surgery

Principles of open surgery are removal of all calcified nodes that may be safely removed without injury to vital structures or parenchymal resection. Broncholithectomy is performed through a bronchotomy, which is carefully repaired and eventually covered with a muscular flap. Nodes that cannot be removed should be incised and their content should be retrieved by cautious curettage.[48] Indications for anatomic resection, most often and preferably lobectomy, are hemoptysis, bronchial obstruction complicated with bronchiectasis or parenchymal destruction, and failed bronchoscopic extraction.[49] However, surgery for massive hemoptysis appears as exceptional.[43] In the series reported by Potaris and colleagues,[43] 64% of patients required combined broncholithectomy and pulmonary resection to some extent. In contrast to the virtually no-complication rate reported by Cerfolio and colleagues,[44] the Mayo experience describes 13% of serious intraoperative complications such as laceration of the pulmonary artery, esophagus, or main bronchus. Similarly, 34% of patients developed postoperative complications. At long-term follow-up 68% of patients remained asymptomatic, whereas broncholithiasis recurred in 13%.[43]

On rare occasions, lithoptysis may lead to spontaneous resolution of symptoms.

In conclusion, the authors wholeheartedly endorse the recommendations presented in Cerfolio's algorithm: in the case of mobile broncholiths, an attempt at bronchoscopic removal should be made; fixed broncholiths should be removed only in symptomatic patients and most often require thoracotomy.[44]

DESTROYED LUNG

A combination of the different elementary lesions described here on grounds of extensive tuberculosis may ultimately lead to a completely destroyed lung. Other classic causes for destroyed lung are congenital malformations such as polycystic lung, acquired bronchiectasis, and radiation pneumonitis following treatment of lung cancer.[50] Destroyed lung seriously compromises long-term survival. In a recent survey of nonoperated patients, overall mortality of such patients was 28%, and median survival was estimated at only 39 months[51]; multivariate analysis identified that the extent of destruction located between 50% and 75% increases the risk of mortality.

Destroyed lung predominates on the left side: 13 of 18 cases reported by Treasure and Seaworth, 21 of 27 cases reported by Rizzi and colleagues, and 116 of 172 cases reported by Bai.[52–54] Ashour and colleagues[55] hypothesized that anatomic features explain this left predominance. The caliber of the left main bronchus is considerably narrower, and the peribronchial space is limited by the aortic arch. Hence, enlarged lymph nodes may determine compression of the bronchus with retention of secretion and chronic infection. Ashour created the concept of left bronchus syndrome, which includes a significant left-to-right shunt owing to hypertrophy of the bronchial arteries.[55]

Surgical Excision

Excision of a destroyed lung is discussed in the presence of various complications such as ongoing pyogenic infection, hemoptysis, bronchopleural fistula, and relapsing tuberculosis, among others. In the case of bilateral disease, chronic respiratory failure may preclude any surgery. Such operations represent a real challenge for both the surgeon and the patient. Since the pioneering years of resectional surgery for tuberculosis, it has been known that presence of granulomatous infection interferes with healing of the bronchial stump, and that active pleuropulmonary sepsis places the pneumonectomy space into serious jeopardy.[56]

There are multiple anatomic complications that appear as additional hazards during operative intervention. Well-vascularized pleural adhesions are the minimum, whereas many patients show extended and even complete obliteration of the pleural space. Calcified pleural peel may be encountered. Troublesome bleeding with diffuse oozing from the extrapleural space may complicate pneumolysis. Perihilar fibrosis is particularly challenging in the setting of completion pneumonectomy, where the time-honored principle of

intrapericardial dissection of vessels should be particularly followed. Dissection of the bronchus is completed in an atmosphere characterized by hyperplasia of bronchial vessels and mediastinal lymph nodes. Reed and colleagues[57] have advocated median sternotomy, which in their opinion carries some advantages over lateral thoracotomy. The main idea was to initiate straightforward cardiopulmonary bypass in the case of injury to a major vessel. In addition, the sternotomy incision is better tolerated when respiratory function is compromised. However, sternotomy offers a poor exposure to the posterior part of the pleural cavity, where adhesions are usually the tightest. In addition, there is a potential risk for sternal sepsis. Accordingly, most thoracic surgeons prefer a lateral thoracotomy.

Although many reports elaborate on the technical challenge of such procedures, postoperative mortality remains within an acceptable range (**Table 4**). In the most recent report by Bai,[54] the mortality is quoted as 2.9%; there was no mortality in a limited pediatric series reported by Kosar and colleagues.[62]

The complication rate varies considerably between areas of low and high prevalence of tuberculosis. In European and North American series, the incidence of empyema and bronchopleural fistula is reported to be in excess of 25%.[50,59] By contrast, in countries with a high prevalence of tuberculosis and a considerably higher case load, such complications occur in fewer than 10% of patients.[54,58,61] In the authors' experience, presence of *Aspergillus* infection has been a risk factor for major complications. In fact, among 7 patients with destroyed lung and aspergilloma, 5 developed empyema or bronchopleural fistula.[50]

BRONCHOESOPHAGEAL FISTULA

Acquired benign BEF is an exceptional condition, which is most often encountered during active tuberculous adenitis or is related to mediastinal

Table 4
Operative risk of pneumonectomy for destroyed lung

Authors,[Ref.] Year	No. of Patients	Deaths (%)	Morbidity (%)	Empyema/Fistula (%)
Blyth,[58] 2000	155	1.2	23	16.7
Conlan,[59] 1995	124	2.4	—	20.9
Halezeroglu et al,[60] 1997	118	5.9	13.2	12
Massard et al,[50] 1996	25	4	—	44
Kim et al,[61] 2003	94	1.1	21.3	15.9

sequelae.[63] During active tuberculous adenitis, the common mechanism is fistulization of the caseous lymph node into both esophagus and bronchus. This condition is outside of the scope of this review; conservative management with stenting and antituberculous chemotherapy is usually successful.[64]

Otherwise, healing of mediastinal tuberculous adenitis may determine a traction diverticulum in the mid-segment of the esophagus; subsequent calcification of the lymph node followed by broncholithiasis eroding into the bronchus may establish BEF. Differential diagnosis with a congenital BEF relies on Brunner's criteria: absence of past or present surrounding inflammation, absence of adherent lymph nodes, presence of mucosa, and definite muscularis mucosae are arguments in favor of a congenital origin.[65]

The median age of patients presenting with BEF is similar to those presenting with symptomatic broncholithiasis, about 56 years. The usual symptoms are intractable cough that worsens after swallowing liquids. Dysphagia seldom occurs. Lithoptysis is reported in up to 67% of patients. The median delay from first symptom to diagnosis is 21 months.[66]

The most proficient diagnostic test is radiocontrast study of the esophagus; identification of the fistula at bronchoscopy or during surgical exploration is also reported. The large majority of BEFs are located on the right side and account for close to 80%; the preferential location is the truncus intermedius.

Principles of repair for BEF are open removal of the calcified nodes, resection of the fistulous tract, repair of both esophagus and bronchus, and interposition of a pericardial or muscular flap to separate both organs.[43] The authors do not recommend simple stapling without division of the tract, because of the potential for spontaneous repermeation.[67]

MASSIVE HEMOPTYSIS

Massive hemoptysis becomes a life-threatening event when flooding of the bronchial tree compromises gas exchange. In addition, acute blood loss can lead to circulatory collapse.[68] In endemic areas, active tuberculosis and sequelae of disease are the leading cause of massive hemoptysis. All of the lesions already described are potential causes of massive hemoptysis, with cavitary tuberculosis and aspergilloma being the most important.[69]

The definition of severe hemoptysis varies from one investigator to another. The following few criteria meet a certain consensus:

- Cumulative amount of bleeding of at least 200 mL within 72 hours
- Acute respiratory failure
- Need for intravenous constrictive agent
- Need for blood transfusion.[70]

The first objective of initial management is to prevent asphyxiation, which may require endobronchial manipulations such as local instillation of cold saline and vasopressors, placement of a bronchial blocking balloon, and use of a rigid endoscope or double-lumen intubation to isolate the healthy lung.[70]

Treatment

Following stabilization of vital functions, there are 3 accepted treatment options:

- Observation
- Bronchial arterial embolization
- Surgical resection.[71]

It is known from historical series that without further treatment, the risk of recurrent bleeding is close to 80%.[72,73] Primary lung resection was considered the gold standard of treatment until the 1980s; however, lung resection was associated with a high mortality and morbidity, especially when performed during active bleeding.[23,72] During the past 2 decades, embolization has become the preferred treatment, especially in patients with tuberculosis.[71,74]

Embolization

Embolization conveys a low complication rate and achieves an immediate control of bleeding in 75% to 94% of patients; however, there is a significant recurrence rate, which is diversely estimated, and ranges from 18% to 42%.[75] Recurrence rate after embolization increases with time: control rate on hemoptysis was an estimated 93% at 2 weeks, 86% at 1 month, 79.5% at 3 months, 63% at 6 months, 51% at 1 year, and 39% at 2 years.[76] These dynamics reflect well the fact that underlying pulmonary inflammation or progressive disease may recruit blood supply and revascularization. In fact, lung cavities, nonbronchial systemic artery collaterals, and systemic-to-pulmonary venous shunts were more common in those who experienced recurrence.[76] When compared with patients with nontuberculous bronchiectasis, patients with previous tuberculosis have considerably more feeding vessels, requiring multiple embolization.

The risk of incomplete embolization may reach up to 30%.[77] Surgical extirpation of the concerned territory may of course secure the patient, but there is a definite subset of patients in whom hemoptysis does not recur. Hence, identification of factors predictive of recurrence becomes an important issue in adequately selecting those patients requiring consolidating surgery.[71,78] Van den Heuvel and colleagues[75] identified 4 risk factors for recurrence following bronchial artery embolization:

- Lack of complete cessation of hemoptysis within 7 days after embolization
- Need for blood transfusion
- Presence of aspergilloma
- Absence of active tuberculosis.

Van den Heuvel and colleagues[75] estimated that patients with no or 1 risk factor had a 10% risk of nonfatal rebleed, whereas patients with 2 to 4 risk factors had a 73% risk of recurrent hemoptysis and a 31% risk of dying from rebleeding. Another publication from this group reported on a prospective evaluation of the latter score. These investigators concluded that patients at low risk and those operated on had an uneventful outcome at 1 year; on the other hand, 2 of 7 inoperable high-risk patients subsequently died.[78]

Another retrospective study analyzed factors predictive of complications or mortality in a series of 111 patients operated on for severe hemoptysis. Although this article did not focus on a population with previous tuberculosis, the conclusions may direct clinical decision making. Half of the operations were performed on an emergency basis after a failed attempt or unsuccessful embolization; another 40% were operated electively a few days after successful embolization to prevent recurrent bleeding. The remaining 10% underwent planned surgery. The following factors were predictive of complications: presence of mycetoma, emergency surgery, and pneumonectomy. Factors predicting mortality were emergency surgery, chronic alcoholism, need of mechanical ventilation and/or vasoactive drugs on admission, and need for blood transfusion before surgery.[70]

LATE COMPLICATIONS OF COLLAPSE THERAPY

Until the advent of modern antituberculous chemotherapy in the early 1960s, collapse therapy was the only active treatment of excavated pulmonary tuberculosis. Although there were various techniques, the common principle was to collapse the excavated lung; external compression of the excavation joined to hypoventilation of the diseased parenchyma allowed for stabilization of the disease in many patients, and sometimes even achieved a permanent cure.

Techniques for Collapsotherapy

The most common treatment was intrapleural pneumothorax. Once the pneumothorax had been created by needle thoracentesis and pressure-controlled insufflation, the patient required re-insufflation every 2 weeks to compensate for pleural resorption. Pleural adhesions present at first insufflation or developing later on were usually taken down by thoracoscopic cauterization.[79] When extensive adhesions precluded intrapleural pneumothorax, extrapleural pneumolysis was performed through a short posterior thoracotomy; again, the collapse was maintained by repeated injections of air.[80] These frequent injections of air, sometimes complicated by empyema, represented a considerable burden to the patient. Hence there was ongoing research for the appropriate substance other than air to fill the space.

Eventually plombage procedures were designed to permanently maintain the collapse with a one-stage procedure. Utilization of Lucite balls was particularly popular between 1948 and 1955.[81] Because extrapleural plombage was often complicated by erosion of the lung, extraperiosteal plombage became the preferred procedure. The space was created through a thoracoplasty incision by stripping the periosteum and intercostal muscles off the ribs; the final appearance was referred to as the bird-cage operation. It was thought that the plombage was facing a more consistent base, which became even more solid owing to subsequent ossification.

Extraperiosteal plombage was credited with several advantages over thoracoplasty, which remained the ultimate collapse procedure: the collapse could be very selective, the cosmetic result was more acceptable, and there was no paradoxic respiration. The procedure could be done in a single stage, whereas thoracoplasty was usually performed in 2 stages. It was applicable in poor-risk patients and in cases of bilateral disease.[82] Thoracoplasty was still required in some patients despite the more refined extraperiosteal plombage, and was even combined with plombage to achieve the so-called mixed collapse in patients with spare muscles.[83]

The expectations placed on extraperiosteal plombage were frustrated by a relatively high complication rate of at least 16%. These complications were mainly infection of the plombage space, bleeding owing to vascular erosion, and breach of the underlying parenchymal cavitation leading to an extrapleural spread of tuberculosis. Consequently, the rule was established that the plombage material should be removed on a routine basis. Removal of plombage required to be combined with a thoracoplasty to obliterate the extrapleural space. Hence, the main advantage of the procedure, namely to avoid thoracoplasty, was eliminated. Eventually the advent of major antituberculous drugs ended the hazards of collapse therapy; however, some patients escaped the routine removal of plombage and presented with long-term complications.[84]

The authors are aware that such patients have become the exception, because collapse therapy for tuberculosis was abandoned more than 50 years ago in Europe and North America. However, some investigators have recommended such procedures in patients with panresistant destructive tuberculosis or atypical mycobacterial infection.[85] Hence, there is still a potential need to care for long-term complications of such treatments.

Late Complications

The usual presentation of late complication after therapeutic pneumothorax is an exudate blowing up the residual pleural or extrapleural pocket. On occasion, the exudate is compressive and causes symptoms such as dyspnea or pain. Cough heralds a bronchopleural fistula, which is further documented by an air-fluid level. While it is thought that such exudates are caused by infection, it is surprising to note that microorganisms are identified in less than half of these patients.[86,87] Most probably, the exudate is related to a transient parenchymal infection in some patients. Even more surprising is the low number of patients with relapsing tuberculosis, given that virtually none of them took major antituberculous drugs: 1 of 15 reported by Schmid and De Haller, and 4 of 28 in the authors' own series.[86,87] Bronchopleural fistula led to colonization by Aspergillus in several patients.[86,88] The presence of a hemorrhagic effusion may occur in patients with pleural metastatic disease; spontaneous bleeding has been reported in a patient treated with coumadin.[89,90]

The ideal treatment of such exudative complications is decortication.[86] Although technically difficult, especially when the pleural peel is calcified, a satisfactory reexpansion of the underlying lung is most often obtained, and this is enough to seal the pleural space. In exceptional cases thoracoplasty is required as a second stage when the lung fails to reexpand. Pneumonectomy should be avoided unless there is a completely destroyed lung. The debate on functional recovery after decortication is ongoing. Historical data are controversial. Some investigators concluded that although a normal radiographic appearance had been restored, there was no gain in lung function;

others demonstrated functional improvement.[91,92] This finding has been challenged by the series of Gorur and colleagues,[93] who conclude that spirometric improvement is significant, with forced expiratory pressure in 1 second increasing from 71.7% to 73.7% and forced vital capacity increasing from 69.6% to 72.8%; although statistically significant, the gain seems rather limited.

Long-term complications of extraperiosteal plombage were usually related to pyogenic or tuberculous infection of the plombage space. The first sign was acute onset of swelling of the collapse space. Owing to the intracavitary tension, the devitalized ribs offer little resistance to the plombage material, which may directly erode the ribs and migrate to the superficial parietal layers. The material typically became palpable either along the thoracoplasty scar or in the supraclavicular area.[84] Spontaneous fistulization to the skin has been reported.[94] Migration to the mediastinum occurred exceptionally, although there are some case reports available. Erosion of the esophagus led to "swallowing" of Lucite balls and intestinal obstruction.[95] Aortic erosion or erosion of intercostal arteries caused pseudoaneurysmal organization of the plombage space.[96] Another exceptional complication is malignant change, such as malignant histiocytofibroma, chondrosarcoma, and lymphoma.[97,98]

Treatment of the standard case with infection requires reopening of the thoracoplasty incision, resection of the devitalized ribs, and removal of all plombage material.[84] There are 2 recommendations. As the operative report indicating the precise number of Lucite balls may be difficult to retrieve, intraoperative use of fluoroscopy may be useful to check whether all plombes have been removed; some of them may be hidden and partly imbedded into the calcified floor of the collapse space. Second, to achieve a fair collapse, the peripheral rim developed peripherally to the calcified floor needs to be trimmed away. In the exceptional event of aortic erosion, femorofemoral bypass needs to be initiated; as the aorta may not be directly cross-clamped, repair may require hypothermic circulatory arrest.[84] In poor-risk patients, a more limited operation with obliteration of the space with a pectoralis flap has been reported.[99]

SUMMARY

Surgery remains an important part of management for sequelae of tuberculosis. When resection is indicated, careful surgical technique, which requires some amount of experience, is mandatory in limiting the risk of complications. To prevent bleeding, preoperative embolization may be used; intraoperatively, special care should be addressed to a careful step-by-step hemostasis while taking down adhesions and dissecting out hilar structures. Because of the increased risk of bronchial fistula, cautious preparation of the bronchial stump and respect of its blood supply is mandatory; the bronchial stump after pneumonectomy should be covered routinely. Historic techniques such as thoracoplasty should be available in the surgeon's armamentarium, because they may be helpful in particularly difficult situations.

As a rule, *Mycobacterium tuberculosis* should be hunted for in any patient through sputum samples and/or bronchial lavage, and in intraoperative samples. Indications for postoperative antituberculous treatment are:

1. Presence of *Mycobacterium tuberculosis* and/ or active granulomas
2. History of tuberculosis in a patient who did not receive modern antituberculous multidrug therapy or who did not comply with it.

The main question remains not how, but when to operate on patients. There is no question as to when significant symptoms are present. The asymptomatic patient represents an ongoing challenge for decision making: should one advocate preventive surgery with a potential for serious morbidity, or wait for symptoms that are related to an increased postoperative morbidity? In the authors' opinion, the decision should favor preventive surgery in the case of aspergilloma only; in most other categories, observation is legitimate.

It is unlikely for the younger generation of thoracic surgeons to be faced with the long-term complications of collapse therapy; however, the experience and expertise of tuberculosis surgeons should be treasured and the information transferred to complete the cultural and scientific training of the youngest surgeons approaching our specialty.

REFERENCES

1. Massard G. Treatment of suppurative lung disease. Eur Respir Mon 2004;29:168–80.
2. Ashour M. Hemodynamic alterations in bronchiectasis: a base for a new subclassification of the disease. J Thorac Cardiovasc Surg 1996;112:328–34.
3. Karakoc GB, Yilmaz M, Altintas DU, et al. Bronchiectasis: still a problem. Pediatr Pneumol 2001;32:175–8.
4. Haciibrahimoglu G, Fazlioglu M, Olcmen A, et al. Surgical management of childhood bronchiectasis due to infectious disease. J Thorac Cardiovasc Surg 2004;127:1361–5.
5. Gursoy S, Ozturk AA, Ucvet, et al. Surgical management of bronchiectasis: the indications and outcomes. Surg Today 2010;40:26–30.
6. Ashour M, Al-Kattan K, Rafay MA, et al. Current surgical therapy for bronchiectasis. World J Surg 1999;23:1096–104.
7. Shoemark A, Ozerovictch L, Wilson R. Aetiology in adult patients with bronchiectasis. Respir Med 2007;101:1163–70.
8. Van der Bruggen-Bogaarts BA, van der Bruggen HM, et al. Assessment of bronchiectasis: comparison of HRCT and spiral volumetric CT. J Comput Assist Tomogr 1996;20:15–9.
9. Munro NC, Cooke JC, Currie DC, et al. Comparison of thin section computed tomography with bronchography for identifying bronchiectatic segments in patients with chronic sputum production. Thorax 1990;45:135–9.
10. Young K, Apestrand F, Kolbenstedt A. High resolution CT and bronchography in the assessment of bronchiectasis. Acta Radiol 1991;32:339–41.
11. Eren S, Esme H, Avci A. Risk factors affecting outcome and morbidity in the surgical management of bronchiectasis. J Thorac Cardiovasc Surg 2007;134:392–8.
12. Mazières J, Murris M, Didier A, et al. Limited operations for severe multisegmental bronchiectasis. Ann Thorac Surg 2003;75:382–7.
13. Mitchell JD, Yu JA, Bishop A, et al. Thoracoscopic lobectomy and segmentectomy for infectious lung disease. Ann Thorac Surg 2012;93:1033–40.
14. Prieto D, Bernardo J, Matos MJ, et al. Surgery for bronchiectasis. Eur J Cardiothorac Surg 2001;20:19–24.
15. Balkanli K, Genc O, Dakak M, et al. Surgical management of bronchiectasis: analysis and short term results in 238 patients. Eur J Cardiothorac Surg 2003;24:699–702.
16. Kutlay H, Cangir AK, Enon S, et al. Surgical treatment in bronchiectasis: analysis of 166 patients. Eur J Cardiothorac Surg 2002;21:634–7.
17. Hiramatsu M, Shiraishi Y, Nakajima Y, et al. Risk factors that affect the surgical outcome in the management of focal bronchiectasis in a developed country. Ann Thorac Surg 2012;93:245–50.
18. Zhang P, Jiang G, Ding J, et al. Surgical treatment of bronchiectasis: retrospective analysis of 790 patients. Ann Thorac Surg 2010;90:246–50.
19. Shim YS. Endobronchial tuberculosis. Respirology 1996;1:95–106.
20. Watanabe Y, Murakami S, Oda M, et al. Treatment of bronchial stricture due to endobronchial stenosis. World J Surg 1997;21:480–7.
21. Um SW, Yoon YS, Lee SM, et al. Predictors of persistent airway stenosis in patients with endobronchial stenosis. Int J Tuberc Lung Dis 2007;11:57–62.

22. So SY, Lam WK, Yu DY. Rapid diagnosis of suspected pulmonary tuberculosis by fiberoptic bronchoscopy. Tubercle 1982;63:195–200.

23. Xue Q, Wang N, Xue X, et al. Endobronchial tuberculosis: an overview. Eur J Clin Microbiol Infect Dis 2011;30:1039–44.

24. Smith LS, Schillaci RF, Sarlin RF. Endobronchial tuberculosis: serial fiberoptic bronchoscopy and natural history. Chest 1987;91:644–7.

25. Hoheisel G, Chan BK, Chan CH, et al. Endobronchial tuberculosis: diagnostic features and therapeutic outcome. Respir Med 1994;88:593–7.

26. Inagaki K, Yamamoto S, Fujii Y, et al. Airway reconstruction for stricture due to tracheobronchial tuberculosis. J Jpn Soc Bronchol 1994;16:830–4.

27. Yano M, Arai T, Inagaki K, et al. Functional results of sleeve lobectomy for tuberculous bronchial stenosis. J Jpn Assoc Bronchol 1995;17:561–5.

28. Low SY, Hsu A, Eng P. Interventional bronchoscopy for tuberculous tracheobronchial stenosis. Eur Respir J 2004;24:345–7.

29. Lee JY, Yi CA, Kim TS, et al. CF scan features as predictors of patient outcome after bronchial intervention in endobronchial TB. Chest 2012;138:380–5.

30. Massard G, Roeslin N, Wihlm JM, et al. Pleuro-pulmonary aspergilloma: clinical spectrum and results of surgical treatment. Ann Thorac Surg 1992;54:1159–64.

31. Belcher J, Plummer N. Surgery in bronchopulmonary aspergillosis. Br J Dis Chest 1960;54:335–41.

32. Daly RC, Pairolero PC, Piehler JM, et al. Pulmonary aspergilloma. Results of surgical treatment. J Thorac Cardiovasc Surg 1986;92:981–8.

33. Faulkner SL, Vernon R, Brown PP, et al. Hemoptysis and pulmonary aspergilloma: operative versus nonoperative treatment. Ann Thorac Surg 1978;25:389–92.

34. Chatzimichalis A, Massard G, Kessler R, et al. Bronchopulmonary aspergilloma: a reappraisal. Ann Thorac Surg 1998;65:927–9.

35. Lejay A, Falcoz PE, Santelmo N, et al. Surgery for aspergilloma: time trend towards improved results. Interact Cardiovasc Thorac Surg 2011;13:392–5.

36. Khan MA, Dar AM, Kawoosa NU, et al. Clinical profile and surgical outcome for pulmonary aspergilloma: 9-year retrospective observational study in a tertiary care hospital. Int J Surg 2011;9:268–71.

37. Brik A, Salem AM, Kamal AR, et al. Surgical outcome of pulmonary aspergilloma. Eur J Cardiothorac Surg 2008;14:882–5.

38. Fraser RS, Muller NL, Colman N, et al. Fraser and Paré's diagnosis of diseases of the chest. 4th edition. Philadelphia: Saunders; 1999. p. 2287–9.

39. Carasso R, Couropmitree C, Heredia R. Egg-shell silicotic calcification causing bronchoesophageal fistula. Am Rev Respir Dis 1973;108:1384–7.

40. Patel S, Kazerooni EA. Case 31: foreign body aspiration: chicken vertebra. Radiology 2001;218:523–5.

41. Zwiebel BR, Austin JH, Grimes MM. Bronchial carcinoid tumors: assessment with CT location and intratumor calcification in 31 patients. Radiology 1991; 179:483–6.

42. Ahn JM, Im JG, Seo JW, et al. Endobronchial hamartoma: CT findings in 3 patients. Am J Roentgenol 1994;163:49–50.

43. Potaris K, Miller DL, Trastek VF, et al. Role of surgical resection in broncholithiasis. Ann Thorac Surg 2000; 70:248–52.

44. Cerfolio RJ, Bryant AS, Maniscalco L. Rigid bronchoscopy and surgical resection for broncholithiasis and calcified mediastinal lymph nodes. J Thorac Cardiovasc Surg 2008;136:186–90.

45. Seo JB, Song KS, Lee JS, et al. Broncholithiasis: review of the causes with radiologic-pathologic correlation. Radiographics 2002;22:S199–213.

46. Cerfolio RJ. Hemoptysis for benign disease. In: Bland KI, Sarr MG, Coffee WG, editors. The practice of general surgery. Philadelphia: WB Saunders; 2002. p. 877–81.

47. Cole FH, Cole FH Jr, Khandekar A, et al. Management of broncholithiasis: is thoracotomy necessary? Ann Thorac Surg 1986;42:255–7.

48. Trastek VF, Pairolero PC, Ceithaml EL, et al. Surgical management of broncholithiasis. J Thorac Cardiovasc Surg 1985;90:842–8.

49. Menivale F, Deslee G, Vallerand H, et al. Therapeutic management of broncholithiasis. Ann Thorac Surg 2005;79:1774–6.

50. Massard G, Dabbagh A, Kessler R, et al. Pneumonectomy for chronic infection is a high risk procedure. Ann Thorac Surg 1996;62:1033–7.

51. Ryu VJ, Lee HJ, Chun EM, et al. Clinical outcomes and prognostic factors in patients with tuberculous destroyed lung. Int J Tuberc Lung Dis 2011;15:246–50.

52. Treasure RL, Seaworth BJ. Current role of surgery in mycobacterium tuberculosis. Ann Thorac Surg 1995;59:1405–9.

53. Rizzi A, Rocco G, Robustellini M, et al. Results of surgical management of tuberculosis. Ann Thorac Surg 1995;59:896–900.

54. Bai L. Surgical treatment efficacy in 172 cases of tuberculosis-destroyed lungs. Eur J Cardiothorac Surg 2012;41:335–40.

55. Ashour M, Pandya L, Mezraqji A, et al. Unilateral posttuberculous lung destruction: the left bronchus syndrome. Thorax 1990;45:210–2.

56. Gale JL, Delarue NC. Surgical history of pulmonary tuberculosis: the rise and fall of various technical procedures. Can J Surg 1969;12:381–8.

57. Reed CE, Parker EF, Crawford FA. Pneumonectomy for chronic infection: fraught with danger? Ann Thorac Surg 1995;59:108–11.

58. Blyth DF. Pneumonectomy for inflammatory lung disease. Eur J Cardiothorac Surg 2000;18:429–34.

59. Conlan AA. Pneumonectomy for infection. Ann Thorac Surg 1995;60:488–90.

60. Halezeroglu S, Keles M, Uysal A, et al. Factors affecting postoperative morbidity and mortality in destroyed lung. Ann Thorac Surg 1997;64:1635–8.

61. Kim YT, Kim HK, Sung SW, et al. Long-term outcomes and risk factor analysis after pneumonectomy for active and sequela forms of pulmonary tuberculosis. Eur J Cardiothorac Surg 2003;23:833–9.

62. Kosar A, Orki A, Kiral H, et al. Pneumonectomy in children for destroyed lung: evaluation of 18 cases. Ann Thorac Surg 2010;89:226–31.

63. Tomiyama K, Ishida H, Miyake M, et al. Benign acquired bronchoesophageal fistula in an adult. Jpn J Thorac Cardiovasc Surg 2003;51:242–5.

64. Erlank A, Goussard P, Androkinou S, et al. Oesophageal perforation as a complication of primary tuberculous lymphadenopathy in children. Pediatr Radiol 2007;37:636–9.

65. Brunner A. Oesophago-bronchial fistula. Munchen Med Wochenschr 1961;103:2181–4.

66. Ford MA, Mueller PS, Morgenthaler TI. Bronchoesophageal fistula due to broncholithiasis: a case series. Respir Med 2005;99:830–5.

67. Massard G, Wihlm JM, Morand G. Benign bronchoesophageal fistula: reopening 4 months after double stapling without division. J Thorac Cardiovasc Surg 1992;103:389–90.

68. Jean-Baptiste E. Clinical assessment and management of massive hemoptysis: a comprehensive review. Crit Care Med 2000;28:1642–7.

69. Brik A, Saalem AM, Shoukry A, et al. Surgery for hemoptysis in various tuberculous lesions: a prospective study. Interact CardioVasc Thorac Surg 2011;13:276–9.

70. Andréjak C, Parrot A, Bazelly B, et al. Surgical lung resection for severe hemoptysis. Ann Thorac Surg 2009;88:1556–65.

71. Haponik EF, Fein A, Chin R. Managing life-threatening hemoptysis: has anything really changed? Chest 2000;118:1431–5.

72. Sehhat S, Oreizie M, Moinedine K. Massive pulmonary hemorrhage: surgical approach as choice of treatment. Ann Thorac Surg 1978;25:12–5.

73. Knott-Craig CJ, Osthuizen JG, Rossouw G, et al. Management and prognosis of massive hemoptysis. Recent experience with 120 patients. J Thorac Cardiovasc Surg 1993;105:394–7.

74. Ramakantan R, Bandekar VG, Gandhi MS, et al. Massive hemoptysis due to pulmonary tuberculosis: control with bronchial artery embolization. Radiology 1996;200:691–4.

75. Van den Heuvel MM, Els Z, Koegelenberg CF, et al. Risk factors for recurrence of haemoptysis following bronchial artery embolization for life-threatening haemoptysis. Int J Tuberc Lung Dis 2007;11:909–14.

76. Anuradha C, Shyamkumar NK, Vinu M, et al. Outcomes of bronchial artery embolization for life-threatening hemoptysis due to tuberculosis and post-tuberculosis sequelae. Diagn Interv Radiol 2012;18:96–101.

77. Lee JH, Kwon SY, Yoon HI, et al. Haemoptysis due to chronic tuberculosis vs. bronchiectasis: comparison of long term outcome of arterial embolisation. Int J Tuberc lung Dis 2007;11:781–7.

78. Gross AM, Diacon AH, van den Heuvel MM, et al. Management of life-threatening haemoptysis in an area of high tuberculosis incidence. Int J Tuberc Lung Dis 2009;13:875–80.

79. Dumarest, Mollard H, Lefevre P, et al. La pratique du pneumothorax thérapeutique. Paris: Masson; 1945.

80. Roberts AT. Extrapleural pneumothorax: a review of 128 cases. Thorax 1948;3:166–73.

81. Wilson NJ, Armada O, Vindzberg WV, et al. Extraperiosteal plombage thoracoplasty: operative technique and results with 161 cases with unilateral surgical problems. J Thorac Surg 1956;32:797–819.

82. Shepherd MP. Plombage in the 1980s. Thorax 1985;40:328–40.

83. Lucas BG, Cleland WP. Thoracoplasty with plombage: a review of the early results in 125 cases. Thorax 1950;5:248–56.

84. Massard G, Thomas P, Barsotti P, et al. Long-term complications of extraperiosteal plombage. Ann Thorac Surg 1997;64:220–5.

85. Jouveshomme S, Dautzenberg B, Bakdach H, et al. Preliminary results of collapse therapy with plombage for pulmonary disease caused by multidrug resistant mycobacteria. Am J Respir Crit Care Med 1998;157:1609–15.

86. Massard G, Rougé C, Ameur S, et al. Decortication is a valuable option for late empyema after collapse therapy. Ann Thorac Surg 1995;60:888–95.

87. Schmid FG, De Haller R. Late exudative complications of collapse therapy for pulmonary tuberculosis. Chest 1986;89:822–7.

88. Krakowka P, Rowinska E, Halweg H. Infection of the pleura by Aspergillus fumigatus. Thorax 1970;25:245–53.

89. Willen R, Bruce T, Dahlstrom G, et al. Squamous epithelial cancer in metaplastic pleura following extrapleural pneumothorax for pulmonary tuberculosis. Virchows Arch 1976;370:225–31.

90. Massard G, Wihlm JM, Roeslin N, et al. Extrapleural hematoma as a late complication of collapse therapy. Chest 1992;101:473–4.

91. Patton WE, Watson TR, Gaengler EA. Pulmonary function before and at intervals after surgical decortication of the lung. Surg Gynecol Obstet 1952;95:477–96.

92. Petty TL, Filley GF, Mitchell RS. Objective functional improvement by decortication after 20 years of artificial pneumothorax for pulmonary tuberculosis. Am Rev Respir Dis 1961;84:572–8.

93. Gorur R, Yildizhan A, Yiyiy N, et al. Spirometric changes after pleural decortication in young adults. ANZ J Surg 2007;77:344–6.

94. Thomas GE, Chandrasekhar B, Grannis FW. Surgical treatment of complications 45 years after extraperiosteal pneumolysis and plombage using acrylic resin balls for cavitary pulmonary tuberculosis. Chest 1995;108:1163–4.

95. Tate CF. Intestinal obstruction in a 55-year old man with previous thoracic surgery (extraperiosteal plombage). JAMA 1980;243:1077–8.

96. Ashour M, Campbell IA, Umachandran V, et al. Late complication of plombage thoracoplasty. Thorax 1985;40:394–5.

97. Fauquert P, Saraux A, Guillermit MN, et al. Histiocytome fibreux malin thoracique. Sem Hop Paris 1989; 65:2181–5.

98. Thompson JR, Entin SD. Primary extraskeletal chondrosarcoma. Cancer 1969;23:936–9.

99. Yadav S, Sharma H, Iyer A. Late extrusion of pulmonary plombage outside the thoracic cavity. Interact Cardiovasc Thorac Surg 2010;10:808–10.

Diagnosis and Management of Lung Infections

Dawn E. Jaroszewski, MD, MBA[a],*, Brandon J. Webb, MD[b],
Kevin O. Leslie, MD[c]

KEYWORDS

- Pulmonary infection • Hemoptysis • Antibiotic therapy for pneumonia • Fungal pneumonia
- Community-acquired pneumonia • Hospital acquired pneumonia • Ventilator associated pneumonia

KEY POINTS

- Thoracic surgeons are often called on to assist in the diagnosis and sometimes treatment of complicated pulmonary and thoracic infections.
- Modern diagnostic techniques used to obtain microbiological and pathologic specimens include bronchoscopy, ultrasound- and electromagnetic-guided endoscopy, transthoracic biopsy, and thoracoscopy.
- Appropriate empiric treatment of bacterial pulmonary infection requires categorization according to risk factors for drug-resistant pathogens; categories include community-acquired, health care–associated, hospital-acquired, and ventilator-associated pneumonia.
- Treatment of fungal and mycobacterial disease is heavily dependent on correct diagnosis; fungal pathogens include endemic fungi, yeast, and invasive molds, whereas mycobacterial infection may be caused *Mycobacterium tuberculosis* complex or nontuberculous mycobacterium.
- Recent advances in treatment, including topical antimicrobial therapy and direct endoscopic intervention, are promising in the treatment of multidrug-resistant infection and hemoptysis.

INTRODUCTION

Thoracic surgeons occasionally must be involved in the diagnosis and treatment of respiratory tract infections. In addition to the complication of postoperative pneumonia in surgical patients, assistance may be needed for diagnosing radiographic abnormalities, community-acquired pneumonia (CAP), nosocomial pneumonia, ventilator-associated pneumonia (VAP), and pneumonia in the immunocompromised host. Although most clinically significant infections can be identified with respiratory cultures and microbiologic analysis, a small percentage of infections require a surgical pathologist for definitive diagnosis.[1]

The spectrum and burden of etiologic organisms are affected by host risk factors and immune status.[2–7] Because organisms are found less often in the lung tissue of patients with normal immunity, diagnosis can be facilitated by cultures, serologic studies, and epidemiologic data.[8] In the immunocompromised host, a broader differential must be considered, including the possibility of multiple simultaneous infections.

In addition to infection, other disorders should be considered, such as pulmonary involvement by

The authors have no disclosures or funding sources.
[a] Division of Cardiothoracic Surgery, Department of Surgery, Mayo Clinic, Arizona, 5777 East Mayo Boulevard, Phoenix, AZ 85054, USA; [b] Department of Internal Medicine, Mayo Clinic Arizona, 5777 East Mayo Boulevard, Phoenix, AZ 85054, USA; [c] Department of Laboratory Medicine and Pathology, Mayo Clinic Arizona, 5777 East Mayo Boulevard, Phoenix, AZ 85054, USA
* Corresponding author.
E-mail address: jaroszewski.dawn@mayo.edu

Thorac Surg Clin 22 (2012) 301–324
doi:10.1016/j.thorsurg.2012.05.002
1547-4127/12/$ – see front matter © 2012 Elsevier Inc. All rights reserved.

preexisting disease, drug-induced or treatment-related injury, noninfectious interstitial pneumonias, and malignancy. Appropriate chest imaging may help narrow the differential. This information, when combined with clinical history and the timing of the disease (acute, subacute, or chronic), is critical to a successful treatment strategy. This article reviews the current diagnostic modalities and medical treatment recommendations for pulmonary infections.

DIAGNOSIS

The successful treatment of pulmonary infections depends on accurate identification of the precipitating pathogen. In contemporary medical practice, distinction of the genus or species of an infectious organism can have important prognostic and therapeutic implications. Suspected pulmonary infections should be defined by (1) signs and symptoms consistent for diagnosing a pneumonia, (2) clinical setting consistent with acquisition of pneumonia, (3) host susceptibility predisposing to pneumonia, and (4) exposure and risk factors of specific pathogens.[9]

For pneumonia, sputum collection with microscopic examination and culture of expectorant is the mainstay of laboratory evaluation. Although simple, quick, and inexpensive, sputum cultures are nonetheless negative for growth 50% of the time despite proven infections. Contamination with oropharynx secretions is also a frequent issue. If sputum evaluation fails to identify causative factors and definitive identification is required for successful patient treatment, more invasive sampling techniques are available, including bronchoscopy, transthoracic needle aspiration or core

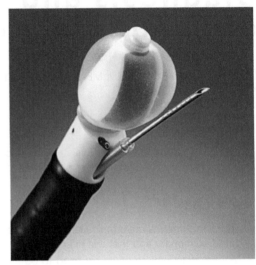

Fig. 2. An Olympus Endoscopic Ultrasound. (*Courtesy of Olympus America, Inc, Center Valley, PA; with permission.*)

biopsy, and surgical wedge biopsy of peripheral lung using a transthoracic approach.[10–17]

Specimens Obtained Through the Flexible Bronchoscope

Current pulmonary endoscopy is dominated by the flexible bronchoscope. Its flexibility provides the advantage of better access to more distal airways.[18,19] Lavage and washings can be

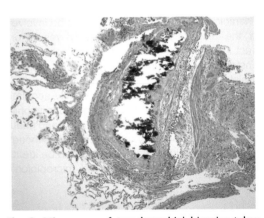

Fig. 3. Microscopy of transbronchial biopsies taken blindly are intended to represent alveolar lung parenchyma. Sometimes these samples are dominated by bronchial mucosa and cartilage if a branch point is directly sampled (a minor carina). This sample shows airway mucosa, lamina propria, and musculature samples with fragments of partially ossified (*dark blue*) cartilage. Scant alveolar parenchyma is present in the lower left of this image. Hematoxylin and eosin stain, original magnification, ×100.

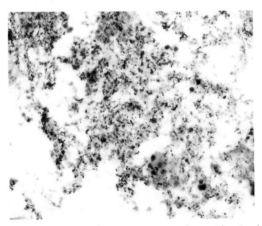

Fig. 1. Microscopy showing acute exudate with mixed gram-positive (*blue*) and gram-negative (*red*) bacterial organisms. Gram stain, original magnification, ×400.

aspirated and the fluid sample of suspended cells can be sent to the laboratory for millipore filtration or cytocentrifuge-type application onto slides (**Fig. 1**).[14,17,20–22] Clinical guidelines confirm the value of a bronchoscopic approach to diagnosis, particularly in patients with VAP, in whom it has been shown to reduce 14-day mortality.[23,24]

Endobronchial ultrasound has also added to the available diagnostic options (**Fig. 2**). Both transbronchial lung biopsy of peripheral pulmonary lesions and sampling of mediastinal and hilar lymph nodes may provide access to infectious pathogens that cannot be identified otherwise.[25,26]

The transbronchial biopsy technique allows obtainment of samples of alveolar lung parenchyma beyond the cartilaginous bronchi.[17,19,20,27] Endoscopic transbronchial biopsies taken blindly are intended to represent alveolar lung parenchyma. Sometimes these samples have bronchial mucosa and cartilage if a branch point, such as a minor carina, is sampled directly (**Fig. 3**). Many types of pulmonary infections can be diagnosed using fine needle aspiration and cytologic evaluation.[28–31] Fine needle aspiration is an especially useful technique, because respiratory secretions (eg, sputum, bronchial washings, brushings, bronchoalveolar lavage) are often limited by the need to differentiate true pathogens from contaminant organisms. Nevertheless, these diagnostic tools are complementary and both remain excellent options in the diagnosis of localized or diffuse pulmonary infection. Electromagnetic navigation bronchoscopy has proven effective in assessing pulmonary nodules accurately with low complication rates. Electromagnetic navigation bronchoscopy uses computer guidance to enable bronchoscopic access to pulmonary lesions (**Fig. 4**).[32,33]

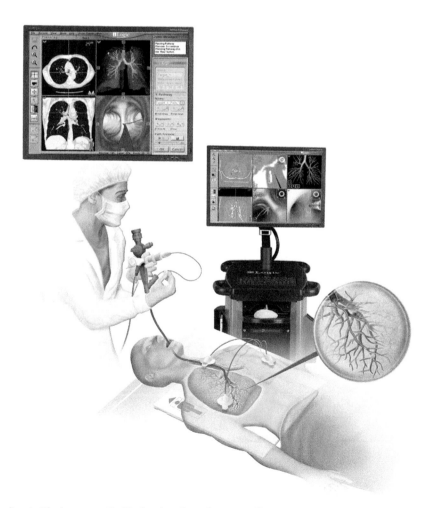

Fig. 4. The iLogic Electromagnetic Navigation Bronchoscopy allows virtual planning and biopsy of pulmonary lesions. (*Courtesy of* SuperDimension, Inc, Minneapolis, MN; with permission.)

Specimens Obtained With Transthoracic Needle Biopsy, Aspiration, and Cores

Contamination can be minimized when the upper respiratory tract can be bypassed. With either transtracheal or transthoracic needle aspiration, the presence of bacteria becomes much more significant, especially when sheets of neutrophils and/or necroinflammatory debris are present (**Fig. 5**), as would be the case with a typical lobar or lobular consolidation, lung abscess, or other complex pneumonia (**Fig. 6**).[34–37] In this context, transthoracic needle aspiration can establish the etiologic diagnosis of CAP and nosocomial pneumonia when coupled with contemporary microbiologic methods.[38–41] In current practice, the use of transthoracic needle aspiration biopsy has become commonplace,[16,42–47] and it is often used to target well-circumscribed nodules when an infectious process must be ruled out (**Fig. 7**). Besides the morphologic features of the microorganism, important cytologic clues to the diagnosis include the accompanying cellular response and the presence and character of any necrotic debris. Anaerobic pulmonary infections, typically in the form of a lung abscess, can also be approached in this way or with transthoracic needle aspiration (**Fig. 8**).[48]

In some cases, core biopsy is preferable to an aspirate. Needle core biopsies may provide better and more abundant diagnostic tissue, whereas aspirate is preferred when evaluating suspected bacterial abscess. Based on the microscopic features of the organism obtained, this technique may yield rapid diagnostic results.[39]

In addition to respiratory samples, pleural fluid can be tapped when effusions are present. Positive cultures of these normally sterile fluids circumvent the interpretive problems associated with bacterial growth in sputum samples. Persistent

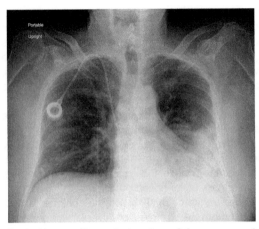

Fig. 6. Chest radiograph showing a lobar pneumonia with consolidation pneumonia in the left lower lobe.

effusions and suspected empyema can be easily analyzed with thoracentesis (**Fig. 9**).[49–51]

Specimens Obtained Through Thoracoscopy

Surgical biopsy of lung parenchyma is indicated to distinguish infection from interstitial and inflammatory lung disease. The introduction of high-resolution video equipment has changed elective thoracic surgery. With small incisions and a thoracoscopic video camera (**Fig. 10**), surgeons can directly biopsy affected lung tissue, with large quantities of parenchyma available for both microbiologic and pathologic evaluation (**Fig. 11**). Video-assisted thoracic surgery has become the standard approach for most surgical biopsies. Mortality is low and length of hospital stay and recovery are improved over those with the standard thoracotomy.[52] When the same thoracic access ports are used,

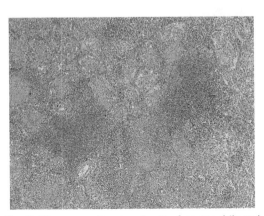

Fig. 5. Microscopy showing sheets of neutrophils and necrotic inflammation.

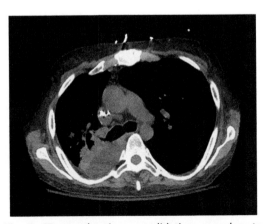

Fig. 7. CT scan showing consolidation secondary to severe lobar pneumonia and consolidation in the right lower lobe.

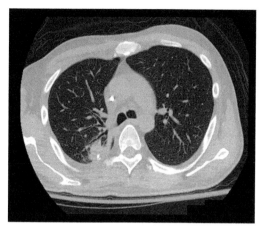

Fig. 8. CT scan showing a nodular abscess in the right lower lobe.

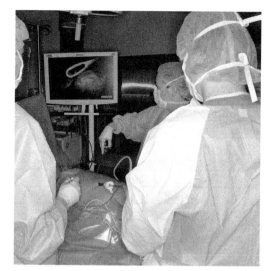

Fig. 10. Minimally invasive surgery with video images allows biopsy of parenchyma and lymph nodes for evaluation.

ipsilateral lymph nodes that may contain disease or abnormalities can be biopsied simultaneously. Before a wedge lung biopsy is performed, consultation among the radiologist, chest physician, and thoracic surgeon is essential to identify ideal locations for biopsy.

CAUSES AND TREATMENT OF PULMONARY INFECTION

Pneumonia may be classified according to several parameters, including pathogenesis, epidemiology, anatomic pattern (see **Fig. 4**), clinical course, and organism.[53] In this article, pulmonary bacterial infection is divided into CAP, health care–associated pneumonia (HCAP), hospital-acquired pneumonia (HAP), and VAP. Mycobacterial, fungal, and viral infections are also addressed because these entities require special diagnostic and treatment considerations. The pathologic patterns and

agents of the most common pulmonary infections are listed in **Table 1**.

CAP

CAP is defined as pneumonia acquired in an outpatient setting by patients in whom common lower respiratory pathogens are suspected. Although viruses (**Fig. 12**) and endemic fungi may cause CAP, the definition and treatment regimens presuppose a bacterial origin. The most common origins are listed in **Table 2** (**Figs. 13** and **14**A, B). Coverage of these agents forms the basis for initial empiric treatment of CAP. However, clinicians must be aware of factors that predispose patients to pneumonia caused by drug-resistant bacteria, such as methicillin-resistant *Staphylococcus*

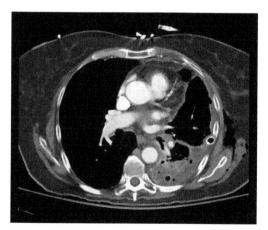

Fig. 9. CT scan showing a large pleural empyema on the left.

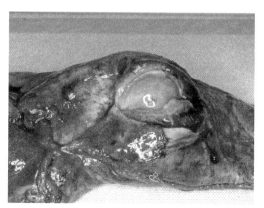

Fig. 11. A wedge biopsy from minimally invasive thoracic surgery shows a large cavitary fungal infection.

Table 1
Pathologic patterns and agents of pulmonary infection

Pattern	Most Common Agents
Airway disease	
Bronchitis/bronchiolitis	Virus; bacteria; mycoplasma
Bronchiectasis	Bacteria; mycobacteria
Acute exudative pneumonia	
Purulent (neutrophilic)	Bacteria
Lobular (bronchopneumonia)	Bacteria
Confluent (lobar pneumonia)	Bacteria
With granules	Botryomycosis; actinomycosis
Eosinophilic	Parasites
Foamy alveolar cast	Pneumocystis
Acute diffuse/localized alveolar damage	Virus; polymicrobial
Chronic pneumonia	
Fibroinflammatory	Bacteria
Organizing diffuse/Localized alveolar damage	Virus
Eosinophilic	Parasite
Histiocytic	Mycobacteria
Interstitial pneumonia	
Perivascular lymphoid	Virus; atypical agents
Eosinophilic	Parasite
Granulomatous	Mycobacteria
Nodules	
Large	
Necrotizing	Fungi; mycobacteria
Granulomatous	Fungi; mycobacteria
Fibrocaseous	Fungi; mycobacteria
Calcified	Fungi; mycobacteria
Miliary	
Necrotizing	Viral; mycobacteria; fungi
Granulomatous	Fungi
Cavities and cysts	Fungi; mycobacteria
Intravascular/Infarct	Fungi
Spindle cell pseudotumor	Mycobacteria
Minimal "Id"type reaction	Polymicrobial

From Jaroszewski DE, Viggiano RW, Leslie KO. Optimal processing of diagnostic lung specimens. In: Leslie KO, Wick MR, editors. Practical pulmonary pathology: a diagnostic approach, 2nd edition. Philadelphia: Elsevier/Saunders; 2011. (Pattern Recognition Series). p. 15–25; with permission.

aureus (MRSA) or *Pseudomonas aeruginosa*; antibiotic selection for these patients should take into consideration additional breadth of spectrum (**Box 1**).[23]

Treatment of CAP

The American Thoracic Society and the Infectious Disease Society of America have published joint guidelines on the diagnosis and management of CAP. **Box 2**[55] summarizes the recommended empiric antibiotics for CAP. Recommended treatment regimens vary based on severity of illness and setting (eg, outpatient, inpatient, intensive care). For empiric inpatient therapy, strong evidence supports use of either a respiratory fluoroquinolone or a combination of a β-lactam plus a macrolide.[56] In patients requiring intensive care, guidelines recommend a β-lactam plus a fluoroquinolone.[55] However, in this critically ill population, in whom

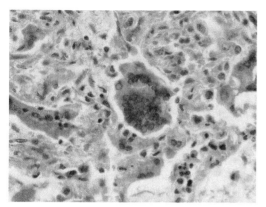

Fig. 12. Multinucleated cell with glassy viral nuclear inclusions consistent with a measles virus are identified in a patient with measles pneumonia. (hematoxylin-eosin, original magnification, ×400).

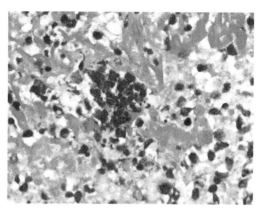

Fig. 13. Staphyloccocal organisms (*center*) in a necrotizing pneumonia. Aggregated bacteria tend to be dark blue in routine stains. Hematoxylin and eosin stain, original magnification, ×400.

the margin for error is low, many clinicians favor an initial broad-spectrum regimen that includes anti-MRSA and antipseudomonal coverage.

If an etiologic agent is identified, antimicrobial therapy should be narrowed to target that pathogen (**Table 3**). Guidelines recommend that before

Table 2
Most common causes of community-acquired pneumonia

Patient Type	Cause
Outpatient	*Streptococcus pneumoniae* *Mycoplasma pneumoniae* *Haemophilus influenzae* *Chlamydophila pneumoniae* Respiratory viruses[a]
Inpatient (non-ICU)	*S pneumoniae* *M pneumoniae* *C pneumoniae* *H influenzae* *Legionella* spp Aspiration Respiratory viruses[a]
Inpatient (ICU)	*S pneumoniae* *Staphylococcus aureus* *Legionella* spp Gram-negative bacilli *H influenzae*

Based on collective data from recent studies.[54]
Abbreviation: ICU, intensive care unit.
[a] Influenza A and B, adenovirus, respiratory syncytial virus, and parainfluenza.
From Mandell LA, Wunderink RG, Anzueto A, et al. Infectious Diseases Society of America/American Thoracic Society consensus guidelines on the management of community-acquired pneumonia in adults. Clin Infect Dis 2007;44:S27–72; with permission.

discontinuation of therapy, a minimum of 5 days of treatment should occur, and patients should have achieved clinical stability as evidenced by the absence of fever for greater than 48 hours, hypoxia, tachypnea, tachycardia, and hypotension. Patients can be safely switched from intravenous to oral therapy when they are hemodynamically stable and able to absorb oral medication.[58,59] A longer duration of therapy may be necessary if the patient does not experience improvement, the identified pathogen was not sensitive to initial empiric therapy, or an extrapulmonary infection is present.

HCAP

A subset of patients presenting with pneumonia acquired in the community will have risk factors for disease caused by drug-resistant pathogens (DRP). In the 2005 guidelines from the American Thoracic Society and the Infectious Diseases Society of America (ATS/IDSA) for HAP and VAP, an additional category, HCAP, was proposed to the existing paradigm.[23] These patients share risk factors for DRP with those susceptible to HAP and VAP, including exposure to *P aeruginosa*, extended spectrum β-lactamase producing *Escherichia coli* and *Klebsiella*, *Acinetobacter*, *Burkholderia*, drug-resistant *Enterobacteriaceae*, and MRSA. Included in the new classification are patients hospitalized within the past 90 days; those receiving chemotherapy, wound care, or intravenous antibiotics; residents of nursing homes or long-term facilities; and patients undergoing hemodialysis. For these patients, the guidelines recommend a more aggressive empiric antibiotic regimen, including an antipseudomonal β-lactam plus either an aminoglycoside or an

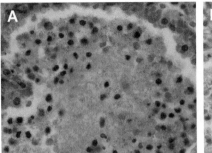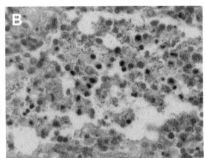

Fig. 14. Streptococcus pneumoniae infection. (*A*). On routine hematoxylin and eosin staining, the organisms present a fine granular blue appearance in a background of more eosinophilic fibrinous exudate. The round blue structure are the nuclei of degenerated inflammatory cells. (*B*) Silver impregnation methods highlight many bacterial forms, making their morphology more discernible in black (Dieterle silver stain). Both images original magnification, ×400.

antipseudomonal fluoroquinolone, plus an agent active against MRSA if risk factors for MRSA are present (**Table 4**).

HAP

Nosocomial pneumonia is generally subdivided into HAP, including postoperative pneumonia, and VAP. HAP is defined as pneumonia occurring in patients hospitalized for longer than 48 hours

<table>
<tr><td>

Box 1
Risk factors for multidrug-resistant pathogens causing HAP, HCAP, and VAP

- Antimicrobial therapy in preceding 90 days
- Current hospitalization of 5 days or more
- High frequency of antibiotic resistance in the community or in the specific hospital unit
- Presence of risk factors for HCAP
  - Hospitalization for 2 days or more in the preceding 90 days
  - Residence in a nursing home or extended care facility
  - Home infusion therapy (including antibiotics)
  - Chronic dialysis within 30 days
  - Home wound care
  - Family member with multidrug-resistant pathogen
- Immunosuppressive disease and/or therapy

Reprinted with permission of the American Thoracic Society. Copyright © 2012 American Thoracic Society. Guidelines for the management of adults with hospital-acquired, ventilator-associated, and health-care-associated pneumonia. Am J Respir Crit Care Med 2005;171:388–416. Official journal of the American Thoracic Society.
</td></tr>
</table>

before onset and is associated with high mortality rates.[23] The treatment algorithm for HAP is based on individual risk for DRP (see **Box 1**) and time of onset. Patients with no preexisting risk factors for DRP in whom early HAP develops (within the first four hospital days) may be treated with a β-lactam such as a third-generation cephalosporin, ampicillin-sulbactam, or ertapenem, or with a respiratory fluoroquinolone such as levofloxacin. Patients with late-onset HAP (five or more inpatient days) or with risk factors for DRP should be treated with a broad-spectrum regimen (see **Table 4**).[23]

VAP

VAP is defined as pneumonia occurring more than 48 hours after initiation of endotracheal intubation and mechanical ventilation.[60] Prior hospitalization within the past 90 days or prior antibiotic therapy predisposes to colonization and infection with antibiotic-resistant pathogens.[61] Suspected cases of VAP should be reviewed for risk factors and signs of antibiotic multidrug resistance (MDR) (**Fig. 15**).

VAP is the most frequently acquired infection in intensive care units (ICUs), with an incidence of 6% to 52%.[60] Generally, VAP is more prevalent in surgical ICUs than in medical ICUs.[60] Risk factors for VAP include both host and intervention factors (**Table 5**). The microbes commonly associated with VAP are similar to those that cause HAP (**Table 6**). VAP caused by more than one pathogen was identified in 30% to 70% of cases.[60,61] Treatment with initial empiric therapy should be guided by the risk for MDR pathogens as described earlier for HCAP and HAP (**Table 7**). A strategy for deescalation from an empiric broad-spectrum, multidrug regimen to a targeted therapy with a narrower

Box 2
Recommended empiric antibiotics for CAP

Outpatient treatment

1. Previously healthy and no use of antimicrobials within the previous 3 months

   A macrolide (strong recommendation; level I evidence)

   Doxycycline (weak recommendation; level III evidence)

2. Presence of comorbidities, such as chronic heart, lung, liver, or renal disease; diabetes mellitus; alcoholism; malignancies; asplenia; immunosuppressing conditions; or use of immunosuppressing drugs; or use of antimicrobials within the previous 3 months (in which case an alternative from a different class should be selected)

   A respiratory fluoroquinolone: moxifloxacin, gemifloxacin, or levofloxacin (750 mg) (strong recommendation; level I evidence)

   A β-lactam plus a macrolide (strong recommendation; level I evidence)

3. In regions with a high rate (>25%) of infection with high-level (minimum inhibitory concentration ≥16 μg/mL) macrolide-resident *Streptococcus pneumoniae*, consider use of alternative agents listed in #2 for patients without comorbidities (moderate recommendation; level III evidence)

Inpatients, non–intensive care unit treatment

A respiratory fluoroquinolone (strong recommendation; level I evidence)

A β-lactam plus a macrolide (strong recommendation; level I evidence)

Inpatients, intensive care unit treatment

A β-lactam (cefotaxime, ceftriaxone, or ampicillin-sulbactam) plus either azithromycin (moderate recommendation; level II evidence) or a respiratory fluoroquinolone (strong recommendation; level I evidence)

   For patients allergic to penicillin, a respiratory fluoroquinolone and aztreonam are recommended

Special concerns

If *Pseudomonas* is a consideration

   An antipneumococcal or antipseudomonal β-lactam (piperacillin-tazobactam, cefepime, imipenem, or meropenem) plus either ciprofloxacin or levofloxacin (750 mg)

   or

   The above β-lactam plus an aminoglycoside and azithromycin

   or

   The above β-lactam plus an aminoglycoside and an antipneumococcal fluoroquinolone (for patients allergic to penicillin, substitute aztreonam for above β-lactam) (moderate recommendation; level III evidence)

If community-acquired MRSA is a consideration, add vancomycin or linezolid (moderate recommendation; level III evidence)

Modified from Mandell LA, Wunderink RG, Anzueto A, et al. Infectious Diseases Society of America/American Thoracic Society consensus guidelines on the management of community-acquired pneumonia in adults. Clin Infect Dis 2007;44:S27–72; with permission.

spectrum is recommended to reduce antibiotic use and the selective pressure for MDR bacteria.[62,63]

Aerosolized Antibiotic Therapy in the ICU

A growing body of data suggests that aerosolized antibiotics may have a role in the treatment of pulmonary infections in mechanically ventilated patients.[64,65] Several aerosolized antibiotics have been described in the literature for off-label use (**Box 3**). Several small randomized controlled trials comparing systemic antibiotics plus aerosolized agents versus systemic treatment alone have recently shown a reduction in clinical pulmonary

Table 3
Recommended antimicrobial therapy for specific pathogens

Organism	Preferred Antimicrobial(s)	Alternative Antimicrobial(s)
Streptococcus pneumoniae		
Penicillin-nonresistant; MIC<2 μg/mL	Penicillin G, amoxicillin	Macrolide, cephalosporins (oral [cefpodoxime, cefprozil, cefuroxime, cefdinir, cefditoren] or parenteral [cefuroxime, ceftriaxone, cefotaxime]), clindamycin, doxycycline, respiratory fluoroquinolone[a]
Penicillin-resistant; MIC≥2 μg/mL	Agents chosen based on susceptibility, including cefotaxime, ceftriaxone, fluoroquinolone	Vancomycin, linezolid, high-dose amoxicillin (3 g/d with penicillin MIC≤4 μg/mL)
Haemophilus influenzae		
Non–β-lactamase–producing	Amoxicillin	Fluoroquinolone, doxycycline, azithromycin, clarithromycin[b]
β-Lactamase–producing	Second- or third-generation cephalosporin, amoxicillin-clavulanate	Fluoroquinolone, doxycycline, azithromycin, clarithromycin[b]
Mycoplasma pneumoniae/ Chlamydophila pneumoniae	Macrolide, a tetracycline	Fluoroquinolone
Legionella spp	Fluoroquinolone, azithromycin	Doxycycline
Chlamydophila psittaci	A tetracycline	Macrolide
Coxiella burnetii	A tetracycline	Macrolide
Francisella tularensis	Doxycycline	Gentamicin, streptomycin
Yersinia pestis	Streptomycin, gentamicin	Doxycycline, fluoroquinolone
Bacillus anthracis (inhalation)	Ciprofloxacin, levofloxacin, doxycycline (usually with second agent)	Other fluoroquinolones; β-lactam, if susceptible; rifampin; clindamycin; chloramphenicol
Enterobacteriaceae	Third-generation cephalosporin, carbapenem[c] (preferred drug if extended-spectrum β-lactamase producer)	β-lactam/β-lactamase inhibitor,[d] fluoroquinolone
Pseudomonas aeruginosa	Antipseudomonal β-lactam[e] plus (ciprofloxacin or levofloxacin[f] or aminoglycoside)	Aminoglycoside plus (ciprofloxacin or levofloxacin[f])
Burkholderia pseudomallei	Carbapenem, ceftazidime	Fluoroquinolone, TMP-SMX
Acinetobacter spp	Carbapenem	Cephalosporin-aminoglycoside, ampicillin-sulbactam, colistin

(*continued on next page*)

Table 3
(continued)

Organism	Preferred Antimicrobial(s)	Alternative Antimicrobial(s)
Staphylococcus aureus		
Methicillin-susceptible	Antistaphylococcal penicillin[g]	Cefazolin, clindamycin
Methicillin-resistant	Vancomycin or linezolid	TMP-SMX
Bordetella pertussis	Macrolide	TMP-SMX
Anaerobe (aspiration)	β-Lactam/β-lactamase inhibitor,[d] clindamycin	Carbapenem
Influenza virus	Oseltamivir or zanamivir	
Mycobacterium tuberculosis	Isoniazid plus rifampin plus ethambutol plus pyrazinamide	Refer to Ref.[57] for specific recommendations
Coccidioides spp	For uncomplicated infection in a normal host, no therapy generally recommended; for therapy, itraconazole, fluconazole	Amphotericin B
Histoplasmosis	Itraconazole	Amphotericin B
Blastomycosis	Itraconazole	Amphotericin B

Choices should be modified based on susceptibility test results and advice from local specialists. Refer to local references for appropriate doses.

Abbreviations: MIC, minimum inhibitory concentration; TMP-SMX, trimethoprim-sulfamethoxazole.

[a] Levofloxacin, moxifloxacin, gemifloxacin (not a first-line choice for penicillin susceptible strains); ciprofloxacin is appropriate for *Legionella* and most gram-negative bacilli (including *H influenza*).

[b] Azithromycin is more active in vitro than clarithromycin for *H influenza*.

[c] Imipenem-cilastatin, meropenem, ertapenem.

[d] Piperacillin-tazobactam for gram-negative bacilli; ticarcillin-clavulanate, ampicillin-sulbactam, or amoxicillin-clavulanate.

[e] Ticarcillin, piperacillin, ceftazidime, cefepime, aztreonam, imipenem, meropenem.

[f] 750 mg/d.

[g] Nafcillin, oxacillin flucloxacillin.

From Mandell LA, Wunderink RG, Anzueto A, et al. Infectious Diseases Society of America/American Thoracic Society consensus guidelines on the management of community-acquired pneumonia in adults. Clin Infect Dis 2007;44:S27–72; with permission.

infection score, facilitation of weaning, and use of systemic antibiotics.[64,66,67] A summary of microbiologic response to aerosolized antibiotics in recent studies is provided in **Table 8**.

With proper delivery, antimicrobial therapy may be targeted directly at the site of infection, increasing concentrations in the lung while minimizing systemic toxicity (**Table 9**).[64] Delivery mechanisms range from atomizers to jet and ultrasonic nebulizers, and vibrating mesh technology. Given the rise in incidence of DRPs in the ICU, large multicenter trials are needed to validate these novel treatment options. The current guidelines from the American Thoracic Society do not recommend routine use of aerosolized antibiotic therapy but do state that aerosolized antibiotics may be considered for treatment of microorganisms with a high minimum inhibitory concentration to parenteral antibiotics.[23]

MYCOBACTERIAL INFECTION

Mycobacterial infection may manifest clinically with vast variation. Pulmonary infection is common and may be diagnostically challenging because of significant overlap in presenting symptoms with other pulmonary infections. Therefore, diagnosis is often delayed until confirmation with an invasive procedure, such as transbronchial biopsy, transthoracic needle biopsy, or surgical lung biopsy.[69,70] Direct acid-fast bacillus smears of respiratory specimens are negative in approximately 50% of cases,[71] and a biopsy may be the first suggestion of a mycobacterial infection (**Fig. 16**).[72] Mycobacterial species can be categorized into two clinically relevant groups: *Mycobacterium tuberculosis* complex and nontuberculous mycobacteria (NTM).

M tuberculosis is the most virulent mycobacterial species and is the etiologic agent of

Table 4
Initial empiric therapy for HAP, VAP, and HCAP in patients with late-onset disease or risk factors for multidrug-resistant pathogens and all disease severity

Potential Pathogens	Combination Antibiotic Therapy[a]
Pathogens listed in **Table 2** and MDR pathogens *Pseudomonas aeruginosa* *Klebsiella pneumoniae* (ESBL+)[b] *Acinetobacter* spp[b]	Antipseudomonal cephalosporin (cefepime, ceftazidime) or Antipseudomonal carbapenem (imipenem or meropenem) or β-Lactam/β-lactamase inhibitor (piperacillin-tazobactam) plus Antipseudomonal fluoroquinolone[b] (ciprofloxacin or levofloxacin) or Aminoglycoside (amikacin, gentamicin, or tobramycin) plus
MRSA *Legionella pneumophila*[b]	Linezolid or vancomycin[c]

Abbreviation: ESBL, extended-spectrum β-lactamase.

[a] Initial antibiotic therapy should be adjusted or streamlined based on microbiologic data and clinical response to therapy.

[b] If an ESBL+ strain, such as *K pneumoniae* or an *Acinetobacter* sp is suspected, a carbapenem is a reliable choice. If *L pneumophila* is suspected, the combination antibiotic regimen should include a macrolide (eg, azithromycin) or a fluoroquinolone (eg, ciprofloxacin or levofloxacin) should be used rather than an aminoglycoside.

[c] If MRSA risk factors are present or there is a high incidence locally.

Reprinted with permission of the American Thoracic Society. Copyright © 2012 American Thoracic Society. Guidelines for the management of adults with hospital-acquired, ventilator-associated, and healthcare-associated pneumonia. Am J Respir Crit Care Med 2005;171:388–416. Official journal of the American Thoracic Society.

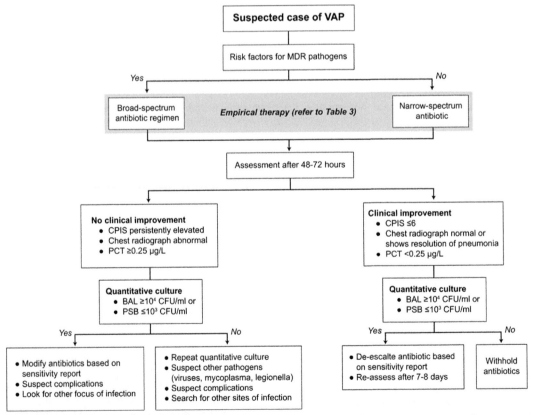

Fig. 15. Algorithm for treatment of VAP. BAL, bronchoalveolar lavage; CPIS, clinical pulmonary infection score; MDR, multi-drug resistant; PCT, procalcitonin; PSB, protected specimen brush. (*From* Joseph NM, Sistla S, Dutta TK, et al. Ventilator-associated pneumonia: a review. Eur J Inter Med 2010;21:360; with permission.)

Table 5	
Risk factors for VAP	
Host Factors	**Intervention Factors**
Oropharyngeal colonization	Emergency intubation
Gastric colonization	Reintubation
Thermal injury (burns)	Tracheostomy
Posttraumatic	Bronchoscopy
Postsurgical	Nasogastric tube
Impaired consciousness	Duration of hospital stay/ICU stay
Immunosuppression	Multiple central venous line insertions
Organ failure	Sedatives
Sinusitis	Stress ulcer prophylaxis
Severity of underlying illness	Prior antibiotics/no antibiotic prophylaxis
Old age ($\geq$60 y)	Immunosuppressives (corticosteroids)
Presence of comorbidities	Supine head position

From Joseph NM, Sistla S, Dutta TK, et al. Ventilator-associated pneumonia: a review. Eur J Intern Med 2010;21:360–8; with permission.

tuberculosis worldwide in its various forms. This organism is responsible for more deaths worldwide than any other single microbe. Postprimary tuberculosis, the most common form in adults, typically involves the apices of the upper lobes, producing granulomatous lesions with cavities and variable degrees of fibrosis and retraction of the parenchyma.[73–75] In a minority of patients, the lesions enlarge and progress secondary to increased necrosis and/or liquefaction.[76]

NTM include more than 125 species[77,78]; however, relatively few cause pulmonary disease.[72,79–81] NTM species are subdivided according to growth rates. Of the rapid growers, *M abscessus* is the most frequently recovered pulmonary pathogen, whereas *M fortuitum* and *M chelonae* are more often associated with wound infection and soft tissue disease.[68] Among the slow growers, *M avium-intracellulare* complex is the most common NTM respiratory pathogen, followed by *M kansasii* in the United States and *M xenopi* in Europe. NTM may cause a wide spectrum of pulmonary and extrapulmonary disease, but most frequently cause fibronodular bronchiectasis or cavitation.[68]

Table 6	
Microbial agents causing VAP	
Common Causes	**Rare/Unusual Causes**
Gram-positive cocci	Gram-positive bacilli
Staphylococcus aureus	*Corynebacterium* spp (diphtheroids)
Streptococcus pneumoniae	*Listeria monocytogenes*
Other streptococci	*Nocardia* spp
Coagulase-negative staphylococci	Aerobic gram-negative bacilli
Enterococci	*Serratia* spp
Aerobic gram-negative bacilli	*Hafnia alvei*
Enteric gram-negative bacilli	*Stenotrophomonas maltophilia*
Escherichia coli	*Burkholderia cepacia*
Klebsiella spp	Gram-negative cocci
Enterobacter spp	*Neisseria* spp
Proteus spp	*Moraxella* spp
Citrobacter spp	Anaerobic bacteria
Nonfermentative	Bacilli
Gram-negative bacilli	*Bacteroides* spp
Pseudomonas spp	*Fusobacterium* spp
Acinetobacter spp	*Prevotella* spp
Haemophilus influenzae	*Actinomyces* spp
Fungi	Cocci
Candida spp	*Veillonella* spp
	Peptostreptococci
	Atypical bacteria
	Legionella spp
	Mycoplasma pneumoniae
	Chlamydia pneumoniae
	Fungi
	Aspergillus spp and other molds
	Pneumocystis jiroveci
	Viruses
	Influenza and other respiratory viruses
	Herpes simplex virus
	Cytomegalovirus
	Miscellaneous causes
	Mycobacterium tuberculosis

From Joseph NM, Sistla S, Dutta TK, et al. Ventilator-associated pneumonia: a review. Eur J Intern Med 2010;21:360–8; with permission.

Table 7
Initial empiric therapy for VAP

VAP With No Risk Factors for MDR Pathogens	VAP With Risk Factors for MDR Pathogens
Ceftriaxone or Levofloxacin, moxifloxacin, or ciprofloxacin or Ampicillin/sulbactam or Ertapenem	Antipseudomonal cephalosporin (cefepime, ceftazidime) or Antipseudomonal carbapenem (imipenem or meropenem) or β-Lactam/β-lactamase inhibitor (piperacillin-tazobactam) plus Antipseudomonal fluoroquinolone (ciprofloxacin or levofloxacin) or Aminoglycoside (amikacin, gentamicin, or tobramycin) plus Linezolid or vancomycin (if risk factors for MRSA are present)

From Joseph NM, Sistla S, Dutta TK, et al. Ventilator-associated pneumonia: a review. Eur J Intern Med 2010;21:360–8; with permission.

Box 3
Aerosolized antibiotics described in the literature: off-label use and U.S. Food and Drug Administration–approved drugs

Cystic fibrosis

  Gentamicin

  Amikacin

  Tobramycin[a]

  Aztreonam lysine[b]

  Liposomal amikacin[c]

Mechanically ventilated patients

  Sisomicin

  Gentamicin

  Amikacin

  Cefuroxime/ceftazidime

  Colistin-polymyxin B

  Vancomycin

  Amikacin proprietary preparation[d]

[a] U.S. Food and Drug Administration (FDA)–approved medication for maintenance therapy for patients with cystic fibrosis who are known to be colonized with P aeruginosa; tobramycin (Tobi, PARI Pharma GmbH, Weilheim, Germany) delivered with PARI LC Plus nebulizer or Pulmo-Aide compressor.
[b] FDA-approved medication for patients with cystic fibrosis for more than 7 years with chronic Pseudomonas infection; aztreonam (Cayston inhalation, PARI Pharma GmbH, Weilheim, Germany) delivery with Altera Nebulizer System using eFlow.
[c] Phase 2 completed. For patients with cystic fibrosis with Pseudomonas infections; liposomal amikacin (Arikace, PARI Pharma GmbH, Weilheim, Germany).
[d] Phase 2 trial completed. Aerosol amikacin, Bayer Healthcare. Delivered with Nektar Therapeutics LPT.
From Palmer LB. Aerosolized antibiotics in the intensive care unit. Clin Chest Med 2011;32:559–74; with permission.

Treatment of Mycobacterial Pulmonary Infection

Treatment of mycobacterial disease is generally more complicated than that for other bacteria because of the slow growth of the organisms, mechanisms of drug resistance (eg, the unique cell wall characteristics of the genus), and poor drug tolerability. Multidrug regimens are required for extended duration. Once the diagnosis of active pulmonary tuberculosis is confirmed, initial recommended treatment comprises a four-drug regimen of isoniazid, rifampin, pyrazinamide, and either ethambutol or streptomycin, according to local patterns of susceptibility.[82] Duration of therapy depends on the drug susceptibility of the isolate, presence of extrapulmonary involvement, and immune status of the patient. Although acquired resistance does occur, the more common cause of treatment failure is medication

nonadherence. For this reason, evidence strongly supports direct observational therapy. Confirmation of clearance of sputum acid-fast bacilli is recommended at 3 months.

Given the increase in MDR and extensively drug-resistant M tuberculosis strains, repeat susceptibility testing is warranted with documented treatment failure. If drug-resistant strains are identified, expert consultation is recommended, and a regimen composed of at least four agents should be selected in a stepwise approach from the following classes: (1) all first-line agents to which the strain is sensitive: isoniazid, rifampin, pyrazinamide, and ethambutol; (2) one fluoroquinolone, if susceptible; (3) one injectable aminoglycoside, such as streptomycin or kanamycin;

Table 8
Microbiological response to aerosolized antibiotics

Authors	Year	Setting	Design	Indication	No of Patients	Method of Aerosolization; Drug	No of Patients on Systemic Antibiotic Use	No of Organisms in Patients	No of Patients with Eradication of Causative Organism	No of Patients with Resistant Organisms
Michalopoulos et al[117]	2005	ICU, Greece	Retrospective chart review	VAP for 6 patients, HAP for 2 patients	8	Aerosolized via Siemens Servo Ventilator; colistin	7/8	Acinetobacter, 7; Pseudomonas, 1	4/5	None
Kwa et al[118]	2005	ICU, Singapore	Retrospective chart review	VAP	21	Aerosolized colistin; no data on method	Yes, but not active against causative organism	Acinetobacter, 17; Pseudomonas, 4	11/11 available cultures	Not described
Berlana et al[119]	2005	ICU, Spain	Retrospective chart review	Pulmonary infection	71	Aerosolized with various compressors; colistin	78% of patients	Acinetobacter, 60; Pseudomonas, 11	Acinetobacter, 33/33; Pseudomonas, 4/7	Not described
Michalopoulos et al[120]	2008	ICU, Greece	Prospective	VAP	60	Aerosolized via Siemens Servo Ventilator; colistin	57	Acinetobacter, 37; Pseudomonas, 12; Klebsiella, 11	50/60	Not described
Palmer et al[65]	2008	ICU, United States	Randomized, double-blind, placebo-controlled	VAT $\geq$2 mL sputum produced over 4 h and organisms on Gram stain	24, placebo; 19, AA	AeroTech jet nebulizer; vancomycin and/or gentamicin	32/43	Multiple species of gram-negative and gram-positive organisms	Placebo, 19; aerosolized, 17	Placebo (8/24), AA (0/19)
Kofferidis et al[121]	2010	ICU, Greece	Retrospective review, matched case control	VAP	43 IV and aerosolized colistin; 43 IV colistin	Aerosolized colistin; no details on method	All patients	Acinetobacter, 66; Klebsiella, 12; Pseudomonas, 8	Placebo, 17 (50%); aerosolized, 19 (45%)	Not described
Korbila et al[122]	2010	ICU, Greece	Retrospective review, matched case control	VAP	43 IV colistin; 78 aerosolized and IV colistin	Aerosolized via Siemens Servo Ventilator; colistin	All patients	MDR gram-negative organisms	Placebo, 26 (60.5%); aerosolized, 62 (79.5%)	Not described

Abbreviations: AA, aerosolized antibiotic; IV, intravenous; VAT, ventilator-associated tracheobronchitis.
From Palmer LB. Aerosolized antibiotics in the intensive care unit. Clin Chest Med 2011;32:559–74; with permission.

Table 9
Toxicity related to aerosolized antibiotics

Drug	Adverse Effects
Aminoglycosides	Bronchial constriction, renal toxicity,[a] tinnitus, vestibular toxicity, hoarseness
Colistin	Nephrotoxicity,[b] bronchospasm,[b] neurologic toxicity
Aztreonam lysine	Cough, bronchoconstriction
Vancomycin	Not well described
Cefotaxime/ceftazidime	Not well described

[a] Renal toxicity rarely seen with tobramycin (Tobi, RARI Pharma GmbH, Weilheim, Germany).
[b] Nephrotoxicity and bronchospasm more severe than with aminoglycosides.
From Palmer LB. Aerosolized antibiotics in the intensive care unit. Clin Chest Med 2011;32:559–74; with permission.

(4) less effective second-line antituberculous drugs, such as ethionamide or cycloserine; and (5) second-line agents for which few data are available: linezolid, clarithromycin, amoxicillin-clavulanate, or clofazamine.[83]

Treatment of pulmonary NTM is less well defined. Although the principles of management are similar to those for *M tuberculosis*, antibiotic regimens vary by species.[68] For *M avium* complex, ATS/IDSA guidelines recommend a combination of clarithromycin, rifampicin, and ethambutol, whereas for *M kansasii*, the initial regimen comprises isoniazid, rifampicin, and ethambutol.[72] For localized pulmonary *M abscessus* infection, medical management alone is not effective and surgical resection is required.

Hemoptysis

Tuberculosis remains the most common cause of hemoptysis worldwide; however, in the United States, invasive fungal infections, chronic

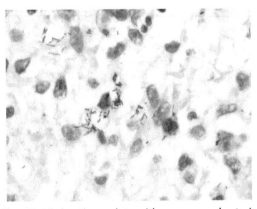

Fig. 16. Histiocytic exudate with many mycobacteria (*red*) in this mycobacterial pneumonia. The relatively large number of organisms seen here and the loose appearance of the histiocytes together suggests an immunocompromised host. Fite mycobacterial stain, original magnification, ×600.

granulomatous disease, bronchiectasis, and bronchitis account for most cases.[84,85] Conservative management can often control bleeding. The current recommended strategy for hemoptysis is initial nonoperative management and stabilization, with surgery reserved for isolated cases.[86–88] For a patient presenting with massive hemoptysis, the immediate goals of the surgeon are to preserve life through protecting the healthy lung from aspiration, to stabilize the patient hemodynamically, and to correct any coagulopathy.[85] Bronchoscopy can often be effective if bleeding is mild.[89]

More than 80% of patients can be treated successfully with bronchoscopic localization.[84,89] The bleeding site can be controlled with balloon tamponade, laser ablation, and local vasopressor therapy. The decision to intervene angiographically should be made based on the clinical examination, imaging results, bronchoscopic findings, and physician expertise. Transcatheter arterial embolization is successful in most patients.[84,85,90–94] Although bronchial embolization is the mainstay of treatment, emergency surgery can be considered if initial attempts to control bleeding and stabilize the patient prove unsuccessful. The decision to take the patient to the operating room requires at a minimum known laterality of the lesion and, optimally, lobar location (**Fig. 17**).[85]

INVASIVE FUNGAL PULMONARY INFECTION

With the rapid increase in bone marrow and solid organ transplantation, invasive fungal infection has become a significant cause of morbidity and mortality. Although nearly 100 fungi have been recovered from respiratory infections,[95] only a small number are consistently implicated as pathogenic (**Box 4**). Broadly, fungal pathogens that infect the lung include yeasts such as *Candida* spp and *Cryptococcus*; endemic dimorphic fungi such as *Histoplasma* and *Coccidioides*; filamentous molds, of which *Aspergillus* is most

Management of Hemoptysis

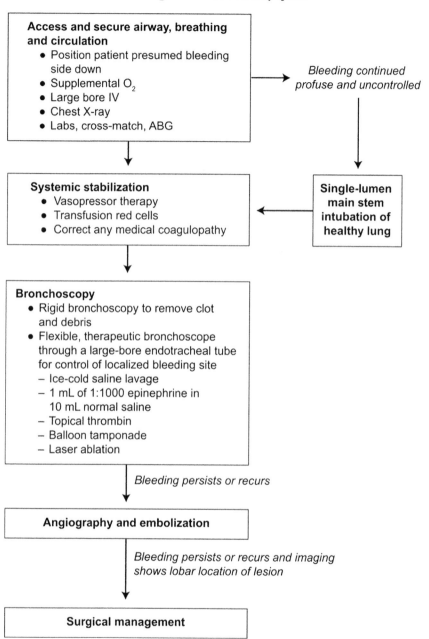

Fig. 17. Algorithm for management of hemoptysis. BG, arterial blood gas.

common; and members of the family Mucorales. The most effective method of diagnosis is often identification of fungi in tissue sections or cyto-logic samples (**Fig. 18**).[31,96,97]

The patient may present with a wide spectrum of radiographic pulmonary disease. In the healthy host, fungal pathogens typically produce one or more nodular lesions (**Fig. 19**), which, in turn,

may become cavitary as the lesions evolve (**Fig. 20**). However, clinical presentation may vary widely and may include solitary or multiple and bilateral nodular lesions; segmental or lobar consolidation; cavitary lesions, fistulas, infarcts; direct extension into mediastinal, thoracic soft tissue, chest wall, and diaphragm; chronic tracheal and endobronchial infection; and fungus

Box 4
Common fungal pathogens in the lung

Dimorphic fungi (mycelia at 25°C–30°C; yeast at 37°C)

Blastomyces dermatitidis

Coccidioides immitis

Histoplasma capsulatum

Paracoccidioides braziliensis

Sporothrix schenckii

Penicillium marneffei

Yeasts

Cryptococcus neoformans

Candida spp

Hyaline (nonpigmented) molds

Aspergillus spp

Zygomycetes organisms

Phaeoid (pigmented; dematiaceous) molds

Bipolaris spp, *Alternaria, Curvularia*

Pseudoallescheria   boydii/Scedosporium apiospermum

Miscellaneous pathogens

Pneumocystis jiroveci

Data from Rosati LA, Leslie KO. Lung infections. In: Leslie KO, Wick MR, editors. Practical pulmonary pathology: a diagnostic approach. Philadelphia: Elsevier/Saunders; 2011.

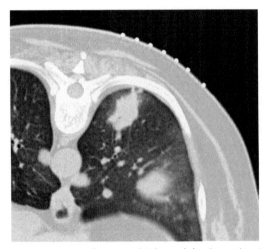

Fig. 19. CT scan shows multiple nodules in patient's lung subsequently shown to be infection with Coccidioidomycosis.

ball such as aspergilloma.[98] Proximal endobronchial disease mimicking a neoplasm has also been described for various fungal species.[99]

Treatment of Fungal Infection

Until recently, effective treatment options for invasive fungal infection were largely limited to amphotericin B deoxycholate, which is well known for its potential for systemic toxicity. However, the development of lipid, liposomal, and aerosolized formulations of amphotericin B, and newer triazole and echinocandin antifungal agents, has greatly expanded treatment options for these diseases. Because of differences in antifungal susceptibility and prognosis between dimorphic endemic fungi, filamentous fungi, and other molds (eg, Mucor), a definitive microbiologic or pathologic diagnosis is strongly preferred before treatment.

For invasive *Aspergillus* infection, a large randomized controlled trial showed the superiority of voriconazole over amphotericin B,[100] and now voriconazole is recommended as the primary

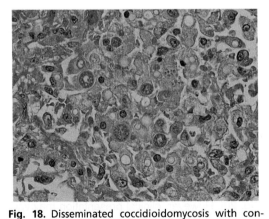

Fig. 18. Disseminated coccidioidomycosis with confluent spherules of Coccidioides immitus. Each spherule has a thick refractile wall and contains numerous tiny endospores. Spherules enlarge and eventually burst, so many sizes are present typically, some of which may be ruptured and empty. Hematoxylin and eosin stain, original magnification, ×200.

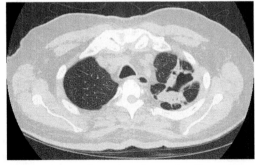

Fig. 20. CT scan shows invasive Aspergilloma fungal ball in the left lower lobe.

treatment of invasive pulmonary aspergillosis in most patients.[101] Limited data suggest that in certain populations, such as heart transplant recipients, voriconazole in combination therapy with caspofungin may contribute to improved outcomes; additional data are anticipated.[102,103] In lung transplant recipients, aerosolized amphotericin B has been used for antifungal prophylaxis and as adjunct therapy in invasive fungal disease.[104]

In pulmonary mucormycosis, however, voriconazole is ineffective. The preferred treatment remains amphotericin B, although some data suggest that liposomal amphotericin B may be more efficacious than the deoxycholate formulation.[105] A novel triazole, posaconazole, has also been approved for salvage therapy, but it is limited by its availability in oral formulation only and its inconsistent bioavailability.[105] Limited evidence also suggests improved outcomes with a combination therapy of amphotericin B and posaconazole or an echinocandin.[105] When empiric therapy is required in critically ill patients in whom hemodynamic instability or cytopenia may prevent invasive diagnostic procedures, the logical approach is combination therapy with voriconazole and amphotericin B.

VIRAL PNEUMONIA

Viruses cause more infections in the respiratory tract than all other types of microorganisms combined.[106] The viruses that commonly infect the lung are presented in **Box 5**. The common

---

Box 5
Viruses linked to CAP in children and adults

- Respiratory syncytial virus
- Rhinovirus
- Influenza A, B, and C viruses
- Human metapneumovirus
- Parainfluenza viruses types 1, 2, 3, and 4
- Human bocavirus[a]
- Coronavirus types 229E, OC43, NL63, HKU1, SARS
- Adenovirus
- Enteroviruses
- Varicella-zoster virus
- Hantavirus
- Parechoviruses
- Epstein-Barr virus
- Human herpesvirus 6 and 7
- Herpes simplex virus
- Mimivirus
- Cytomegalovirus[b]
- Measles[b]

[a] Mostly in children.
[b] Mostly in developing countries.
  Data from Ruuskanen O, Lahti E, Jennings LC, et al. Viral pneumonia. Lancet 2011;377:1264–75.

Table 10
Possibilities for antiviral treatment and prevention of severe viral pneumonia

	Treatment	Prevention
Influenza A and B viruses	Oseltamivir (oral); zanamivir (inhalation, intravenous); peramivir (intravenous)	Vaccines (inactivated, live); oseltamivir; zanamivir
Influenza A virus	Amantadine (oral); rimantadine (oral)	Vaccines (inactivated, live); oseltamivir; zanamivir
Respiratory syncytial virus	Ribavirin (inhalation, intravenous)	Palivizumab (intramuscular)
Adenovirus	Cidofovir (intravenous)	Vaccine for types 4 and 7[a]
Rhinovirus	Pleconaril[b]	Alfa interferon (intranasal)
Enteroviruses	Pleconaril[b]	Alfa interferon (intranasal)
Human metapneumovirus	Ribavirin (intravenous)	Alfa interferon (intranasal)
Hantavirus	Ribavirin (intravenous)	Alfa interferon (intranasal)
Varicella-zoster virus	Acyclovir (intravenous)	Vaccine

[a] Long successful use in U.S. military conscripts, no production now.
[b] Has been used for compassionate cases.
  Data from Ruuskanen O, Lahti E, Jennings LC, et al. Viral pneumonia. Lancet 2011;377:1264–75.

respiratory viruses (eg, influenza, parainfluenza, respiratory syncytial virus, adenovirus) cause outbreaks of respiratory illness in the general population each year. Fortunately, most viral respiratory infections are mild and self-limited. However, viruses are also capable of producing serious or life-threatening infections, such as in the case of primary varicella-zoster pneumonia[107] or respiratory disease caused by highly pathogenic strains of influenza.[108,109] In addition, viral-mediated bronchial epithelial damage predisposes susceptible patients to secondary bacterial infection, which is associated with significant morbidity and mortality.[110] Recent outbreaks of the H1N1 strain of influenza A have served to highlight the increased risk of mortality associated with influenza complicated by secondary bacterial infection, especially with S aureus.[111,112]

In immunocompromised hosts, less common viral agents may cause severe clinical disease. In these patients, diagnosis may be made through respiratory cytologic specimens, from which herpes simplex, *Cytomegalovirus,* and adenovirus are the most commonly identified viral pathogens.[113] The cytologic features of viral infections in the respiratory tract are most likely to be found in exfoliative specimens, such as bronchial washings and bronchoalveolar lavage.[114,115]

Treatment of Viral Pulmonary Infection

In most respiratory infection caused by viruses, no treatment is necessary. No consensus exists on prophylactic antibiotic treatment of influenza-like illness. However, when secondary bacterial pneumonia is suspected, antibacterial agents targeting the most common causative pathogens (S pneumoniae and S aureus, including MRSA) should be initiated. Treatment options for primary viral respiratory tract infections are limited. For influenza A, early treatment with oseltamivir or zanamivir within 48 hours of the onset of symptoms has been shown to decrease complications, especially in the very young, elderly individuals, and patients with impaired immune status or comorbid conditions. **Table 10**[116] summarizes the possible for antiviral treatments for prevention of severe viral pneumonia.

REFERENCES

1. Chandler F. Approaches to the pathologic diagnosis of infectious diseases. In: Connor D, Chandler F, Schwartz D, et al, editors. Pathology of infectious disease, vol. 1. 1st edition. Stamford (CT): Appleton and Lange; 1997. p. 3.
2. Colby TV, Weiss RL. Current concepts in the surgical pathology of pulmonary infections. Am J Surg Pathol 1987;11(Suppl 1):25.
3. Dichter JR, Levine SJ, Shelhamer JH. Approach to the immunocompromised host with pulmonary symptoms. Hematol Oncol Clin North Am 1993;7:887.
4. Dunn DL. Diagnosis and treatment of opportunistic infections in immunocompromised surgical patients. Am Surg 2000;66:117.
5. Levine SJ. An approach to the diagnosis of pulmonary infections in immunosuppressed patients. Semin Respir Infect 1992;7:81.
6. Travis WD. Surgical pathology of pulmonary infections. Semin Thorac Cardiovasc Surg 1995;7:62.
7. Wilson WR, Cockerill FR 3rd, Rosenow EC 3rd. Pulmonary disease in the immunocompromised host (2). Mayo Clin Proc 1985;60:610.
8. Khoor A, Leslie KO, Tazelaar HD, et al. Diffuse pulmonary disease caused by nontuberculous mycobacteria in immunocompetent people (hot tub lung). Am J Clin Pathol 2001;115:755.
9. Donowitz GR, Mandell GL. Acute pneumonia. In: Mandell GL, Bennett JE, Dolin R, editors. Principles and practice of infectious diseases, vol. 1. 5th edition. Philadelphia: Churchill Livingstone Elsevier; 2000. p. 717.
10. Burt ME, Flye W, Webber BL, et al. Prospective evaluation of aspiration needle, cutting needle, transbronchial and open lung biopsy in patients with pulmonary infiltrates. Ann Thorac Surg 1981;32:146.
11. Danes C, Gonzalez-Martin J, Pumarola T, et al. Pulmonary infiltrates in immunosuppressed patients: analysis of a diagnostic protocol. J Clin Microbiol 2002;40:2134.
12. Leslie K, Lanza L, Helmers R, et al. Diagnostic sampling of lung tissues and cells. In: Davis G, Marcey T, Seward E, editors. Medical management of pulmonary diseases. 1st edition. New York: Marcel Dekker; 1999. p. 213.
13. Muscedere J, Dudek P, Keenan S, et al. Comprehensive evidence-based clinical practice guidelines for ventilator- associated pneumonia: diagnosis and treatment. J Crit Care 2008;23:132.
14. Popp W, Rauscher H, Ritschka L, et al. Diagnostic sensitivity of different techniques in the diagnosis of lung tumors with the flexible fiberoptic bronchoscope-comparison of brush biopsy, imprint cytology of forceps biopsy, and histology of forceps biopsy. Cancer 1991;67:72.
15. Rea-Neto A, Youssef N, Tuche F, et al. Diagnosis of ventilator-associated pneumonia: a systematic review of the literature. Crit Care 2008;12:R56.
16. Yang P, Lee Y, Yu C, et al. Ultrasonographically guided biopsy of thoracic tumors—a comparison of large-bore cutting biopsy with fine-needle aspiration. Cancer 1992;69:2553.
17. Zavala D. Diagnostic fiberoptic bronchoscopy: techniques and results of biopsy in 600 patients. Chest 1975;68:12.

18. Joos L, Patuto N, Chhajed PN, et al. Diagnostic yield of flexible bronchoscopy in current clinical practice. Swiss Med Wkly 2006;136:155.

19. Kovnat DM, Rath GS, Anderson WM, et al. Maximal extent of visualization of bronchial tree by flexible fiberoptic bronchoscopy. Am Rev Respir Dis 1974;110:88.

20. Mitchell D, Emerson C, Collins J, et al. Transbronchial lung biopsy with the fibreoptic bronchoscope: analysis of results in 433 patients. Br J Dis Chest 1981;75:258.

21. Robb J, Melello C, Odom C. Comparison of cyto-shuttle and cytocentrifuge as processing methods for nongynecologic cytology specimens. Diagn Cytopathol 1996;14:305.

22. Willcox M, Kervitsky A, Watters L, et al. Quantification of cells recovered by bronchoalveolar lavage. Comparison of cytocentrifuge preparations with the filter method. Am Rev Respir Dis 1988;138:74.

23. Guidelines for the management of adults with hospital-acquired, ventilator-associated, and healthcare-associated pneumonia. Am J Respir Crit Care Med 2005;171:388.

24. Fagon JY, Chastre J, Wolff M, et al. Invasive and noninvasive strategies for management of suspected ventilator-associated pneumonia. A randomized trial. Ann Intern Med 2000;132:621.

25. Franke KJ, Bruckner C, Szyrach M, et al. The contribution of endobronchial ultrasound-guided forceps biopsy in the diagnostic workup of unexplained mediastinal and hilar lymphadenopathy. Lung 2012;190(2):227–32.

26. Triller N, Dimitrijevic J, Rozman A. A comparative study on endobronchial ultrasound-guided and fluoroscopic-guided transbronchial lung biopsy of peripheral pulmonary lesions. Respir Med 2011; 105(Suppl 1):S74.

27. Andersen H. Transbronchoscopic lung biopsy for diffuse pulmonary diseases. Results in 939 patients. Chest 1978;73:734.

28. Al-Za'abi A, MacDonald S, Geddie W, et al. Cytologic examination of bronchoalveolar lavage fluid from immunosuppressed patients. Diagn Cytopathol 2007;35:710.

29. DeMay RM. A micromiscellany. In: DeMay R, editor. The art and science of cytopathology: exfoliative cytology. Chicago: ASCP Press; 1996. p. 53.

30. Johnson W, Elson C. Respiratory tract. In: Bibbo M, editor. Comprehensive cytopathology. Philadelphia: Saunders; 1991. p. 340.

31. Powers C. Diagnosis of infectious disease: a cytopathologists perspective. Clin Microbiol Rev 1998; 11:341.

32. Minnich S, Taubert K. [The combined application of ultrasound and impulse current]. Zeitschrift fur arztliche Fortbildung 1991;85:668 [in German].

33. Pearlstein DP, Quinn CC, Burtis CC, et al. Electromagnetic navigation bronchoscopy performed by thoracic surgeons: one center's early success. Ann Thorac Surg 2012;93:944.

34. Grinan N, Lucerna F, Romero J. Yield of percutaneous aspiration in lung abscess. Chest 1990;97:69.

35. Ruiz- Gonzales A, Falquera M, Nogues A. Is Streptococcus pneumoniae the leading cause of pneumonia of unknown etiology? Am J Med 1999;106:385.

36. Vera-alverez J, Marigil-Gomez M, Garcia-Prats M, et al. Primary pulmonary botryomycosis diagnosed by fine needle aspiration biopsy. Acta Cytol 2006; 50:331.

37. Yang PC, Luh KT, Lee YC, et al. Lung abscesses: US examination and US-guided transthoracic aspiration. Radiology 1991;180:171.

38. Garg S, Handa U, Mohan H, et al. Comparative analysis of various cytohistological techniques in diagnosis of lung diseases. Diagn Cytopathol 2007;35:26.

39. Granville L, Laucirica R, Verstovek G. Clinical significance of cultures collected from fine-needle aspirates. Diagn Cytopathol 2008;36:85.

40. Mayer J. Laboratory diagnosis of nosocomial pneumonia. Semin Respir Infect 2000;15:119.

41. Vuori-Holopainen E, Salo E, Saxen H, et al. Etiological diagnosis of childhood pneumonia by use of transthoracic needle aspiration and modern microbiological methods. Clin Infect Dis 2002;34:583.

42. Bocking A, Klose K, Kyll H, et al. Cytologic versus histologic evaluation of needle biopsy of the lung, hilum and mediastinum-sensitivity, specificity and typing accuracy. Acta Cytol 1995;39:463.

43. Lohela P, Tikkakoski T, Ammala K, et al. Diagnosis of diffuse lung disease by cutting needle biopsy. Acta Radiol 1994;35:251.

44. Milman N. Percutaneous lung biopsy with semi-automatic, spring-driven fine needle-preliminary results in 13 patients. Respiration 1993;60:289.

45. Sanders C. Transthoracic needle aspiration. Clin Chest Med 1992;13:11.

46. Smyth R, Carty H, Thomas H, et al. Diagnosis of interstitial lung disease by a percutaneous lung biopsy sample. Arch Dis Child 1994;70:143.

47. Williams A, Santiago S, Lehrman S, et al. Transcutaneous needle aspiration of solitary pulmonary masses: how many passes? Am Rev Respir Dis 1987;136:452.

48. Verma P. Laboratory diagnosis of anaerobic pleuropulmonary infections. Semin Respir Infect 2000;15:114.

49. Berquist TH, Bailey PB, Cortese DA, et al. Transthoracic needle biopsy: accuracy and complications in relation to location and type of lesion. Mayo Clin Proc 1980;55:475.

50. Crosby JH, Hager B, Hoeg K. Transthoracic fine-needle aspiration. Experience in a cancer center. Cancer 1985;56:2504.

51. Larscheid RC, Thorpe PE, Scott WJ. Percutaneous transthoracic needle aspiration biopsy:

a comprehensive review of its current role in the diagnosis and treatment of lung tumors. Chest 1998;114:704.

52. Jaklitsch MT, DeCamp MM Jr, Liptay MJ, et al. Video-assisted thoracic surgery in the elderly. A review of 307 cases. Chest 1996;110:751.

53. Travis WD. Lung infections. In: King D, editor. Non-neoplastic disorders of the lower respiratory tract atlas of non tumor pathology. Washington, DC: American Registry of Pathology; 2002. p. 539.

54. File TM. Community-acquired pneumonia. Lancet 2003;362:1991.

55. Mandell LA, Wunderink RG, Anzueto A, et al. Infectious Diseases Society of America/American Thoracic Society consensus guidelines on the management of community-acquired pneumonia in adults. Clin Infect Dis 2007;44(Suppl 2):S27.

56. McCabe C, Kirchner C, Zhang H, et al. Guideline-concordant therapy and reduced mortality and length of stay in adults with community-acquired pneumonia: playing by the rules. Arch Intern Med 2009;169:1525.

57. American Thoracic Society/Centers for Disease Control and Prevention/Infectious Diseases Society of America: controlling tuberculosis in the United States. Am J Respir Crit Care Med 2005;172:1169.

58. Athanassa Z, Makris G, Dimopoulos G, et al. Early switch to oral treatment in patients with moderate to severe community-acquired pneumonia: a meta-analysis. Drugs 2008;68:2469.

59. Halm EA, Fine MJ, Marrie TJ, et al. Time to clinical stability in patients hospitalized with community-acquired pneumonia: implications for practice guidelines. JAMA 1998;279:1452.

60. Napolitano LM. Hospital-acquired and ventilator-associated pneumonia: what's new in diagnosis and treatment? Am J Surg 2003;186:4S.

61. Joseph NM, Sistla S, Dutta TK, et al. Ventilator-associated pneumonia: a review. Eur J Inter Med 2010;21:360.

62. Niederman MS. De-escalation therapy in ventilator-associated pneumonia. Curr Opin Crit Care 2006; 12:452.

63. Porzecanski I, Bowton DL. Diagnosis and treatment of ventilator-associated pneumonia. Chest 2006; 130:597.

64. Palmer LB. Aerosolized antibiotics in the intensive care unit. Clin Chest Med 2011;32:559.

65. Palmer LB, Smaldone GC, Chen JJ, et al. Aerosolized antibiotics and ventilator-associated tracheobronchitis in the intensive care unit. Crit Care Med 2008;36(7):2008–13.

66. Niederman M, Chastre J, Corkery K. Inhaled amikacin reduces IV antibiotic use in intubated mechanically ventilated patients [abstract]. Am J Respir Crit Care Med 2007;175:A326.

67. Rattanaumpawan P, Lorsutthitham J, Ungprasert P, et al. Randomized controlled trial of nebulized colistimethate sodium as adjunctive therapy of ventilator-associated pneumonia caused by Gram-negative bacteria. J Antimicrobial Chemother 2010;65:2645.

68. McGrath EE, McCabe J, Anderson PB. Guidelines on the diagnosis and treatment of pulmonary non-tuberculous mycobacteria infection. Int J Clin Pract 2008;62:1947.

69. Kunimoto D, Long R. Tuberculosis: still overlooked as a cause of community-acquired pneumonia—how not to miss it. Respir Care Clin N Am 2005;11:25.

70. Storla D, Yimer S, Bjune GA. A systematic review of delay in the diagnosis and treatment of tuberculosis. BMC Public Health 2008;8:15.

71. Gardiner DF, Beavis KG. Laboratory diagnosis of mycobacterial infections. Semin Respir Infect 2000;15:132.

72. Griffith DE, Aksamit T, Brown-Elliott BA, et al. An official ATS/IDSA statement: diagnosis, treatment, and prevention of nontuberculous mycobacterial diseases. Am J Respir Crit Care Med 2007; 175:367.

73. Dehda K, Booth H, Huggett J, et al. Lung remodeling in pulmonary tuberculosis. J Infect Dis 2005; 192:1201.

74. Lack E, Connor D. Tuberculosis. In: Chandler F, Connor D, Schwartz D, editors. Pathology of infectious disease. Stamford (CT): Appleton & Lange; 1997. p. 857.

75. Van Dyke P, Hoenacker F, Van Den Brande P, et al. Imaging of pulmonary tuberculosis. Eur Radiol 2003;13:1771.

76. Brantianos P, Swanson J, Torbenson M, et al. Tuberculosis-associated hemophagocytic syndrome. Lancet Infect Dis 2006;6:447–54.

77. Primm T, Lucero C, Falkinham J. Health impacts of environmental mycobacteria. Clin Micro Rev 2004; 17:98.

78. Tortoli E. Impact of genotypic studies on mycobacterial taxonomy: the new mycobacteria of the 1990s. Clin Microbiol Rev 2003;16:319.

79. Field S, Cowie R. Lung disease due to more common mycobacteria. Chest 2006;129:1653.

80. Glassroth J. Pulmonary disease due to nontuberculous mycobacteria. Chest 2008;133:243.

81. Johnson M, Waller E, Leventhal JP. Non tuberculous mycobacterial pulmonary disease. Curr Opin Pulm Med 2008;14:203.

82. Horsburgh CR Jr, Feldman S, Ridzon R. Practice guidelines for the treatment of tuberculosis. Clin Infect Dis 2000;31:633.

83. Caminero JA, Sotgiu G, Zumla A, et al. Best drug treatment for multidrug-resistant and extensively drug-resistant tuberculosis. Lancet Infect Dis 2010;10:621.

84. Dave BR, Sharma A, Kalva SP, et al. Nine-year single-center experience with transcatheter arterial embolization for hemoptysis: medium-term outcomes. Vasc Endovascular Surg 2011;45:258.

85. Kapur S, Louie BE. Hemoptysis and thoracic fungal infections. Surg Clin North Am 2010;90:985.

86. Andrejak C, Parrot A, Bazelly B, et al. Surgical lung resection for severe hemoptysis. Ann Thorac Surg 2009;88:1556.

87. Jougon J, Ballester M, Delcambre F, et al. Massive hemoptysis: what place for medical and surgical treatment. Eur J Cardiothorac Surg 2002;22:345.

88. Shigemura N, Wan IY, Yu SC, et al. Multidisciplinary management of life-threatening massive hemoptysis: a 10-year experience. Ann Thorac Surg 2009;87:849.

89. Karmy-Jones R, Cuschieri J, Vallieres E. Role of bronchoscopy in massive hemoptysis. Chest Surg Clin N Am 2001;11:873.

90. Kato A, Kudo S, Matsumoto K, et al. Bronchial artery embolization for hemoptysis due to benign diseases: immediate and long-term results. Cardiovasc Intervent Radiol 2000;23:351.

91. Rabkin JE, Astafjev VI, Gothman LN, et al. Transcatheter embolization in the management of pulmonary hemorrhage. Radiology 1987;163:361.

92. Remy-Jardin M, Wattinne L, Remy J. Transcatheter occlusion of pulmonary arterial circulation and collateral supply: failures, incidents, and complications. Radiology 1991;180:699.

93. Uflacker R, Kaemmerer A, Neves C, et al. Management of massive hemoptysis by bronchial artery embolization. Radiology 1983;146:627.

94. Yoon W, Kim JK, Kim YH, et al. Bronchial and nonbronchial systemic artery embolization for life-threatening hemoptysis: a comprehensive review. Radiographics 2002;22:1395.

95. Saubolle MA. Fungal pneumonias. Semin Respir Infect 2000;15:162.

96. Haque A, McGinnis MR. Fungal infections. In: Tomashefski J, Cagle P, Farver C, et al, editors. Dail and Hammar's pulmonary pathology. New York: Springer; 2008. p. 349.

97. Sabonya R. Fungal disease, including pneumocystis. In: Churg A, Meyers J, Tazelaar H, et al, editors. Thurlbeck's pathology of the lung. New York: Thieme; 2005. p. 283.

98. Irwin R, Rinaldi M, Walsh T. Zygomycosis of the respiratory tract. In: Sarosi G, Davies S, editors. Fungal diseases of the lung. 3rd edition. Philadelphia: Lippincott Williams & Wilkins; 2000. p. 163.

99. Karnak D, Avery R, Gilder T, et al. Endobronchial fungal disease: an under recognized entity. Respiration 2007;74:88.

100. Herbrecht R, Denning DW, Patterson TF, et al. Voriconazole versus amphotericin B for primary therapy of invasive aspergillosis. N Engl J Med 2002;347:408.

101. Walsh TJ, Anaissie EJ, Denning DW, et al. Treatment of aspergillosis: clinical practice guidelines of the Infectious Diseases Society of America. Clin Infect Dis 2008;46:327.

102. Marr KA, Boeckh M, Carter RA, et al. Combination antifungal therapy for invasive aspergillosis. Clin Infect Dis 2004;39:797.

103. Singh N, Limaye AP, Forrest G, et al. Combination of voriconazole and caspofungin as primary therapy for invasive aspergillosis in solid organ transplant recipients: a prospective, multicenter, observational study. Transplantation 2006;81:320.

104. Sole A. Invasive fungal infections in lung transplantation: role of aerosolised amphotericin B. Int J Antimicrobial Agents 2008;32(Suppl 2):S161.

105. Rogers TR. Treatment of zygomycosis: current and new options. J Antimicrobial Chemother 2008; 61(Suppl 1):i35.

106. Treanor J. Respiratory infections. In: Richman D, Whitley R, editors. Clinical virology. New York: Churchhill-Livingston; 1997. p. 5.

107. Storch GA. Diagnostic virology. Clin Infect Dis 2000;31:739.

108. Gilliam-Ross L. Emerging respiratory viruses: challenges and vaccine strategies. Clin Microbiol Rev 2006;19:614.

109. Kahn J. Newly identified respiratory viruses. Pediatr Infect Dis J 2007;26:745.

110. Hidron AI, Low CE, Honig EG, et al. Emergence of community-acquired methicillin-resistant Staphylococcus aureus strain USA300 as a cause of necrotising community-onset pneumonia. Lancet Infect Dis 2009;9:384.

111. Hageman JC, Uyeki TM, Francis JS, et al. Severe community-acquired pneumonia due to Staphylococcus aureus, 2003-04 influenza season. Emerg Infect Dis 2006;12:894.

112. Rabella N, Rodriguez P, Labeaga R, et al. Conventional respiratory viruses recovered from immunocompromised patients: clinical considerations. Clin Infect Dis 1999;28:1043.

113. Ruuskanen O, Putto A, Sarkkinen H, et al. C-reactive protein in respiratory virus infections. J Pediatr 1985;107:97.

114. Anjuna V, Colby T. Pathologic features of lung biopsy specimens from influenza pneumonia cases. Hum Pathol 1994;25:47.

115. Taubenberger J, Morens D. The pathology of influenza virus infections. Ann Rev Pathol 2008;3:499.

116. Harper SA, Bradley JS, Englund JA, et al. Seasonal influenza in adults and children—diagnosis, treatment, chemoprophylaxis, and institutional outbreak management: clinical practice guidelines of the Infectious Diseases Society of America. Clin Infect Dis 2009;48:1003.

117. Michalopoulos A, Kasiakou SK, Mastora Z, et al. Aerosolized colistin for the treatment of nosocomial pneumonia due to multidrug-resistant Gram-negative bacteria in patients without cystic fibrosis. Crit Care 2005;9(1):R53–9.

118. Kwa AL, Loh C, Low JG, et al. Nebulized colistin in the treatment of pneumonia due to multidrug-resistant Acinetobacter baumannii and Pseudomonas aeruginosa. Clin Infect Dis 2005;41(5):754–7.

119. Berlana D, Llop JM, Fort E, et al. Use of colistin in the treatment of multiple-drug-resistant gram-negative infections. Am J Health Syst Pharm 2005;62(1):39–47.

120. Michalopoulos A, Fotakis D, Virtzili S, et al. Aerosolized colistin as adjunctive treatment of ventilator-associated pneumonia due to multidrug-resistant Gram-negative bacteria: a prospective study. Respir Med 2008;102(3):407–12.

121. Kofteridis DP, Alexopoulou C, Valachis A, et al. Aerosolized plus intravenous colistin versus intravenous colistin alone for the treatment of ventilator-associated pneumonia: a matched case-control study. Clin Infect Dis 2010;51(11):1238–44.

122. Korbila IP, Michalopoulos A, Rafailidis PI, et al. Inhaled colistin as adjunctive therapy to intravenous colistin for the treatment of microbiologically documented ventilator-associated pneumonia: a comparative cohort study. Clin Microbiol Infect 2010;16(8):1230–6.

Indications for Surgery in Patients with Localized Pulmonary Infection

Robert E. Merritt, MD[a], Joseph B. Shrager, MD[a,b],*

KEYWORDS

- Localized pulmonary infection • Aspergilloma • Mucormycosis • Surgical resection

KEY POINTS

- The indications for surgical therapy for localized pulmonary infections can be broken down into 4 broad categories: (1) failure of medical therapy; (2) no medical therapy available that is effective as monotherapy; (3) development of complications such as hemoptysis, empyema, and/or bronchopleural fistula; (4) inability to rule out malignancy in a mass lesion.
- The common localized pulmonary infections that are encountered in adult thoracic surgical practice in the developed world include bacterial lung abscess, aspergilloma, multidrug-resistant tuberculosis, and mucormycosis.
- The principles of surgical therapy, when indicated, are: resection consisting ideally of either lobectomy or sublobar resection; decortication, tissue flap transposition, or other modalities to obliterate any residual pleural space; and coverage of bronchial stumps. Pneumonectomy is avoided if at all possible because of its high morbidity and mortality rates in this patient population.

INTRODUCTION

The availability of effective antibiotic and antifungal therapy has altered the natural history of some of the infections that can involve the lung parenchyma in a localized manner, such as bacterial abscess and infection with nonresistant tuberculosis strains. In these diseases, the need for surgical intervention has become rare. However, other localized pulmonary infections, for example aspergilloma and mucormycosis, are highly resistant to nonsurgical therapy, and in these diseases there are no generally successful options that do not include surgical resection. Furthermore, vulnerable patient populations, such as those who are immunocompromised secondary to chemotherapy or corticosteroid therapy, may require surgical therapy even for infections that in normal patients are typically responsive to antibiotics. Any patient with a localized pulmonary infection can develop life-threatening complications, such as massive hemoptysis or bronchopleural fistula with associated empyema, which will dictate the need for surgical intervention.

The localized pulmonary infections that are encountered with some regularity in adult thoracic surgical practice in the developed world include:

- Bacterial lung abscess
- Aspergilloma
- Mucormycosis
- Multidrug-resistant tuberculosis.

This article reviews the indications for surgical intervention in the treatment of each of these common infections involving the lung. Because each of these topics will be covered in more detail

a Division of Thoracic Surgery, Department of Cardiothoracic Surgery, Stanford University School of Medicine, Stanford, CA, USA; b Division of Thoracic Surgery, VA Palo Alto Health Care System, Palo Alto, CA, USA
* Corresponding author. Stanford Medical Center, 300 Pasteur Drive, Second Floor Falk Building, Stanford, CA 94305.
E-mail address: Shrager@stanford.edu

Thorac Surg Clin 22 (2012) 325–332
doi:10.1016/j.thorsurg.2012.05.005
1547-4127/12/$ – see front matter Published by Elsevier Inc

in articles elsewhere in this issue, the authors focus here on the general approaches to management rather than the details of that management.

GENERAL APPROACHES TO MANAGEMENT

To generalize, the indications for surgical therapy for localized pulmonary infections can be broken down into 4 categories:

1. Failure of medical therapy
2. No medical therapy available that is effective as monotherapy
3. Development of complications such as hemoptysis, empyema, and/or bronchopleural fistula
4. Inability to rule out malignancy in a mass lesion.

Other than in cases in category 3, where surgical therapy is usually urgent and cannot be avoided, there is much "art" that comes into the decision making about when and how to surgically intervene in each of these other categories. These patients are often critically ill (immunosuppressed, few platelets, and so forth), and one must always be sure that the surgical "cure" is not worse than the disease and that one is not operating on a patient with minimal chance of survival. On the other hand, one must realize that in many of these patients, despite the substantial risk of operation, surgery is the only chance of cure. It is therefore often appropriate to be surgically aggressive.

BACTERIAL LUNG ABSCESS

A bacterial lung abscess results from necrosis of the pulmonary parenchyma caused by a microbial infection that creates a cavity which then fills with purulent fluid and debris. Aspiration of oropharyngeal flora is the most common mechanism for the development of a bacterial lung abscess. Patients with altered mental status, esophageal motility disorders, recurrent nerve palsy, immunocompromised states, and poor oral hygiene are at particular risk for the development of this problem. The posterior segment of the right upper lobe and the superior segment of the right lower lobe are the most common locations for the development of lung abscesses, because of their dependent locations.

The common microbial pathogens involved with lung abscesses include[1]:

- *Peptostreptococcus*
- *Bacteroides*
- *Prevotella*
- *Streptococcus pneumoniae*
- *Haemophilus influenzae*
- *Klebsiella pneumoniae*
- Mycobacteria.

The symptoms of bacterial lung abscess are similar to the symptoms of pneumonia, which include:

- Malaise
- Productive cough
- Night sweats
- Fevers
- Weight loss.

Patients can also present with hemoptysis when the lung abscess involves the pulmonary vasculature. A chest radiograph will often demonstrate the distinctive appearance of a lung abscess, with an air-fluid level resulting from communication with the airway (**Fig. 1**). A computed tomography (CT) scan of the chest will often demonstrate a cavitary lesion with associated consolidation (**Fig. 2**). Because a cavitary lung carcinoma can have a similar appearance to a lung abscess on CT scan, and may in fact become infected, separating benign from malignant disease can occasionally be challenging. Flexible fiberoptic bronchoscopy can be performed to rule out an obstructing or associated tumor or foreign body. Transthoracic needle biopsy of the thickest part of the cavity's wall may be indicated when malignancy seems possible.

Medical Treatment

The implementation of appropriate antimicrobial therapy is the cornerstone of medical treatment of bacterial lung abscess.[2,3] In addition to initially broad antimicrobial therapy, which can subsequently be narrowed based on culture results, patients should receive chest physiotherapy with postural drainage and nutritional supplementation as supportive therapy.

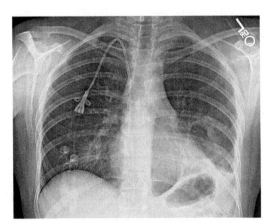

Fig. 1. Chest radiograph demonstrating a left lower lobe lung abscess with air-fluid level.

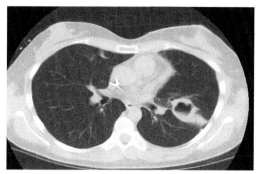

Fig. 2. Chest computed tomography scan demonstrating a left lower lobe cavitary lung abscess with associated infiltrate.

Invasive Therapy

The introduction of effective antimicrobial therapy for bacterial lung abscess has significantly affected the natural history of the disease process and has limited the role of invasive therapy. Furthermore, when invasive therapy is required, first-line management is typically placement of a drainage catheter under radiologic guidance, a procedure typically performed by interventional radiologists. In general, surgical resection has been indicated when medical therapy with or without interventional drainage for bacterial lung abscess fails because of the following situations:

- Persistent infection secondary to bronchial obstruction from neoplasm or foreign body
- A multidrug-resistant pathogen
- A large abscess greater than 6 cm
- Significant hemoptysis
- Rupture of the abscess cavity with formation of empyema, and often an associated bronchopleural fistula
- A cavitary lung cancer or inability to rule out lung cancer, or underlying pulmonary sequestration.

The surgical management of a bacterial lung abscess includes either external drainage or surgical resection. External drainage of lung abscess can be accomplished with either tube thoracostomy or, rarely, surgical cavernostomy. Tube drainage is appropriately attempted first, and ultrasound-guided or CT-guided percutaneous drainage of lung abscess is certainly preferred now to unguided, bedside placement of a chest tube. The effectiveness of external drainage has been reported to be between 73% and 100%.[4,5] The potential complications of percutaneous drainage of a bacterial lung abscess that may dictate surgical therapy include empyema (often with creation of a bronchopleural fistula), hemorrhage, and pneumothorax. These

complications are relatively rare, and the morbidity and mortality associated with percutaneous drainage is generally encountered only in critically ill patients.[4] For these reasons, external tube drainage is generally attempted before moving toward resection or cavernostomy, if tube drainage fails.

Cavernostomy would typically only be performed in situations where antibiotics and percutaneous drainage have failed, and resection is not possible because of the poor condition of the patient. Resection essentially eliminates the chance of recurrent infection, and thus it is preferred to cavernostomy in those who would seem to be able to tolerate it. Cavernostomy with immediate closure, consisting of operative debridement of the cavity and immediate filling with a vascularized soft tissue flap, is the next best option. In those who are thought to be too compromised for even the limited thoracotomy required for this procedure, an open cavernostomy, or marsupialization of the cavity to the atmosphere via limited rib resection, can be performed. The downside of the chronic wound left by this latter approach must be balanced against the greater acute risks of the more definitive approaches.

One unusual situation in which cavernostomy may be preferred to resection is when resection can be achieved only by pneumonectomy. Pneumonectomy in the setting of lung abscess (or any lung infection, for that matter) greatly increases morbidity. The risk of bronchopleural fistula is higher, as is the risk of empyema without fistula. Pneumonectomy in the setting of a lung abscess, which despite the surgeon's best efforts may occasionally be entered and spilled into the pleural space during the resection, is a setup for a disastrous postpneumonectomy empyema. For these reasons, when medical therapy and percutaneous drainage fail for a large lung abscess that cannot be encompassed by lobectomy, cavernostomy may be the preferred approach.

In the modern era, surgical resection is required in fewer than 10% of cases of bacterial lung abscess.[5] The most common indication for surgical resection is the inability to rule out a cavitary lung cancer. Patients who present with a thick-walled lung cavity, lack of fever and leukocytosis, and no response to antibiotic therapy should be suspected of having a necrotic lung carcinoma rather than an abscess, and they must be managed as such. Furthermore, in patients who resolve a clinical lung abscess with nonsurgical therapy, but who on subsequent follow-up have growth of what would be expected to be a slowly resolving scar, there must be a concern for an associated occult malignancy. This aspect highlights the need to continue to follow patients who have had a lung abscess successfully treated (particularly those with a history of cigarette smoking) with serial radiographic examinations following the resolution of the acute infection.

Substantial hemoptysis is another occasional indication for surgical resection. Although this has been reported to occur in approximately 15% of cases of lung abscess, in the authors' experience it is rare to have hemoptysis with a bacterial lung abscess that is sufficient on its own to mandate resection.[6]

When surgical resection is required for management of lung abscess, a lobectomy is required in most cases. The use of a double-lumen endotracheal tube or a bronchial blocker is very important in preventing contamination of the contralateral lung with purulent debris or blood during the procedure. In addition, an intercostal muscle flap or other vascularized soft tissue should be used for coverage of the bronchial stump to reduce the risk of bronchopleural fistula. In situations where there is a concern for a residual pleural space, such as when the interlobar staple line must be carried into an adjacent lobe to complete the resection, or when the remaining lobe(s) are relatively nonexpansile owing to chronic inflammation associated with the abscess, bulkier soft-tissue pedicles such as the latissimus dorsi muscle or omentum may be used to both cover the bronchial stump and fill residual space.

ASPERGILLUS INFECTION

Aspergillus is a ubiquitous fungus that can form lung infections after the inhalation of spores by the host. The manifestations of pulmonary *Aspergillus* infection includes localized infection (or aspergilloma), allergic bronchopulmonary aspergillosis, and disseminated aspergillosis seen in immunocompromised patients. The indications for surgical resection for *Aspergillus* infections are shown in **Box 1**.

Aspergilloma

An aspergilloma can be defined as a conglomeration of *Aspergillus* hyphae that are intertwined with fibrin, mucous debris, and cellular debris. Patients who develop aspergilloma usually have underlying pulmonary disease, such as bullous emphysema, fibrotic lung disease, cavitary tuberculosis, or sarcoidosis with bullae.[7] Aspergilloma may also develop in immunocompromised hosts in whom invasive *Aspergillus* infection rapidly destroys a region of lung parenchyma, forming a cavity, which subsequently harbors an aspergilloma. The majority of pulmonary aspergillomas are

---

Box 1
Indications for surgical resection for *Aspergillus* infections

- Recurrent hemoptysis
- Massive hemoptysis
- Inability to rule out a cavitary lung carcinoma
- Resection of complex aspergilloma
- Chronic cough
- Systemic symptoms
- Localized infection in an immunocompromised host

---

asymptomatic; therefore, the management often hinges on the development of life-threatening symptoms.

Massive hemoptysis is the most common potentially life-threatening symptom of aspergilloma, and can cause death from asphyxiation in up to 26% of patients.[7] In addition, there are certain risk factors that portend a poor prognosis for aspergilloma and that dictate consideration of surgical resection even in the absence of hemoptysis or other symptoms:

- Increasing size of aspergilloma on imaging studies
- Immunosuppression
- Increasing *Aspergillus*-specific immunoglobulin G titers
- Human immunodeficiency virus (HIV) infection.

At present, there is no consensus of opinion for the optimal treatment of aspergilloma, and there are certainly no randomized trials that provide evidence to guide treatment. Because life-threatening hemoptysis occurs in a minority of patients with aspergilloma, and because hemoptysis is rarely massive at its first presentation, surgical resection has not been recommended in asymptomatic patients given the significant morbidity and mortality associated with surgical therapy. The decision to perform surgical resection is a balance between the risks of complications of the aspergilloma weighed against the risk of the procedure.

Embolization of feeding bronchial arteries by interventional radiologists will often stop an acute episode of bleeding from an aspergilloma. However, this is only a temporizing maneuver, as the aspergilloma will almost invariably recruit a new blood supply over the next several months and the patient will bleed again in the future. Thus, once an episode of hemoptysis has occurred, surgical resection is clearly indicated in patients who would be predicted to have adequate postoperative pulmonary function.

Unfortunately, many of these patients have severe underlying lung disease, rendering this decision difficult even if only a lobectomy appears to be required. It is only in uncommon circumstances that a pneumonectomy is reasonable therapy for an aspergilloma.[8–13] Some of the most difficult decisions making ever encountered by general thoracic surgeons is that surrounding the unfortunately not infrequent, bleeding patient with complex, pleuropulmonary aspergilloma who may require a pneumonectomy for resection. Inevitably these patients will have pulmonary function that will leave them, at best, marginally compensated following a pneumonectomy. These patients are at high risk for postoperative respiratory failure, bronchopleural fistula, and empyema, and have an approximately 15% perioperative mortality rate. There is no good solution for such patients, although small series suggest some efficacy with placement of amphotericin paste into the aspergilloma cavity.[14,15]

The ideal treatment for aspergilloma when surgery is required is surgical resection with either lobectomy or sublobar resection.[8] Lobectomy with additional wedge or anatomic segmentectomy of an adjacent lobe is also commonly required. Surgical resection prevents recurrent hemoptysis, controls infection, and almost certainly increases overall survival. Even lobectomy for aspergilloma, however, is often difficult because of dense vascular adhesions and pleural fibrosis, which result in relatively high intraoperative blood loss and transfusion rates.[9,11] The overall operative mortality rates reported for resection of aspergilloma range from 5.6% to 22.6%.[9,11–13,16] Even after lobectomy, the potential postoperative complications that contribute to mortality include hemorrhage, empyema, bronchopleural fistula, and respiratory failure.

A persistent pleural space is common after resection of aspergilloma. The inflammatory fibrosis of the lung parenchyma limits the reexpansion of the remaining pulmonary parenchyma, which can result in persistent air leaks and empyema.[17] As a result various techniques, such as pleural tent, pneumoperitoneum, decortication, and muscle flaps, have been recommended after resection of aspergilloma.[12] The authors believe that one should enter these operations preparing to harvest whatever healthy, vascularized tissue is available to assure both coverage of the bronchial stump and complete obliteration of the anticipated residual pleural space. In the authors' experience, pedicled latissimus muscle is the minimum tissue flap that is required for a lobectomy for anything other than the smallest, least complex aspergilloma. Frequently, the authors harvest both latissimus and serratus anterior, and for lower lobectomies omental transposition may be required.

Despite the technical challenges and potential for postoperative complications, surgical resection for aspergilloma is clearly indicated for patients with hemoptysis and reasonable pulmonary functional reserve. Jewkes and colleagues[16] demonstrated a 5-year survival of 84% for resection of aspergilloma in patients with hemoptysis compared with a 5-year survival of 41% for medical therapy alone. Similarly, Kim and colleagues[17] reported a 10-year actuarial survival rate of 80% following resection of aspergilloma.

Invasive Aspergillosis

Invasive pulmonary aspergillosis is a serious but unfortunately common infection encountered in patients who are immunocompromised, most often secondary to bone marrow transplantation or solid organ transplants. This disease is completely different from aspergilloma. *Aspergillus* infections in this patient population often present as multifocal infiltrates with vascular invasion and dissemination to other solid organs. Despite optimal medical therapy with amphotericin B alone, the mortality rate for invasive pulmonary aspergillosis in patients who receive bone marrow transplants can be as high as 94%.[18]

The decision making as to when to operate with invasive *Aspergillus* is even more difficult than for localized aspergilloma. When confined to resectable portions of lung, without evidence of spread to other organs, aggressive, early surgical resection does have a role in selected immunocompromised patients with invasive pulmonary aspergillosis. It appears from small series that complete surgical resection of localized disease combined with intravenous antifungal therapy can substantially improve survival in this high-risk patient population.[18] These patients are difficult to manage and generally require platelet transfusion, tissue flaps for bronchial coverage, and prolonged recovery requiring the close involvement of several subspecialties. The risks of this approach in these fragile patients, which are substantial, must be weighed against the likelihood that without surgical resection they will have a high probability for mortality.

MUCORMYCOSIS

Mucormycosis is a rare fungal infection caused by *Rhizopus* or *Mucor* species.[19] The spores are inhaled and then germinate forming hyphal elements. Pulmonary mucormycosis infections typically occur in immunocompromised hosts, which include patients on high-dose chemotherapy or patients on chronic corticosteroid therapy. The mucorales are saprophytic fungi that thrive in acidic environments; therefore, patients with diabetic ketoacidosis or renal failure are also susceptible.

Mucor hyphae are characterized as being highly angioinvasive. The invasion into blood vessels by the *Mucor* hyphae often results in hemorrhage, thrombosis, infarction, and tissue necrosis. Pulmonary mucormycosis is thus a rapidly spreading infection that occurs when the spores settle into the bronchioles and alveoli. A diffuse consolidative pneumonia forms resulting in infarction and pulmonary parenchymal necrosis. As a result of the rapid progression of mucormycosis, the mortality rate is high if treatment is not introduced promptly. The in-hospital mortality rate for patients with isolated pulmonary mucormycosis is 65%, and 96% for patients with disseminated disease.[19]

The initial treatment of mucormycosis consists of amphotericin B therapy and control of blood glucose levels. The most common cause of death is fungal sepsis related to widely disseminated disease. Operative intervention is indicated in patients with isolated mucormycosis involving one lung. Sublobar resection or lobectomy with complete resection/debridement of infected surrounding pleural and chest wall tissue is recommended, and should be performed early in patients who can tolerate the procedure.[20] Tedder and colleagues[20] reported a 9.4% mortality rate in patients treated with surgical resection for isolated mucormycosis compared with a 50% mortality rate in similar patients treated with medical therapy alone. Of the 36 patients who underwent surgical therapy, 61% underwent lobectomy, 11% underwent pneumonectomy, and 8% underwent wedge resection. The investigators concluded that patients with isolated mucormycosis limited to one lung benefit more from aggressive surgical resection than from medical therapy alone.

ACTINOMYCOSIS/NOCARDIA

Actinomyces and *Nocardia* are gram-positive bacterial organisms that, because of their filamentous appearance, were once misclassified as fungi and considered together with *Mucor*. Actinomycosis most commonly infects the skin and can generally be treated with medical therapy alone, although bulky disease may be benefited by surgical resection. *Nocardia* can occur in the skin in normal hosts, but most often involves the lung in immunocompromised hosts. In the latter situation, *Nocardia*, if resectable, should be treated like *Mucor* with early surgical resection in combination with antibiotics to gain the best chance of cure.

TUBERCULOSIS

Tuberculosis (TB) is a pulmonary infection caused by the pathogen *Mycobacterium tuberculosis*. The incidence of TB cases in the United States had increased between 1980 and 1992 because of the HIV/AIDS epidemic, the emergence of multidrug-resistant TB, and a decline in TB treatment program infrastructure which had occurred.[21] Surgical treatment of TB has been mostly replaced by medical therapy for pulmonary TB, including isoniazid, rifampin, ethambutol, and pyrazinamide. In cases of cavitary disease and multidrug-resistant TB, however, surgical resection still has an essential role. The current indications for surgical intervention for TB in the modern era are shown in **Box 2**.

Surgical resection of infected lung parenchyma, the clearance of the pleural space infection, and decortication for pleural disease are the cornerstones of surgical therapy for TB. Traditional surgical therapy for TB, such thoracoplasty and other forms of collapse therapy, have been largely supplanted by anatomic pulmonary resections, along with filling of any residual pleural spaces with vascularized soft-tissue flaps (muscle and/or omentum).[22] There are still rare cases in which a residual space cannot be filled with available soft tissue, and in these cases thoracoplasty may still be indicated.

In the modern era, medical therapy has largely obviated surgical management of standard, drug-sensitive TB. The only operations performed with any frequency at all for standard TB today are situations whereby cavities or areas of destroyed lung occur that become superinfected or become sites of hemoptysis. One also encounters the occasional

---

Box 2
Indications for surgical intervention for TB

- Ruling out malignancy in pulmonary nodules or mediastinal lymphadenopathy
- Persistent cavitary disease
- Massive hemoptysis
- Bronchial stenosis
- Aspergilloma in a TB cavity
- Multidrug-resistant *M tuberculosis* with localized disease
- Destroyed lung parenchyma

residual bronchial stenosis, requiring sleeve bronchial resection or sleeve lobectomy, following successful drug treatment of TB with an endobronchial component. All of these operations, however, are relatively rare in industrialized nations.

For multidrug-resistant TB, however, this is not the case, and surgical intervention is more frequent. Patients with multidrug-resistant TB present more commonly than patients with sensitive TB strains with destroyed lung parenchyma and persistent cavitary lesions that are symptomatic and resistant to medical therapy. Furthermore, it has been established that with multidrug-resistant TB, surgical resection of localized pulmonary disease, even if not complicated by cavitation, combined with medical therapy, can improve the cure rate.[22] Pomerantz and colleagues[23] reported a large series of patients undergoing pulmonary resection for multidrug-resistant TB. Over a 17-year period, 98 lobectomies and 82 pneumonectomies were performed, with an operative mortality rate of only 3.3% and a morbidity rate of 12%. The investigators recommended the use of vascularized muscle flaps to cover the bronchial stump to minimize the rate of residual pleural space and bronchopleural fistula. Another modern surgical series reported the results of pulmonary resection for multidrug-resistant TB with no early operative mortality.[24] Patients should receive at least 3 months of the best possible antituberculosis medical therapy (based on in vitro sensitivities) with the goal of clearing the sputum of active infection before the planned surgical resection. In multidrug-resistant TB, this goal cannot always be reached.

SUMMARY

The surgical management of localized lung infections can be challenging for thoracic surgeons. Many of these patients are immunocompromised owing to chemotherapy received for various forms of cancer, or they are receiving immunosuppressive therapy following solid organ or bone marrow transplantation. In addition, patients with underlying lung destruction caused by emphysema or bullous sarcoidosis are at risk for many of these lung infections, and such patients frequently lack adequate pulmonary reserve to tolerate the required anatomic pulmonary resection. Nonetheless, surgical resection does have a defined role in the management of localized lung infection in select groups of patients with bacterial lung abscess, aspergilloma/aspergillosis, mucormycosis, and tuberculosis.

In general, surgical resection is indicated when medical therapy is incapable of, or has failed in,

clearing active disease, or when patients develop life-threatening complications such as hemoptysis or bronchopleural fistula with associated empyema. Resection consisting of either lobectomy or sublobar resection is usually sufficient, with decortication and/or tissue-flap transposition to obliterate any residual pleural space, and certainly coverage of all bronchial stumps. Pneumonectomy is rarely undertaken because of its high morbidity and mortality rates in this patient population. Although there are occasional circumstances whereby even pneumonectomy might need to be undertaken, this can generally be avoided by nonresectional procedures such as cavernostomy. Some of these patients are too critically ill to tolerate even surgical cavernostomy, and in these rare instances surgeons are sometimes forced to concede defeat at the hands of disease.

REFERENCES

1. Bartlett JG. The role of anaerobic bacteria in lung abscess. Clin Infect Dis 2005;40:923–5.
2. Allewelt M, Shuler P, Boleskei PL, et al. Ampicillin + sulbactam vs clindamycin +/- cephalosporin for treatment of aspiration pneumonia and primary lung abscess. Clin Microbiol Infect 2004;10:163–70.
3. Guidiol F, Manresa F, Pallares R, et al. Clindamycin vs penicillin failures associated with penicillin-resistant *Bacteroides melaninogenicus*. Arch Intern Med 1990;150:2525–9.
4. Liambiase RE, Deyoe L, Cronan JJ, et al. Percutaneous drainage of 335 consecutive abscesses: results of primary drainage with 1 year followup. Radiology 1992;184:167–79.
5. Wiedemann HP, Rice TW. Lung abscess and empyema. Semin Thorac Cardiovasc Surg 1995;7: 119–28.
6. Darling G, Downey GP, Herridge MS. Bacterial infections of the lung. Pearson's thoracic and esophageal surgery. 3rd edition. Philadelphia: Elsevier; 2008. p. 479–98.
7. Stevens DA, Kan VL, Judson MA, et al. Practice guidelines for diseases caused by *Aspergillus*. Clin Infect Dis 2000;30:696–709.
8. Park CK, Jheon S. Results of surgical treatment of pulmonary aspergilloma. Eur J Cardiothorac Surg 2002;21:918–23.
9. Massard G, Roeslin N, Wihlm JM, et al. Pleuropulmonary aspergilloma: clinical spectrum and results of surgical treatment. Ann Thorac Surg 1992;54: 1159–64.
10. Shirakusa T, Ueda H, Suito T, et al. Surgical treatment of pulmonary aspergilloma and *Aspergillus* empyema. Ann Thorac Surg 1989;48:779–82.

11. Regnard JF, Icard P, Nicolosi M, et al. Aspergilloma: a series of 89 surgical cases. Ann Thorac Surg 2000;69:898–903.

12. Daly RC, Pairolero PC, Piehler JM, et al. Pulmonary aspergilloma. Results of surgical treatment. J Thorac Cardiovasc Surg 1986;92:981–8.

13. Karas A, Hankins JR, Attar S, et al. An analysis of 41 patients. Ann Thorac Surg 1976;22:1–7.

14. Munk PL, Vellet AD, Rankin RN, et al. Intracavitary aspergilloma: transthoracic percutaneous injection of amphotericin gelatin solution. Radiology 1993; 188(3):821–3.

15. Giron JM, Poey CG, Fajadet PP, et al. Inoperable pulmonary aspergilloma: percutaneous CT-guided injection with glycerin and amphotericin B paste in 15 cases. Radiology 1993;188(3):825–7.

16. Jewkes J, Kay PH, Paneth M, et al. Pulmonary aspergilloma: analysis of prognosis in relation to haemoptysis and survey of treatment. Thorax 1983;38: 572–8.

17. Kim YT, Kang MC, Sung SW, et al. Good long-term outcomes after surgical treatment of simple and complex pulmonary aspergilloma. Ann Thorac Surg 2005;79:294–8.

18. Robinson LA, Reed EC, Galbraith TA, et al. Pulmonary resection for invasive *Aspergillus* infections in immunocompromised patients. J Thorac Cardiovasc Surg 1995;109:1182–96.

19. Bigby T, Serota ML, Tierney LM, et al. Clinical spectrum of pulmonary mucormycosis. Chest 1986;89: 435–9.

20. Tedder M, Spratt JA, Anstadt MP, et al. Pulmonary mucormycosis: results of medical and surgical therapy. Ann Thorac Surg 1994;57:1044–50.

21. Corbett EL, Watt CJ, Walker N, et al. The growing burden of tuberculosis: global trends and interactions with the HIV epidemic. Arch Intern Med 2003; 163:1009–21.

22. Mouroux J, Maalouf J, Padovani B, et al. Surgical management of pleuropulmonary tuberculosis. J Thorac Cardiovasc Surg 1996;111:662–70.

23. Pomerantz BJ, Cleveland JC Jr, Olson HK, et al. Pulmonary resection of multi-drug resistant tuberculosis. J Thorac Cardiovasc Surg 2001;121:448–53.

24. Shiraishi Y, Nakajima Y, Katsuragi N, et al. Resectional surgery combined with chemotherapy remains the treatment of choice for multidrug resistant tuberculosis. J Thorac Cardiovasc Surg 2004;128:523–8.

Results of Surgery for Bronchiectasis and Pulmonary Abscesses

Thirugnanam Agasthian, MBBS

KEYWORDS

- Noncystic bronchiectasis • Lung abscess • Surgery • Outcomes

KEY POINTS

- Best surgical outcomes are obtained when complete resection of localized bronchiectasis is done.
- Palliative resections benefit those with localized severely diseased cystic bronchiectasis on a background of mild cylindrical diffuse bronchiectasis.
- Most lung abscesses respond to antibiotics and percutaneous drainage.

SURGERY FOR NONCYSTIC FIBROSIS BRONCHIECTASIS

Introduction

Noncystic fibrosis bronchiectasis remains an important cause of respiratory disease especially in developing countries. One study reports a prevalence of bronchiectasis as being 4.2 per 100,000 persons aged 18 to 34 years and 272 per 100,000 in those older than 75 years.[1] There is also an association with chronic obstructive pulmonary disease (COPD), with 2 studies reporting an incidence of bronchiectasis in COPD as being 29% to 50%.[2,3] Although medical therapy remains the mainstay of treatment, surgery offers the only form of cure for this disease in selected cases. In some instances, it may help palliate symptoms and help delay progression of disease.

Pathology

Bronchiectasis is defined as irreversible dilatation of peripheral airways secondary to damage of the structural components of the bronchial wall (elastin, muscles, and cartilage). The main mechanisms responsible for bronchiectasis are bronchial wall injury, bronchial lumen obstruction, and traction from adjacent fibrosis seen in end-stage lung fibrosis. The most widely known model of the development of bronchiectasis is Cole's[4] "vicious cycle" hypothesis in which after the initial infection, often against a background of genetic susceptibility and impaired mucosal clearance, results in persistence of microorganisms in the bronchial tree. Microbial colonization in the crypts of dilated airways with overproduction of thick viscid mucus, which acts as a fertile medium together with impairment of the mucociliary escalator mechanisms, causes a vicious cycle of repeated and prolonged episodes of chronic inflammation resulting in progressive airway and lung damage.

Detailed pathologic study of 200 operated bronchiectasis lung specimens by Whitwell[5] demonstrated the presence of enlarged lymphoid follicles and marked inflammation in the bronchial wall of the small airways. This small airway inflammation causes the release of elastases and inflammatory cytokines, causing intense transmural airway inflammation, which damages the large airways resulting in bronchial dilation, increase in submucosal glands, loss of ciliary-lined epithelium, and neovascularisation.[6,7] With progression of the disease, lymphoid follicles enlarge further

Department of Cardiothoracic Surgery, National University Hospital, 1E Kent Ridge Road, NUHS Tower Blk Level 9, Singapore 119228, SGP
E-mail address: agasthian@singnet.com.sg

Thorac Surg Clin 22 (2012) 333–344
doi:10.1016/j.thorsurg.2012.04.008
1547-4127/12/$ – see front matter © 2012 Elsevier Inc. All rights reserved.

in size, causing obstruction to the small airways. The inflammation eventually spreads from the airways to lung parenchyma, causing fibrosis and end-stage lung failure. High-resolution computed tomography (HRCT) and lung function studies show airflow obstruction in bronchiectasis to be predominantly a result of small and medium airway involvement. The small airway constrictive bronchiolitis is diagnosed by the presence of a mosaic pattern on expiratory HRCT films.[8] Although the large airways become dilated in bronchiectasis, it is the inflammatory process affecting the predominant small and medium airways that gives rise to airflow obstruction. With progression of the disease, however, the pattern would be a mixed one of obstructive and restrictive.

Acquired bacterial and viral infections still rank first in the etiology of bronchiectasis in developing countries. With the reemergence of tuberculosis, an increased incidence of postinfectious bronchiectasis is also increasing noted. About 11% of patients with tuberculosis develop bronchiectasis.[9] In developed countries, immune deficiency syndromes (hypogammaglobulinemia and leukocyte dysfunctions), metabolic defects (cystic fibrosis, alpha-1 antitrypsin deficiency), ultrastructural defects (primary ciliary dyskinesia, Young syndrome, Kartegener syndrome, congenital defects of cartilage), and pulmonary sequestrations are more common causes.[6,10]

Bronchiectasis can be localized (confined to one lobe or segment) or diffuse, which is more common. The rate of localized involvement has been reported as 3.6% to 19.0%.[11] Distribution of bronchiectasis in the lung may vary according to etiology. The left lung tends to be more involved than the right lung in 55% to 80% of cases.[11] This may be because the left main bronchi are narrower and longer than the right and subject to greater compression pressures, especially by the aortic arch. The left lower lobe is the commonest lobe affected (30%) followed by the middle lobe and lingular segments. The lower lobes are commonly affected owing to gravity-dependent retention of infected secretions. The upper lobes are usually affected secondary to post tuberculosis infection and allergic bronchopulmonary aspergillosis (ABPA). Central airway bronchiectasis is seen in ABPA, cystic fibrosis, and Mournier Kuhn syndrome. Right middle lobe and lingular segment bronchiectasis has been associated with nontuberculosis mycobacterial infections. Enlarged tuberculous lymph nodes around the proximal middle lobe bronchus may also lead to obstruction and secondary bronchiectasis.[12,13]

Reid[14] categorized bronchiectasis into 3 main anatomic, morphologic types: tubular or cylindrical, characterized by smooth dilation of the bronchi; varicose, in which the bronchi are dilated with multiple indentations; and cystic or saccular, in which dilated bronchi terminate in blind ending sacs of pus with no communication with the rest of lung. Cylindrical bronchiectasis is frequently associated with tuberculosis and immune disorders and communicates with the lung parenchyma. Cystic is associated with severe infections, and following airway obstruction. Varicose consists of alternating areas of cylindrical and saccular types. Pseudo-bronchiectasis is temporary cylindrical dilatation of bronchi after an acute infection that resolves with clearing of the infection. Cylindrical bronchiectasis is the commonest form seen on HRCT.

Another significant classification to emerge in the past decade is the functional classification of bronchiectasis. Ashour[15] described 2 types of bronchiectasis based on functional hemodynamic perfusion studies: perfused and nonperfused types. The perfused type has cylindrical bronchiectatic changes with intact pulmonary artery flow based on ventilation/perfusion (V/Q) scans, where the nonperfused type involves cystic bronchiectasis with an absent pulmonary artery flow with retrograde filling of the pulmonary artery through the systemic circulation.

Therefore, based on the morphologic and functional classifications, tubular or cylindrical bronchiectasis tends to have better prognosis than cystic/varicose varieties, as it is an early bronchiectatic change that can be reversible. Areas affected by cylindrical bronchiectasis tend to have good function and perfusion and rarely progress to severe forms of the disease. Cystic bronchiectasis tends to be a completely destroyed, nonfunctioning, and nonperfused lung.[15,16] All parameters of respiratory function are worse in the saccular type as compared with the tubular type. They tend to be the main harbingers of the greatest bacterial load with virulent strains, such as *Pseudomonas*, thereby contributing mainly to the symptomatology and more importantly to crossover contamination of healthier lung with progression of disease. Surgical removal of these completely destroyed diseased segments helps improve quality of life and may delay progression of disease.[17]

The clinical course of noncystic fibrosis bronchiectasis is variable, as some have few symptoms and others exhibit symptoms with progressive loss of lung function over time with loss of forced expiratory volume in 1 second (FEV1) at 50 mL per year.[16,18,19] One large clinical trial showed a frequency of 1.5 exacerbations per year in patients.[6] Factors associated with an accelerated rate of decline of lung function include cystic bronchiectasis, colonization by *Pseudomonas aeruginosa*, and history of repeated severe exacerbations.[16] Patients with no pathogens isolated from their sputum had the mildest disease. Alzeer and colleagues[20] showed that noncystic fibrosis bronchiectasis was associated with cardiac abnormalities, including right ventricular and left ventricular systolic and diastolic dysfunction.

Microbiology

Haemophilus influenzae is the commonest pathogen isolated in bronchiectasis (range 29%–70%) followed by *P aeruginosa* (range 12%–31%).[21,22] Despite being purulent, 30% to 40% of sputum samples will fail to grow any pathogenic bacteria, in spite of bronchoscopy with protected brush and bronchoalveolar lavage being used.[21,22] *H influenzae* has the capacity to cause direct damage to airway epithelium and is also able to invade into the bronchial wall and interstitium of the lung. *P aeruginosa* is associated with more sputum, more extensive bronchiectasis, frequent exacerbations, more hospitalizations, accelerated decline in lung function, and worse quality of life. It also has the capacity to form biofilms. Biofilms occur particularly in advanced disease and form an impenetrable matrix around the bacterial wall, shielding it from the immune system and antibiotics.[23]

Other common organisms include *Klebsiella pneumoniae*, *Streptococcus pneumoniae*, *Staphylococcus aureus*, and *Mycobacterium tuberculosis*. The presence of *S aureus* should raise the presence of cystic fibrosis. The bronchi also have a dynamic turnover of pathogens. A 2-year prospective study found that a proportion of patients colonized by *Moxarella catarrhalis* had continuous turnover of strains every 2 to 3 months. There also appears to be a change in microbial flora with severity of disease.[21,22] Typically, subjects with the best preserved lung function are most likely to have no pathogenic bacteria isolated. As lung function declines, *H influenzae* becomes predominant. Finally, in patients with the most severe disease, the usual pathogen isolated is *P aeruginosa*.[21]

Nontuberculous mycobacterial (NTM) infections are also important in bronchiectasis, with prevalence rates of 2% to 10%.[24] These infections are associated with bronchiectasis, particularly in older women, where the combination of mycobacterium avium complex (MAC) infections with right middle lobe and lingular bronchiectasis is a well-described syndrome.[13] It should also be remembered that NTM infections are opportunistic and may cause infection in other chronic lung diseases, such as COPD, and therefore infection with NTM may be secondary to bronchiectasis. It is not clear what the effect of secondary MAC colonization is on the progression of bronchiectasis. Although medical therapy remains the primary treatment modality for patients with pulmonary NTM disease, the selective use of pulmonary resection may reduce the incidence of symptomatic disease recurrence.[13,24,25]

Radiological Imaging

Precise preoperative imaging of the severity, distribution, and type of bronchiectasis is important in the planning of surgery, as completeness of surgery is the most important factor for successful surgical outcome. Since 1996, HRCT has supplanted bronchography as the radiological imaging of choice in the diagnosis of bronchiectasis.[26] HRCT or thin-sliced CT is a sensitive noninvasive method for the detection of bronchiectasis, especially in early mild disease with only 2% false-negative and 1% false-positive rates.[26–29] Besides assessing the degree and extent of airway disease, it is also useful in defining the morphologic types (saccular vs cylindrical), which are important in predicting the prognosis and functional severity of the disease. It also allows for noninvasive monitoring of disease progression, regression, or response to therapy.[28]

The HRCT technique with the simplest and lowest radiation dose remains at narrow collimation (1 mm) sections obtained at 10-mm intervals from lung apex to base, with the patient in supine position, and breath holding at maximum inspiration. With such protocol, clinically important bronchiectasis is unlikely to be missed in the gaps between the thin sections. The use of multidetector CT scanners, which allow an almost infinite variety of CT sections (no gap between slices), is becoming more common despite the risk of increased irradiation, and may eventually supplant HRCT scanning as the optimal imaging technique for bronchiectasis.[30] Because of concern for radiation exposure from HRCT, especially in children, magnetic resonance imaging (MRI) has been recently studied in bronchiectasis and has been found to be a promising alternative to HRCT.[31]

The main CT diagnostic features are as follows:

- Internal diameter of a bronchus is 1.5 times wider than its adjacent pulmonary artery (signet ring sign)
- Failure of the bronchi to taper
- Visualization of bronchi in the outer 1 to 2 cm of the lung field.

In early stages of disease, the HRCT signs are more subtle, such as bronchial wall thickening, small airway trapping with areas of decreased attenuation of the lung parenchyma, or mosaic attenuation may coexist, suggestive of constrictive bronchiolitis. Sections taken at end-expiration enhance the feature of decreased attenuation, the extent of which correlates with functional indices of airway obstruction. This finding is most prevalent in lobes with severe bronchiectasis but may be seen in some lobes in which there are no CT features of bronchiectasis. The extent and severity of bronchiectasis seen on HRCT scans has been correlated with functional change and clinical outcomes and degree of airflow obstruction.[29]

Pulmonary Function Test

Baseline pulmonary function tests should be obtained to assess functional status and to assess deterioration in lung function with progression of disease, as this may help in the timing of surgery. As a marker for disease severity, however, pulmonary function tests are relatively insensitive, especially in young children. With increasing age, FEV1 values in patients with bronchiectasis decline more rapidly and are used as a prognostic marker.[19]

Preoperative lung function, together with differential lung perfusion scan, would give a reasonable idea of the postoperative predicted FEV1, which should be at least 40% to 45% of the predicted value. This would allow the surgeon to decide whether complete resection of all diseased segments is possible or if only the most diseased segments can be removed. Pulmonary function tests may be performed routinely in older children (>5 years) and all adult patients. Children younger than 5 years were evaluated by an exercise-tolerance test.[30]

Pulmonary V/Q scans are performed to estimate the postoperative predicted lung function. Functional status is evaluated by physical examination, spirometry, arterial blood gases, quantitative ventilation measurements, and perfusion scans.

In one study, there was no significant change between preoperative and postoperative lung function (FEV1), especially if little or nonfunctioning lung is removed.[32] In another study, however, where more than 90% of patients improved in symptoms after surgery, there was a decrease in FEV1 in 68% of patients postoperatively, whereas exercise tolerance decreased in only 20%, reflecting that FEV1 is not an accurate assessment of postoperative surgical outcomes.[33]

INDICATIONS FOR SURGERY

For most cases of bronchiectasis, the mainstay of treatment remains medical therapy, which includes antibiotic therapy and postural drainage with vibratory massage. The indications for surgery have not changed much since the 1930s, and include the following:

- Failed medical therapy
- Chronic cough with copious fetid sputum
- Frequent infective exacerbations requiring antibiotic therapy
- Complications of bronchiectasis (hemoptysis, lung abscess, and empyema).[34]

Newer indications include the following:

- Prevention of possible progression of disease secondary to contamination from severely diseased segments to normal lung
- Colonization by nontuberculous mycobacterium that is resistant to prolonged medical therapy.[13]

The history of bronchiectasis parallels that of thoracic surgery. Since the 1930s, the role of surgery has been mainly confined to unilateral localized bronchiectasis, which has failed medical therapy and offered the only form of potential cure for this disease in a small group of patients.[30] Therefore, the goals of surgery were to remove localized destroyed lung completely with low morbidity and mortality and to offer a possible cure and improve quality of life. Whenever possible, early surgery is recommended to prevent further progression of disease secondary to spillage and contamination of adjacent healthy lung. The single most important prognostic factor for favorable surgical outcomes is completeness in eradicating all diseased lung.[11,35–39] Therefore, diffuse and bilateral bronchiectasis was considered a contraindication to surgery. Furthermore, bilateral resections used to be fraught with higher morbidity and mortality with risk of respiratory compromise.[40] As most patients fell into the diffuse group with varying severity of bronchiectasis in both lungs, they were treated medically to palliate symptoms and eventually progress to respiratory failure with cor pulmonale, with the only option of bilateral sequential lung transplantation; however, transplantation has not been an ideal alternative in this group because of long waiting times, donor shortage, and significant morbidity with modest long-term survival. Many die while waiting for transplantation.[41]

Over the past decade, with better understanding of the natural history of bronchiectasis based on morphologic and functional classifications, surgery has been extended to selected multisegmental, bilateral, and diffuse disease. Although cure rates (30%) are lower in this group than in localized disease, as complete resections are not possible, there has been significant improvement of disabling symptoms, reduction in hospital stay, and antibiotic usage, with improved quality of life and, more importantly, delay in the progression of disease by preventing contamination of adjacent lung.[42–46] The higher mortality and morbidity associated with bilateral resections reported in earlier series has been superceded by better outcomes in more recent studies owing to better antibiotics, more refined imaging techniques, and improved perioperative and postoperative care.[42–46]

Therefore, patients considered for surgery for bronchiectasis can be divided into

- Homogeneous bronchiectasis, in which there is diffuse, predominantly cystic or saccular bronchiectasis affecting most parts of lung with no good intervening functional lung on V/Q scan. Most of these patients are in respiratory failure and will progress to end-stage lung disease requiring lung transplantation.
- Heterogeneous bronchiectasis, which can be further subdivided into the following:
  - Unilateral localized bronchiectasis: Bronchiectasis localized to a segment, lobe, or whole lung (completely destroyed lung) and has the best surgical outcomes. This group would benefit the most from surgery, as complete resection with good chance for potential cure is usually possible in most cases.[9,36,37,47]
  - Bilateral localized bronchiectasis: Mutilsegmental bilateral disease with intervening normal lung or minimally diseased lung. This pattern is commonly seen in nontuberculous infections.[10] Complete resection is possible if all diseased segments can be removed without respiratory compromise. Resections include combinations of lobectomy with segmentectomy or wedge resections. Complete resection is possible with a high chance of improvement in symptoms. Surgery can be staged by bilateral lateral thoracotomy or done at same sitting by median sternotomy, bilateral clam shell anterior thoracotomy, or bilateral video-assisted thorascopic surgery (VATS).[13,40]
  - Bilateral diffuse bronchiectasis: In bilateral diffuse bronchiectasis, there are multiple or single segments of cystic, severely diseased nonfunctioning lung on a background of cylindrical, perfused, functioning segments. Therefore, in selected cases, limited resection of the most diseased lungs, usually cystic, may help improve symptoms and slow progression of disease. The extent of improvement and persistence of symptomatology after surgery will depend on the type and severity of background residual bronchiectasis in the rest of the lungs. The best would be minimal cylindrical residual bronchiectasis, which is nonprogressive with residual low-grade symptoms that can be controlled effectively by medical therapy.[42–46]

Preoperative Surgical Management

History, general physical examination, and investigations on possible etiology should be elucidated, as this can affect management and prognosis. An underlying cause can be determined in up to 50% to 74% of patients with a change in management in 37% of patients.[10,48] Comorbidities, such as sinusitis and hypogammaglobulinemia, which have negative bearing on surgical outcomes, should be ruled out preoperatively.

Preoperative bronchoscopy is indicated when bronchiectasis is localized to a single lobe where a proximal obstruction, such as a foreign body (especially in children), stricture, or neoplasm, needs to be excluded. For patients in whom serial testing of sputum does not yield microbiological information and who are not responding well to treatment, bronchoscopic sampling of lower respiratory tract secretions may be indicated. Whenever NTM infection is suspected on HRCT, and sputum cultures are negative, bronchoscopic-protected sputum collection may be required.[30]

Preoperative identification of target areas to be resected is crucial to successful surgical outcomes. Ideal targets areas would be localized, completely destroyed, nonfunctioning, nonperfused lung amenable to complete resection. Although recognition of patients with localized unilateral bronchiectasis is relatively straightforward, the selection of patients who may benefit from surgery with bilateral and diffuse disease is more difficult. A combination of information based on HRCT, V/Q scans, and lung function studies is required to identify target areas.[44] HRCT recognition of the various types and distribution of bronchiectasis is crucial to selection of patients for surgery. Target areas suitable for surgery identified by HRCT should be correlated closely with V/Q scans. In bilateral multiple bronchiectasis, V/Q scans may identify nonperfusing and nonfunctioning segments of lung among the various diseased segments that may be amenable to surgical resection. Studies have shown good correlation between anatomic morphology and V/Q scans.[44]

Proper baseline preoperative lung function, together with differential lung perfusion scan, would give a reasonable idea of the postoperative predicted FEV1, which should be at least 40% to 45% of the predicted value. This would allow the surgeon to decide whether complete resection of all diseased segments is possible or only the most diseased segments can be removed.

Active and acute infections should be treated aggressively before surgery with antibiotics, based on sputum cultures. Surgery should be done between exacerbations when the disease is quiescent and the bacterial load is minimal, as this decreases the surgical morbidity, especially of empyema and bronchopleural fistula (BPF). Mucoid sputum has less elastase than purulent sputum and is less injurious to the lung and airway.[7] Although complete bacterial eradication is not possible, aims of antibiotic therapy are to reduce the volume and color of the sputum. Therefore, patients with purulent and copious sputum production, chest physiotherapy, and antibiotics are continued until the sputum volume is decreased to a minimum and the color is mucoid. This may take a minimum of 2 weeks. They are then admitted 48 hours before surgery for intensive chest physiotherapy and postural drainage with vibratory massage. This is continued into the postoperative period. Prophylactic antibiotics are given at induction and continued postoperatively for 48 hours.[37,47] Chronic antibiotic treatment is currently not recommended, except macrolide therapy, which has an anti-inflammatory effect. Patients treated with a long-term low-dose macrolidelike azithromycin showed decrease in exacerbations and sputum volume with improvement in lung function.[49]

Surgical Technique

Anesthetic management
Anesthetic management is crucial for the safe conduct of surgery for bronchiectasis. Bronchoscopic suctioning of secretions in the airway and accurate lung isolation under bronchoscopic guidance is mandatory before commencement of surgery. As surgery for bronchiectasis is fraught by dense chest wall and hilar adhesions as a result of repeated infections, good lung isolation ensures exposure to all parts of the chest, especially the apex and diaphragm, which are the most inaccessible through a thoracotomy. More importantly, it prevents spillage and contamination of secretions from infected lung segments to normal lung caused by manipulation and positioning at time of surgery.[50,51]

In diffuse bilateral bronchiectasis, it is important to prevent accumulation of secretions from the nonoperative diseased lung during surgery, which can cause troublesome oxygen desaturation. This can be prevented by frequent bronchoscopic bronchial toilet by the anesthesiologist. A left-sided double-lumen endotracheal tube is routine, except during a left pneumonectomy when a right-sided tube is used. In children and small adults, in whom the double-lumen endotracheal tube is too big to be used, a bronchial blocker is used.[50]

In bilateral resections, whether staged or same sitting, anesthetic considerations are important in choosing the side to be operated on first. Based on V/Q scan, the least diseased part or the better functioning side should be operated on first to allow for safe single-lung ventilation when operating on the more disease side subsequently. In some cases in which there has been a previous contralateral lobectomy, the patient may not be able to tolerate single-lung ventilation and may need ancillary measures, such as continuous positive airway pressure (5–10 mm Hg) application to the operated lung or selective bronchial blockage of the intermediated bronchus, to allow ventilation of the right upper lobe while surgery is conducted on either the middle or lower lobes.[50]

Approaches

Posterolateral thoracotomy continues to be the standard approach of choice for most bronchiectasis. Anesthetically it is well tolerated and offers good exposure to all parts of the chest and allows for major complications that may arise to be tackled through the same incision. Staged operations can also be done through posterolateral thoracotomy; however, in bilateral cases, the surgery needs to be staged rather than done simultaneously because of the pain and impairment of postoperative lung function. Staged bilateral resections through thoracotomy are usually done after an interval of 6 weeks. Whenever possible, especially in bilateral resections, a muscle-sparing thoracotomy should be done to minimize shoulder and chest wall dysfunction.[32,37,47]

Bilateral anterior thoracotomy and median sternotomy can be used if simultaneous resections are to be done, especially of the middle lobe and lingular segments. Median sternotomy gives excellent exposure to all lobes except the left lower lobe, which may then need a left hemi–clam shell extension to the sternotomy. It is also a good option for completion pneumonectomy after previous lobectomy, as it allows early and safe intrapericardial ligation of the bronchus and vascular structures through relatively unscarred tissue. Lysis of dense posterior chest wall adhesions can be a problem through this incision, however. Bilateral anterior thoracotomy gives exposure to all parts of the lung but causes considerable pain with greater chest wall trauma and impairment of lung capacity. Single-lung ventilation is also less well tolerated in the supine position.[45,50]

Video-assisted thorascopic surgery

With increasing experience of VATS for lung cancer, it is increasingly used for inflammatory conditions like bronchiectasis. Its advantages over thoracotomy are the optics, magnification, and lighting, which give excellent exposure to all parts of the chest cavity. It should be attempted only by experienced VATS surgeons, however, as the surgery is much more demanding than when operating for cancers. In one report, the conversion rate of VATS to thoracotomy was 3.0% to 14.0%, with up to 28.8% of patients having dense adhesions.[45] There were no differences in blood loss and mean operative time over open thoracotomy.[45] Shorter hospital stay, fewer complications, and equally good symptom improvement rates were also reported. It may be ideal for selected single-stage bilateral resections, as it is better tolerated owing to less chest wall injury and better preservation of postoperative lung function.[9] At the present time, VATS should probably be suitable for localized bronchiectasis with minimal scarring and absence of calcified nodes in the proximity of major vessels; however, with ongoing experience its role may expand to more challenging cases.[13,25,33,52]

Management of possible intraoperative technical problems

Dense vascular chest wall and hilar adhesions need to be carefully and meticulously taken down with cautery. Meticulous hemostasis of hypertrophied tortuous bronchial arteries needs to be maintained, which can be a source of major bleeding. Injury to the pulmonary artery can occur owing to fibrosis at the hilum from repeated infections with encasement of the pulmonary artery by calcified nodes. This can be avoided by obtaining proximal control of the main pulmonary artery or by intrapericardial dissection of the structures.

When possible, bronchus should be clamped and divided early to minimize risk of spillage of infection secretions to healthy segments of the same lung. Risk of BPF is minimized by avoiding extensive bronchial dissection to preservation of peribronchial tissues. The bronchial stump should be kept short and should be routinely covered by vascularized tissue to prevent bronchopleural

and bronchovascular fistulas. When pneumonectomy is to be performed in the background of empyema, extrapleural pneumonectomy should be done again to prevent contamination of the postpneumonectomy space.

Types of resections

In more than 80% of patients, the surgery is for unilateral disease, and in fewer than 20%, it is for bilateral disease. Lobectomy was the commonest performed procedure, followed by segmentectomies and pneumonectomies. The incidence for lobectomies varies from 54% to 74%, segmentectomies from 22% to 34%, and pneumonectomies from 3% to 15%.[11,37–39] Pneumonectomies are more common where tuberculosis is prevalent. Less common resections include bilobectomy, lobectomy with segmentectomy, and wedge resections (mainly for lingular segments); 8% to 10% are repeat resections for recurrent progressive disease.[37] Lower lobes were the commonest to be resected (60%–70%), followed by lingular and middle lobes.[11,32–38] Completion pneumonectomy for bronchiectasis constitutes about 6% of patients.[37] Whenever a lower lobectomy is contemplated, the apical segment should be spared if not involved.

Postoperative Management

At the end of the surgery, bronchoscopy is done routinely to check the bronchial suture and for bronchial toilet. Patients in whom bronchoscopy was not performed had a significantly higher rate of postoperative complications, such as atelectasis, pneumonia, and sputum retention.[49] Most can be extubated in the operating room. Postoperative pain control is treated with epidural or patient-controlled analgesia. Antibiotics were administered for 5 days after surgery, or longer if the patient had inflammatory symptoms. Percussive chest physiotherapy was performed 3 to 4 times daily by respiratory therapists. The fluids of some elderly patients, especially those who had undergone pneumonectomy, were restricted to 1500 mL/day, and diuretic therapy was administered to maintain a negative fluid balance. Early ambulation is encouraged.

Mortality and Morbidity

Surgical mortality in the modern era has been low, varying from 0% to 2.2%.[32–34,42–46] Similarly, low mortality has been reported in children and in bilateral diffuse disease.[42–46] Mortality is higher when surgery is performed as an emergency and in the presence of sepsis.[53] There is increased risk for major morbidity and mortality when pneumonectomy is performed for benign conditions of the lung.[54–58] Although completion pneumonectomy for benign conditions is a high-risk procedure, with mortality rates of 20% to 30% and morbidity of greater than 40%,[54–57] Sirmali and colleagues[58] reported 0% mortality and 45% morbidity in completion pneumonectomy for bronchiectasis.

Morbidity is about 18% to 23%,[9,11,32–47,59] with no significant differences in mortality and morbidity between bilateral diffuse and localized disease.[40,42,45,46] Common complications include prolonged air leak, atelectasis, supraventricular arrhythmias, and retention of secretions. Major complications (1%–3%) include reexploration for bleeding, empyema, and BPF.[53]

Postoperative empyema usually responds to intercostal drainage and antibiotic treatment. Prolonged air leak is usually secondary to parenchymal injury from lysis of adhesions and almost always responds to conservative treatment with outpatient Heimlich valve chest tube management. BPF is usually treated with an Eloesser flap in the early postoperative period with subsequent delayed closure with a muscle flap and subsequent window closure. The key to low morbidity is proper selection of patients and timing of surgery, adequate preoperative preparation, meticulous anesthesia and surgical techniques, and good postoperative care.[25,33,53]

Clinical Outcomes and Prognostic Factors

Most series quote overall surgical outcomes in which 45% to 83% were cured or asymptomatic, 22% to 38% had symptom improvement, and 3% to 16% had no improvement or worsening of symptoms. All series conclude that those with complete resections had better outcomes than those with incomplete resections, however.[25,32–34,42–46] Complete resection was defined as an anatomic resection of all affected segments assessed preoperatively by HRCT and V/Q scans. More than 90% of patients had improvement in their symptoms with a higher than 60% cure rate in those who had complete resection, as opposed to 70% symptom improvement and less than 20% cure rate in those with incomplete resections.[37] This also explains the variable improvement outcomes in different series depending on the ability to achieve complete resections.

As complete resections are more possible in localized disease, the surgical outcomes were also more favorable in this group. Complete resection was achievable in 60% to 80% of unilateral disease, as opposed to 4% to 20% in bilateral disease.[25,37] There is 59% to 75% improvement

in symptoms in those with localized disease, as opposed to 35% to 50% in those with diffuse disease.[25,32–34,42–46] Unifocal unilateral disease does better than unilateral multifoci disease, as the former is an earlier form of disease more amenable to complete resections.[33]

In diffuse disease in which complete resection is not possible, preoperative extent of bronchiectasis and degree of residual disease after surgery are important prognostic factors. Although cure rates are lower in this group, there is improvement of disabling symptoms, reductions in hospitalizations and antibiotic usage, and improved quality of life in 75% to 83% of patients.[40,42–46] One study showed that in those with residual disease, there is only 33% improvement in symptoms with up to 50% showing progression of disease and symptoms[46]; however, this depends on the predominant type of residual background bronchiectasis, as patients with cylindrical bronchiectasis do better, as they have fewer symptoms, harbor less-virulent organisms, and tend not to progress. Therefore, in bilateral diffuse disease, those who do best with surgery are those with localized cystic bronchiectasis with minimal residual disease, especially of the cylindrical type.[15,33,44,45]

Other factors that predicted good postoperative surgical outcomes include minor airway obstruction, absence of sinusitis or hypogammaglobulinemia, early age at the time of operation, cylindrical bronchiectasis, and absence of colonization by *Pseudomonas* or *Mycobacterium* organisms.[60] The presence of *Pseudomonas* colonization, sinusitis, or hypogammaglobulinemia, even with complete resection, may lead to development of new bronchiectasis, thus leading to poorer surgical outcomes. Adequate preoperative control of these conditions is mandatory before lung surgery.[13,53]

Management of complications of bronchiectasis that may need surgical intervention are hemoptysis, empyema, and lung abscess.[33] Hemoptysis is a common symptom in bronchiectasis and is more common in cases with dry bronchiectasis.[33,37,47] It originates from collaterals between hypertrophied bronchial arteries and pulmonary vessels or aneurysms of the bronchial artery. It is seen in 50% of cases with bronchiectasis.[61,62] Surgical indications for bronchiectasis with hemoptysis are massive hemoptysis or recurrent episodes of significant hemoptysis. Massive hemoptysis is generally defined as more than 600 mL of blood within 24 hours.[61,62] In all patients with hemoptysis, a rigid or flexible bronchoscopy should be done early to localize the bleeding site, especially if the scans show bilateral disease, as there has been little correlation between severity of disease and site of bleeding.[61] In massive hemoptysis, whenever there is a risk of contralateral spillage of blood, the bleeding bronchus may temporarily be tamponaded with a bronchial blocker at the same sitting until surgery or embolization is done.[63]

Emergency operations in patients who are unstable with bronchiectasis and ongoing life-threatening hemoptyses are associated with high mortality of up to 37%.[61,62] Therefore, bronchial artery angiography and embolization should always be attempted first as a temporizing measure, as it allows the patient to be clinically stabilized before undergoing definitive surgery on a semi-elective basis. Angiography in hypotensive patients may cause low flow or vasospasm, leading to cessation of bleeding in some vessels that may resume bleeding when the patient's hemodynamic status improves. Overall embolization success rates are about 85% to 100%, with recurrences in 10% to 33%, 1 week to 1 month postembolization owing to recanalization of embolized vessels.[63] Therefore, as most patients will have a significant chance of recurrence postembolization, definitive surgery should be offered early if they are fit. Those unfit for pulmonary resection may require multiple courses of embolization.[61–63]

For patients with concomitant lung abscess or empyema, antibiotics and drainage are the main first-line treatments. Surgery should be delayed until sepsis is completely controlled, which usually takes about 6 to 8 weeks. Surgery may be considered early if there is an increase in abscess size or unremitting sepsis despite medical treatment.

SUMMARY

Current goals of surgical therapy for bronchiectasis are to offer possible cure and better quality of life after failed medical treatment and to resolve complications, such as empyema, severe or recurrent hemoptysis, and lung abscess. The best surgical outcomes are obtained with complete resections of localized bronchiectasis. Palliative resections benefit those with localized severely diseased cystic bronchiectasis on a background of mild diffuse bronchiectasis.

SURGERY FOR LUNG ABSCESS
Introduction

The incidence of lung abscess has generally decreased with the advent of effective antibiotic therapy; however, in the modern era, it remains an important cause of mortality in the elderly and immunocompromised patients. This is because of the increased use of immunosuppressive and chemotherapeutic drugs, which has changed the natural flora of the oropharyngeal cavity, giving rise to increased frequency of opportunistic lung abscesses.[64,65] The current mainstay of treatment is still medical therapy, with surgery undertaken only after failed medical therapy.

Pathology

Lung abscess usually begins as a necrotizing pneumonia progressing to liquefactive necrosis of the lung parenchyma. The liquefied necrotic material eventually empties into a draining bronchus, forming a necrotic cavity containing an air-fluid level. With rupture, the infection may extend into the pleural space, producing an empyema.

Abscesses can be acute or chronic (>6 weeks). They can also be primary when they arise in a previously healthy individual or secondary to underlying cause. The commonest cause of primary abscess is aspiration owing to impaired consciousness or neuromuscular or esophageal diseases. Secondary causes include bronchial obstruction, necrotizing pneumonia (S aureus, K pneumoniae), septicemia, and immunocompromised states. Bloodborne infections give rise to multiple lung abscesses in the periphery of the lung and are secondary to septic emboli from bacteremia, endocarditis, septic thrombophlebitis, or subphrenic infection. In children, hematogenous lung abscesses are usually caused by staphylococcal bacteremia from infected skin pustules.[65] As aspiration is the commonest cause, most lung abscesses are polymicrobial with predominance of anaerobic organisms (Peptostreptococcus, Bacteroides fragilis, and Fusobacterium). This explains the predominance of lung abscess to right lung in 60% to 75% of cases, especially in the dependent posterior segment of the right upper lobe and superior segment of the lower lobe owing to gravitation of the infectious material from the oropharynx. They can frequently be recurrent too.[66]

Over the years, however, as the incidence of lung abscess secondary to immunocompromised states has increased, anaerobes now comprise only 31%, with other virulent aerobes, such as Klebsiella (33%), Pseudomonas, Proteus, Enterobacter, and S aureus comprising the rest. Gram-negative lung abscess occurs in elderly and immunocompromised patients with nosocomial pneumonia.[67] Other less common organisms include amebiasis, fungal (Aspergillus, mucormycosis), actinomycosis, and nocardiosis. Seven percent to 17% of patients with squamous cell bronchogenic carcinomas can present with cavitations simulating a lung abscess; however, the wall of the carcinomatous abscess is usually thicker (>11 mm) and more irregular than that of an infective abscess.[64,66–68]

Clinical Features

Symptom presentation can be subacute or chronic depending on the underlying etiology and symptoms are usually present for at least 2 weeks. The clinical features overlap with pneumonia. Common presenting symptoms are usually those of cough, fever, putrid sputum, chest pain, and weight loss. Hemoptyis occurs in 31% of patients. Raised serum inflammatory markers with leukocytosis are often present. Chest radiograph and CT scan of the thorax are usually sufficient to aid diagnosis and differentiate between empyema and abscess. Cavitation is generally apparent on chest radiographs 2 weeks after the onset of symptoms. Radiological resolution lags behind clinical and biochemical improvements. Only 13% resolution of cavitation is seen in 2 weeks and takes 3 months for resolution in up to 70%. Microbiological cultures before commencing antibiotics can be obtained by sputum culture, pleural fluid, or transthoracic aspiration.[64]

Management

First-line treatment is with antibiotics, having both aerobic and anaerobic coverage for a period of 4 to 6 weeks. If there is no clinical improvement with antibiotic therapy by 1 to 2 weeks, then radiologically guided percutaneous lung drainage may be considered in a solitary abscess. Other indications for drainage are progressively enlarging lung abscess in imminent danger of rupture, failure to wean from mechanical ventilation, and contamination of the opposite lung. Although radiological guidance can be accomplished by ultrasound or fluoroscopy, most are drained under CT guidance, as this give the highest accuracy in 79% to 94% of cases. In addition to drainage, it also allows for microbiological sampling of the aspirated pus, which allows for more accurate antimicrobial therapy. In up to 47% of patients, initial antibiotics may have to be changed because of antimicrobial sensitivity of pus obtained after percutaneous aspiration. A common complication of this procedure is pneumothorax, which occurs in 15% of patients.[69]

Bronchoscopy can also facilitate abscess drainage by aspiration of the appropriate bronchus through the bronchoscope; however, there are reports of therapeutic bronchoscopy-induced spillage of purulent material from the involved lung segment into other parts of the lung. Recently, lasers have been used for endobronchial drainage of lung abscess by artificially perforating

the wall though the airways to provide a route for catheter drainage.[70]

Antibiotics given over 4 to 6 weeks with percutaneous drainage is effective in 85% to 95% of patients.[64] Surgery is indicated when there is failure of clinical or radiological improvement after 4 to 6 weeks of antibiotic therapy, usually with abscesses larger than 6 cm, life-threatening hemoptysis (4%), persisting sepsis after 2 weeks in spite of antibiotics and percutaneous drainage, suspicion of malignancy, and for complications like BPF and empyema (4%). In addition, if after 4 to 6 weeks of medical treatment a notable residual cavity remains and the patient is symptomatic, surgical resection is advocated.[64]

The surgical and anesthetic management for surgery for lung abscess is similar to bronchiectasis. Owing to the high risk of spillage of the abscess into the contralateral lung, a double-lumen tube is mandatory to protect the airway, with rapid clamping of the bronchus to prevent spillage into the trachea.[50,51] Routine buttressing of the bronchial stump with vascularized tissue is routine to prevent BPF. Although thoracotomy is the approach of choice, recently VATS has been successfully used in the treatment of lung abscesses in children. A study by Nagasawa and Johnson[71] has shown that thoracoscopic surgery can lead to effective drainage of pediatric lung abscess without major complications. In addition, other benefits of thoracoscopy include rapid recovery, less pain, and minimal morbidity. Lobectomy is the commonest procedure performed for lung abscess and is done with low mortality (0%–2%) and morbidity.[72]

Mortality for lung abscess has decreased from 30% to 40% in the preantibiotic era to 10% in the present era.[72] Mortality is highest in elderly individuals, immunocompromised patients, abscesses larger than 6 cm, bronchial obstruction, multiple abscesses, necrotizing pneumonia, and gram-negative pneumonia. The prognosis associated with amebic lung abscess is good when treatment is prompt. Fungal abscesses are difficult to treat; antifungal and surgical drainage remain the only modalities of treatment, often with only limited success.[72]

SUMMARY

Most lung abscesses can be successfully treated medically, provided the diagnosis and treatment are prompt.

REFERENCES

1. Weycker D, Edelsberg J, Oster G, et al. Prevalence and economic burden of bronchiectasis. Clin Pulm Med 2005;4:205–9.

2. O'Brien C, Guest PJ, Hill SL, et al. Physiological and radiological characterisation of patients diagnosed with chronic obstructive pulmonary disease in primary care. Thorax 2000;55:635–42.

3. Patel IS, Vlahos I, Wilkinson TM, et al. Bronchiectasis, exacerbation indices, and inflammation in chronic obstructive pulmonary disease. Am J Respir Crit Care Med 2004;170:400–7.

4. Cole PJ. Inflammation: a two-edged sword—the model of bronchiectasis. Eur J Respir Dis Suppl 1986;147:6–15.

5. Whitwell F. A study of the pathology and pathogenesis of bronchiectasis. Thorax 1952;7:213–9.

6. King PT, Holdsworth SR, Freezer NJ, et al. Characterisation of the onset and presenting clinical features of adult bronchiectasis. Respir Med 2006; 100:2183–9.

7. Tsang KW, Chan K, Ho P, et al. Sputum elastase in steady-state bronchiectasis. Chest 2000;117(2):420–6.

8. Roberts HR, Wells AU, Milne DG, et al. Airflow obstruction in bronchiectasis: correlation between computed tomography features and pulmonary function tests. Thorax 2000;55:198–204.

9. Ashour M, Al-Kattan KM, Jain SK, et al. Surgery for unilateral bronchiectasis: results and prognostic factors. Tuber Lung Dis 1996;77:168–72.

10. Shoemark A, Ozerovitch L, Wilson R. Aetiology in adult patients with bronchiectasis. Respir Med 2007;101:1163–70.

11. Kutlay H, Cangir AK, Enon S, et al. Surgical treatment in bronchiectasis: analysis of 166 patients. Eur J Cardiothorac Surg 2002;21:634–7.

12. Kwon KY, Myers JL, Swensen SJ, et al. Middle lobe syndrome: a clinicopathological study of 21 patients. Hum Pathol 1995;26:302–7.

13. Yu JA, Pomerantz M, Bishop A. Lady windermere syndrome revisited. Treatment with thoracoscopic lobectomy/segmentectomy for right middle and lingular bronchiectasis associated with non tuberculous mycobacterial disease. Eur J Cardiothorac Surg 2011;40:671–5.

14. Reid L. Reduction in bronchial subdivisions in bronchiectasis. Thorax 1950;5:223–47.

15. Ashour M. Hemodynamic alterations in bronchiectasis. A basis for a new subclassification of the disease. J Thorac Cardiovasc Surg 1996;112:328–34.

16. Cobanoglu U, Yalcinkaya I, Er M, et al. Surgery for bronchiectasis: the effect of morphological types to prognosis. Ann Thorac Med 2011;6:25–32.

17. Ashour M, Al-Kattan K, Rafay MA, et al. Current surgical therapy for bronchiectasis. World J Surg 1999;23:1096–104.

18. Martinez-Garcia MA, Soler-Cataluna JJ, Perpina-Tordera M, et al. Factors associated with lung function decline in adult patients with stable non-cystic fibrosis bronchiectasis. Chest 2007;132:1565–72.

19. King PT, Holdsworth SR, Freezer NJ, et al. Outcome in adult bronchiectasis. COPD 2005;2:27–34.

20. Alzeer AH, Al-Mobeirek AF, Al-Otair HA, et al. Right and left ventricular function and pulmonary artery pressure in patients with bronchiectasis. Chest 2008;133:468–73.

21. King PT, Holdsworth SR, Freezer NJ, et al. Microbiologic follow-up study in adult bronchiectasis. Respir Med 2007;101:1633–8.

22. Nicotra MB, Rivera M, Dale AM, et al. Clinical, pathophysiologic, and microbiologic characterization of bronchiectasis in an aging cohort. Chest 1995;108: 955–61.

23. Davies JC, Bilton D. Bugs, biofilms, and resistance in cystic fibrosis. Respir Care 2009;54:628–40.

24. Wickremasinghe M, Ozerovitch LJ, Davies G, et al. Non-tuberculous mycobacteria in patients with bronchiectasis. Thorax 2005;60:1045–51.

25. Hiramatsu M, Shiraishi Y, Nakajima Y. Risk factors that affect the surgical outcome in the management of focal bronchiectasis in a developed country. Ann Thorac Surg 2012;93:245–50.

26. Young K, Aspestrand F, Kolbenstvedt A. High resolution CT and bronchography in the assessment of bronchiectasis. Acta Radiol 1991;32:439–41.

27. Hansell DM. Bronchiectasis. Radiol Clin North Am 1998;36:107–28.

28. Lynch DA, Newell J, Hale V, et al. Correlation of CT findings with clinical evaluations in 261 patients with symptomatic bronchiectasis. AJR Am J Roentgenol 1999;173:53–8.

29. Javidan-Nejad C, Bhalla S. Bronchiectasis. Radiol Clin North Am 2009;47:289–306.

30. British Thoracic Society guideline for non-cystic fibrosis bronchiectasis. Thorax 2010;65:11–158.

31. Montella S, Santamaria F, Salvatore M, et al. Assessment of MRI in children and young adults with non cystic fibrosis bronchiectasis. Invest Radiol 2009; 44:532–8.

32. Prieto D, Bernardo J, Matos MJ, et al. Surgery for bronchiectasis. Eur J Cardiothorac Surg 2001;20:19–24.

33. Ricardo Giovannetti R, Alifano M, Stefani A, et al. Surgical treatment of bronchiectasis: early and long-term results. Interact Cardiovasc Thorac Surg 2008;7:609–12.

34. Etiene T, Spiliopoulos A, Megevand R. Bronchiectasis: indication and timing for surgery. Ann Chir 1993;47:729–35.

35. Oschner A, DeBakey M, DeCamp PT. Bronchiectasis: its curative treatment by pulmonary resection. Surgery 1949;25:518–32.

36. Vejlsted H, Hjelms E, Jacobsen O. Results of pulmonary resection in cases of unilateral bronchiectasis. Scand J Thorac Cardiovasc Surg 1982;16:81–5.

37. Agasthian T, Deschamps C, Trastek VF, et al. Surgical management of bronchiectasis. Ann Thorac Surg 1996;62:976–80.

38. Balkanli K, Genç O, Dakak M, et al. Surgical management of bronchiectasis: analysis and

short-term results in 238 patients. Eur J Cardiothorac Surg 2003;24(5):699–702.

39. Zhang P, Jiang G, Ding J, et al. Surgical treatment of bronchiectasis: a retrospective analysis of 790 patients. Ann Thorac Surg 2010;90:246–50.

40. George SA, Leonardo HK, Overholt RH. Bilateral pulmonary resections for bronchiectasis: a 40 year experience. Ann Thorac Surg 1979;28:48–53.

41. Beirne PA, Banner NR, Khaghani A, et al. Lung transplantation for non-cystic fibrosis bronchiectasis: analysis of a 13-year experience. J Heart Lung Transplant 2005;24:1530–5.

42. Mazières J, Murris M, Didier A, et al. Limited operation for severe multisegmental bilateral bronchiectasis. Ann Thorac Surg 2003;75:382–7.

43. Schneiter D, Meyer N, Lardinois D, et al. Surgery for non-localized bronchiectasis. Br J Surg 2005;92:836–9.

44. Al-Kattan KM, Essa MA, Hajjar WM, et al. Surgical results for bronchiectasis based on hemodynamic (functional and morphologic) classification. J Thorac Cardiovasc Surg 2005;130(5):1385–90.

45. Aghajanzadeh M, Sarshad A, Amani H, et al. Surgical management of bilateral bronchiectases: results in 29 patients. Asian Cardiovasc Thorac Ann 2006;14:219–22.

46. Stephen T, Thankachen R, Madhu AP, et al. Surgical results in bronchiectasis: analysis of 149 patients. Asian Cardiovasc Thorac Ann 2007;15:290–29 6.

47. Fujimoto T, Hillejan L, Stamatis G. Current strategy for surgical management of bronchiectasis. Ann Thorac Surg 2001;72:1711–5.

48. Drain M, Elbond JS. Assessment and investigation of adults with bronchiectasis. Eur Respir Monogr 2011;52:32–43.

49. Anwar GA, Bourke SC, Afolabi G, et al. Effects of long-term low-dose azithromycin in patients with non-CF bronchiectasis. Respir Med 2008;102:1494–6.

50. Benumof JL, Alfery DD. Anesthesia for thoracic surgery. In: Miller RD, editor. Anesthesia. 5th edition. Philadelphia: Churchill Livingstone; 2000. p. 1665–75.

51. Cheong KF, Koh KF. Placement of left-sided double-lumen endobronchial tubes: comparison of clinical and fibreoptic-guided placement. Br J Anaesth 1999;82:920.

52. Zhang P, Zhang F, Jiang S, et al. Video-assisted thoracic surgery for bronchiectasis. Ann Thorac Surg 2011;91:239–43.

53. Eren S, Esme H, Avci A. Risk factors affecting outcome and morbidity in the surgical management of bronchiectasis. J Thorac Cardiovasc Surg 2007;134(2):392–8.

54. Miller DL, Deschamps C, Jenkins GD, et al. Completion pneumonectomy: factors affecting operative mortality and cardiopulmonary morbidity. Ann Thorac Surg 2002;74(3):876–84.

55. Jungraithmayr W, Hasse J, Olschewski M, et al. Indications and results of completion pneumonectomy. Eur J Cardiothorac Surg 2004;26(1):189–96.

56. Chataigner E, Fadel B, Yildizeli A, et al. Factors affecting early and long-term outcomes after completion pneumonectomy. Eur J Cardiothorac Surg 2008;33(5):837–43.

57. Shapiro M, Swanson SJ, Wright CD, et al. Predictors of major morbidity and mortality after pneumonectomy utilizing the Society For Thoracic Surgeons general thoracic surgery database. Ann Thorac Surg 2010;90(3):927–35.

58. Sirmali M, Karasu S, Gezer S, et al. Completion pneumonectomy for bronchiectasis: mortality, morbidity and management. Thorac Cardiovasc Surg 2008;56(4):221–5.

59. Haciibrahimoglu G, Fazlioglu M, Olcmen A, et al. Surgical management of childhood bronchiectasis due to infectious disease. J Thorac Cardiovasc Surg 2004;127:1361–5.

60. Ripe E. Bronchiectasis: a followup study after surgical treatment. Scand J Respir Dis 1971;52:96–101.

61. Garzon A, Gourin A. Surgical management of massive hemoptysis: a 10-year experience. Ann Surg 1978;187:267–71.

62. Lim YP, Wong D, Agasthian T. Management of life threatening hemoptysis. Asian Cardiovasc Thorac Ann 2001;9:2000–203.

63. Mal H, Rullon I, Mellot F, et al. Immediate and long-term results of bronchial artery embolization for life-threatening hemoptysis. Chest 1999;115:996–1001.

64. Davis B, Systrom DM. Lung abscess: pathogenesis, diagnosis and treatment. Curr Clin Top Infect Dis 1998;18:252–73.

65. Magalhaes L, Valadares D, Oliveira JR, et al. Lung abscesses: review of 60 cases. Rev Port Pneumol 2009;15(2):165–78.

66. Shinzato T. [Effects and management of odontogenic infections on pulmonary infections]. Yakugaku Zasshi 2009;129(12):1461–4 [in Japanese].

67. Bartlett JG, Gorbach SL, Tally FP, et al. Bacteriology and treatment of primary lung abscess. Am Rev Respir Dis 1974;109(5):510–8.

68. Adebonojo SA, Grillo IA, Osinowo O, et al. Suppurative diseases of the lung and pleura: a continuing challenge in developing countries. Ann Thorac Surg 1982;33(1):40–7.

69. VanSonnenberg E, D'Agostino HB, Casola G, et al. Lung abscess: CT-guided drainage. Radiology 1991;178(2):347–51.

70. Shlomi D, Kramer MR, Fuks L, et al. Endobronchial drainage of lung abscess: the use of laser. Scand J Infect Dis 2010;42(1):65–8.

71. Nagasawa KK, Johnson SM. Thoracoscopic treatment of pediatric lung abscesses. J Pediatr Surg 2010;45(3):574–8.

72. Hirshberg B, Sklair-Levi M, Nir-Paz R, et al. Factors predicting mortality of patients with lung abscess. Chest 1999;115:746–9.

Pulmonary Aspergilloma
Clinical Aspects and Surgical Treatment Outcome

Eliseo Passera, MD[a],*, Adriano Rizzi, MD[a],
Mario Robustellini, MD[b], Gerolamo Rossi, MD[c],
Claudio Della Pona, MD[b], Fabio Massera, MD[d],
Gaetano Rocco, MD, FRCSEd[e]

KEYWORDS

- Aspergilloma • Pulmonary mycetoma • Tuberculosis • Hemoptysis • Fungal infections
- Thoracic surgery

KEY POINTS

- Neither the size of aspergilloma nor associated clinical features predict the development of life-threatening hemoptysis; therefore, an aggressive approach toward patients with pulmonary mycetomas is justified independently of the symptoms.
- Early surgical resection of pulmonary aspergilloma in all patients with good lung function is the best therapeutic option and offers clear benefits: the aspergilloma is removed; hemoptysis is controlled; clinical symptoms are attenuated; quality of life is improved; life is prolonged.
- Complex mycetoma is usually related to patients whose general condition is poor with heavily compromised lungs; a conservative surgical approach (cavernostomy) is preferable in these cases. Other conservative treatments should be considered.
- Postoperative empyema is a catastrophic event; to minimize this risk, extrapleural dissection is recommended, and additional procedures to reinforce bronchial stump and to obliterate pleural space are advocated.
- For the best outcome, avoid operating as an emergency (massive hemoptysis); stabilize respiratory and hemodynamic conditions first.

INTRODUCTION: THE NATURE OF THE PROBLEM

Between 1932 and 1940 in the Alps of northern Italy, at 1200 m above sea level, a 3000-bed hospital was built on the pioneering pattern of Davos, the sanatorium in Thomas Mann's famous novel "The Magic Mountain." Eugenio Morelli Hospital was considered the biggest sanatorium in Europe, with 9 wings for each of its 10 floors and covering an area of 350,000 m², on a road network of 12.5 km and occupying a volume of 650,000 m³ (**Fig. 1**).[1]

When tuberculosis no longer presented a major public health threat, Eugenio Morelli Hospital became a regional hospital. However, because

The authors have nothing to disclose.

[a] Division of Thoracic Surgery, Humanitas Gavazzeni Hospital, via Gavazzeni, 21, 24123 Bergamo, Italy; [b] Division of Thoracic Surgery, E. Morelli Hospital, via Zubiani, 33, 23039 Sondalo, Italy; [c] Division of Thoracic Surgery, Valduce Hospital, via Alighieri, 11, 22100 Como, Italy; [d] Division of Thoracic Surgery, Maggiore della Carità Hospital, Corso Mazzini, 18, 28100 Novara, Italy; [e] Division of Thoracic Surgery, Department of Thoracic Surgery and Oncology, National Cancer Institute, Pascale Foundation, Via Semmola 81, 80131 Naples, Italy
* Corresponding author.
E-mail address: eliseo.passera@gavazzeni.it

Thorac Surg Clin 22 (2012) 345–361
doi:10.1016/j.thorsurg.2012.04.001
1547-4127/12/$ – see front matter © 2012 Elsevier Inc. All rights reserved.

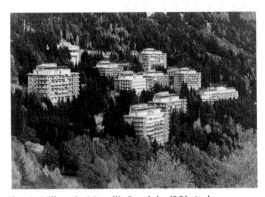

Fig. 1. Villaggio Morelli, Sondalo (SO), Italy.

Box 1
Clinical conditions related to mycetoma

1. Former tuberculosis (tuberculosis cavity)
2. Advanced sarcoidosis
3. Pneumoconioses
4. Bullous emphysema
5. Acute or chronic infections
6. Bronchiectasis
7. Lung abscess
8. Malignant lesions (lung cancer, hematologic disease)
9. Pulmonary infarcts
10. Postradiation pulmonary cavity
11. Radiofrequency ablation
12. Ankylosing spondylitis
13. Congenital cyst

of its background as a sanatorium, the hospital has retained a mission to cure infective diseases.

Sondalo, where Eugenio Morelli Hospital is located, is like Davos; 2 places that share the wonderful landscape of the Alps, the clearness arising from the intense green belt all around, the daylight springing over the terraced meadows and the shining sunlight gathered as if in a bright amphitheatre.

The authors of this article all worked together for at least a decade as staff surgeons at the Division of Thoracic Surgery (Chair, Dr A. Rizzi) of the Morelli Hospital in Sondalo (Valtellina), Italy. For these reasons and because of the specific referral pattern for infectious patients originating from all over Italy and North Africa, lung mycotic infections have frequently been managed at the Morelli Hospital.

"La meraviglia, quasi straniante, coglie chiunque affronti il Villaggio Morelli e lascia perdutamente incantati" ("the wonder, alienating almost anyone, captures whoever takes leave to address the Villaggio Morelli and remains spellbound").[1]

Definition

A pulmonary mycetoma is a mycotic colonized preexisting cavity or cyst (fungus ball) of the lung. Cavities and cysts are partly filled by growing mycelia and septate hyphae.[2] Other than open-state negative and positive cavities in granulomatous infections, in advanced sarcoidosis, and in histoplasmosis, bullae and bronchiectasis may be the site of fungal colonization (**Box 1**). The imaging findings in the lungs adjacent to or remote from the mycetoma may be influenced by the underlying disease. Despite a usually solitary aspect, multiple and bilateral lesions can be observed. Upper lobes and apical segments of lower lobes represent the predominant sites. In contrast, patients with impaired immunity and normal lung structure can have mycetomas in any part of the lung.

Apart from *Mucor* or yeast fungi, such as *Candida* species, which are rarely described as causal agents of mycetoma, species of the genus *Aspergillus* (ie, *Aspergillus fumigatus* and *Aspergillus niger*) are the most common colonizing fungi.[3] Among the sites of *Aspergillus* infection, the lung is the most common organ of involvement.[3]

Epidemiology

Pulmonary aspergillosis is reported with increasing frequency, and pulmonary aspergilloma is the best recognized form of the clinical syndromes caused by *Aspergillus*. Until the 1980s, the most common preexisting condition was tuberculosis. The Research Committee of the British Tuberculosis Association[4] found that patients with an open negative posttubercular cavity had a higher risk of mycotic colonization. Up to 17% of patients had radiologic evidence of mycetoma. The interval between the diagnosis of pulmonary tuberculosis and development of mycetoma varied from 1 to 30 years. The introduction of antituberculous agents and the extensive use of antifungal agents[5] have reduced the incidence of mycetoma. However, 2 groups of patients are still at risk of developing saprophytic mycotic infection:

1. Patients with impaired immunity:
   a. Congenital: immune deficiency syndromes
   b. Acquired: transplant recipients on immunosuppressive therapy, patients with cancer receiving chemotherapy (invasive pulmonary aspergillosis occurs in up to 20% of patients who undergo treatment of

acute leukemia)[6] or radiotherapy, prolonged corticosteroid use for any reason, chronic diabetes, severely debilitated patients in the intensive care unit (long intubation, long-lasting courses of broad-spectrum antibiotic coverage)
2. Patients with chronically diseased or destroyed lungs: these patients have impaired local bronchopulmonary defense mechanisms

Classification

Other than allergic bronchopulmonary aspergillosis (ABPA) and invasive pulmonary aspergillosis (chronic necrotizing pulmonary aspergillosis [CNPA]), Hinson and colleagues[7] defined aspergilloma as the saprophytic infection of preexisting lung cavities. The variability of circumstances surrounding host encounters with *Aspergillus* results in a spectrum of aspergillus disease that ranges from allergic to infectious in nature (**Box 2**).[8,9]

Furthermore, clinical crossover between infectious and hypersensitivity aspergillus syndrome often occurs and clinical overlap among these syndromes can arise (**Fig. 2**).

Belcher and Plummer[10] classified pulmonary mycetoma into:

Box 2
Respiratory diseases related to *Aspergillus*

- Hypersensitivity:
  - Obstructive bronchopulmonary aspergillosis
    - Extrinsic asthma
    - Extrinsic allergic alveolitis
    - ABPA
- Invasive aspergillosis:
  - Acute (generalized) (IPA)
  - CNPA (localized)
- Noninvasive infection (saprophytic colonization):
  - Aspergilloma (mycetoma):
    - Endobronchial
    - Pleural
    - Pulmonary
  - Mucoid impaction of the airways
  - Tracheobronchitis
  - Ulcerative bronchitis
  - Pseudomembranous tracheobronchitis

- Simple mycetoma: neoformed cavitation of limited volume with thin walls in a normal lung or minimal associated pleuroparenchymal sequelae
- Complex mycetoma: preexisting cavitation with thick walls in an impaired lung, often connected to the thoracic wall through thick and extremely vascularized adhesions

Relevant Anatomy/Pathophysiology

The natural history of mycotic infection is not well documented. Few long-term follow-up reports have been published, and, in many of the reports, it is difficult to distinguish between the course of the underlying disease and the aspergilloma.[11] Furthermore, a possible sharing of the different pathologic features related to *Aspergillus* infection has been described (see **Fig. 2**).[8,9] Dobbertin and colleagues[12] found that CNPA and ABPA are sometimes associated with endobronchial aspergillosis. However, up to 60% of pulmonary aspergillomas grow in poorly drained and avascular posttuberculous cavities shaping independent necrotic masses of matted hyphae, inflammatory cells, fibrin, and blood (so-called fungus ball) (**Fig. 3**). In chronically diseased lungs, old bronchiectasis can give rise to mycetomas. There is usually thickening of the pleura adjacent to the cavity. In contrast, in immunocompromised patients, the *Aspergillus* is able to hollow out the lung affected by consolidation (ie, radiation pneumonitis). Furthermore, mycotic infection may extend into the residual pleural space after lung resection, or after collapse therapy as a consequence of bronchopleural fistulas. Direct manifestation of invasive aspergillosis has also been described.[13]

Clinical Presentation

The clinical picture of aspergilloma ranges from patients who are asymptomatic with an incidental radiologic finding to life-threatening hemoptysis. The size of aspergilloma is variable and is not usually related to the severity of hemoptysis.[14] Mycetomas remain one of the common causes of massive hemoptysis (together with tuberculosis and lung abscess) in both developed and undeveloped countries. Weight loss, chronic cough, and malaise may occur. Fever is rare (**Box 3**). Aspergilloma may become stable or may grow, causing pneumonia, pulmonary fibrosis and disseminated infections (ie, invasive aspergillosis) in addition to the obvious symptom of hemoptysis.

In reported series,[15,16] the incidence of hemoptysis in patients with aspergilloma has ranged from 54% to 87.5% and could be massive in

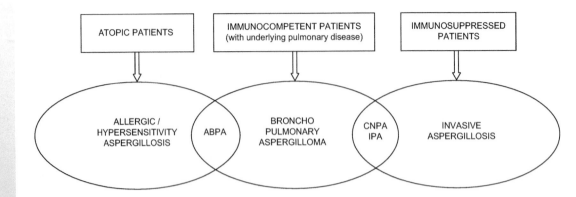

ABPA: ALLERGIC BRONCHOPULMONARY ASPERGILLOSIS
CNPA: CHRONIC NECROTIZING PULMONARY ASPERGILLOSIS
IPA: INVASIVE PULMONARY ASPERGILLOSIS

Fig. 2. Patients with mycetoma (noninvasive infection) may develop a bronchopulmonary aspergillosis compo-nent (hypersensitivity) to their disease. Rapidly invasive pneumonia may suddenly arrest and manifest as a myce-toma. A chronic mycetoma may suddenly break down and become a rapidly invasive pulmonary infection.

up to 10%.[17] Bleeding classically occurs from the erosion of bronchial arteries and usually stops spontaneously. Several mechanisms for the he-moptysis have been proposed, included erosion of the vascular cyst wall by friction from the fungus ball, elaboration of endotoxin by the fungus, and the patient's underlying disease.

Neither the size, the complexity of the lesion, the presence of a warning minor hemoptysis, nor the type of underlying disease can predict those patients who will progress to life-threatening hemoptysis.[14] Hemoptysis can turn into a fatal hemorrhage in up to 30% of patients with pulmo-nary mycetoma.[18] Systemic antifungal agents, which have been shown to be effective in superfi-cial infections and in some systemic fungal infec-tions, have shown no consistent success in alleviating symptoms or treating the disease process.[17]

Bronchial aspergilloma occurs frequently as a pseudotumor and is usually characterized by few, if any, symptoms. Patients with pleural asper-gilloma are usually debilitated, if not in obvious cachexia.

Diagnosis of Aspergilloma

Preoperative diagnosis should be attempted to plan the correct surgical treatment; the pulmo-nary involvement of *Aspergillus*, the distinction between simple and complex aspergilloma, and the evaluation of the underlying pulmonary diseases are essential features that may guide surgeons to predict the potential for postoperative complications.

Excluding cavitating hematoma, lung cancer, metastatic lesions, lung abscess, and hydatid cyst,[19] an aspergilloma should be suspected in patients with chronic lung disease showing an in-cavity mass lesion on radiology. The diagnosis of aspergilloma is made incidentally on a routine chest roentgenogram or during evaluation of hemoptysis. A chest radiograph is usually suffi-cient to suspect a pulmonary aspergilloma through the classic picture of an in-cavity, moveable, and homogeneous mass surrounded by a halo or a crescent of air (**Fig. 4**).

Computed tomography (CT) (**Fig. 5**) is able to confirm the morphologic diagnosis and define the size of the mycetoma, the internal structure of cavitation with the growing ball, the cavity wall thickness and make up, the details of the sur-rounding parenchyma and pleura, and the relation-ship with close vessels (pulmonary and bronchial arteries, neovascularization both in the paren-chyma near the lesion and in the parietal pleura with an intricate network of vessels). In the case of tuberculosis as the underlying disease of myce-toma, CT offers (unlike chest radiography) a clear image of contrast-enhanced pulmonary arteries in the wall of a pulmonary cavity with possible evidence of Rasmussen pseudoaneurysm.[20] In the early stages of aspergilloma, CT scan may show subtle cavitation within known nodules and irregular spongelike networks filling the cavity (**Box 4**).[21]

Before the introduction of CT, Metras or Thomp-son catheters were used to fill segmental bronchi for selective bronchography (**Fig. 6**); these tech-niques are now obsolete.

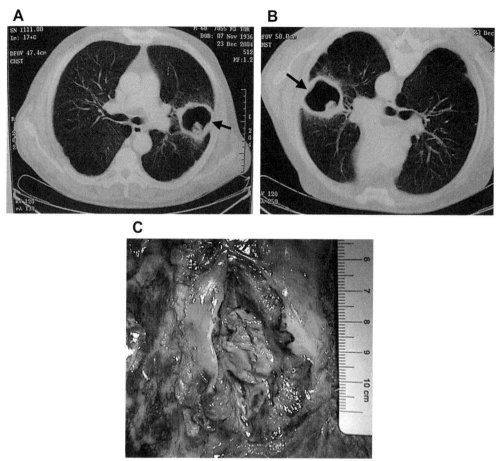

Fig. 3. Aspergilloma: demonstration of mobility of fungus ball on axial computed tomography (CT). (*A*) Supine image from axial CT reveals a left upper lobe cavity with a fungus ball (*arrow*) with healthy lung tissue (patient with chronic obstructive pulmonary disease). (*B*) Prone image (same level) shows that the internal opacity is mobile (*arrow*), characteristic of mycetoma. (*C*) Gross surgical specimen (same patient) shows a cavity with necrotic internal debris (fungus ball).

Diagnosis currently relies on cultivation of *Aspergillus* species from respiratory tract secretions (isolated sputum culture is negative in 50% of cases) or visualization of hyphae in biopsied tissue (transbronchial biopsies through a fiberoptic bronchoscopy or CT-guided percutaneous transthoracic lung biopsies).

To improve the relative insensitivity of bronchoalveolar lavage fluid culture (40%–50%), serum precipitating *Aspergillus* antibodies, bronchial galactomannan enzyme immunoassay, and quantitative polymerase chain reaction assay add sensitivity to the procedure (94%–98%).[22]

Box 3
Symptoms in aspergilloma

1. Hemoptysis
2. Pneumothorax
3. Cough
4. Fever
5. Weight loss
6. Sputum
7. Chest pain
8. Dyspnea
9. Asymptomatic

THERAPEUTIC OPTIONS AND SURGICAL TECHNIQUES

In contrast with other mycotic and aspergillus diseases (apart from selected patients with an invasive aspergillosis who could undergo surgical resection),[23] pulmonary aspergilloma is a condition to be evaluated surgically (**Fig. 7**).

Although there is controversy concerning the optimal management of aspergilloma,[14,24]

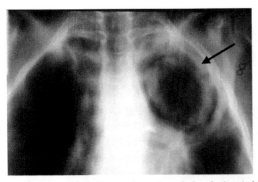

Fig. 4. Linear tomogram (stratigraphy) of the left upper lobe reveals a mass of soft tissue opacity (*arrow*) with an air-crescent sign.

nonoperative treatment has a limited role.[25] The efficacy of medical therapy varies considerably from case to case and does not affect the size of the fungus ball, the entity of hemoptysis, and the patient's death.[26] The risk of evolving complications argues for an invasive approach: after hemoptysis, observed 5-year survival is 84% for operated patients and 41% for nonoperated patients.[14] Rafferty and colleagues[19] observed the development of invasive aspergillosis in 20% of non–surgically treated mycetoma. Accordingly, Babatasi and colleagues,[15] in a 39-year series of 80 patients, concluded that pulmonary resection was the best option whenever the diagnosis of mycetoma has been confirmed and the patient is a suitable candidate for operation. Furthermore, Massard and colleagues[25] advocated the prophylactic resection of all pulmonary aspergillomas because of the risk of massive hemoptysis (operation on an elective basis). However, a careful evaluation of the cost/benefit ratio must be made when a surgical option is contemplated because of the high incidence of postoperative complications.[27] Accordingly, Daly and colleagues[28] preferred surgical treatment after hemoptysis alone. Bronchial artery embolization has been largely unsuccessful because of the usual complexity of the neovascularization (**Fig. 8**) and the difficulty in identifying the bleeding artery.

Surgical Techniques

The size of aspergilloma and the underlying pulmonary disease should be considered in planning the surgical procedure. The main goal is to resect the mycotic cavity including in-going pulmonary vessels. At the same time, because most patients have decreased pulmonary reserve, the parenchymal resection should be limited as much as possible to avoid impairing lung function. Moreover, preoperative planning should be

attempted to differentiate simple from complex mycetoma and to qualify performance status.

In pulmonary mycetoma, the standard surgical approach includes anatomic pulmonary resections such as segmentectomies or lobectomies; conversely, wedge parenchymal resections should be reserved for small, simple mycetomas,[25] and pneumonectomies for overlapping destroyed lung[29] (**Fig. 9**).

Despite its benign nature, pulmonary mycetoma has to be treated according to the same rigorous surgical rules that every surgeon should follow against a neoplasia. Consequently, manipulation of mycetoma should be reduced to a minimum to limit the risk of spreading the fungus; a radical resection can be improved by an extrapleural dissection; an anatomic resection is usually necessary to obtain a complete resection both under an anatomic and biologic profile; accurate hemostasis and evaluation of the pleural space and air leaks should be highly favored to limit the recurrence of infection.

Pneumonectomy for aspergilloma

Pneumonectomy could be a result of widespread-disease (megamycetoma, multiple unilateral aspergillomas), surrounding destroyed lung tissue, an intraoperative incident (eg, injury of the pulmonary artery), or a second-stage completion pneumonectomy (ie, lobar torsion). It is the type of operation that should be avoided[30] as far as possible: first, most patients (with complex mycetoma) do not have an adequate performance status; second, pneumonectomy regularly leads to major complications, including death. Furthermore, mycetoma is a benign disease, so the risk of early postoperative death should be avoided.

Cavernostomy/cavernoplasty

Introduced by Monaldi[31] in 1938 in the treatment of tuberculous cavities,[20] open cavernostomy allows removal of the fungus ball, packing of the cavern with gauze containing antiseptic solutions or antifungal substances,[20,32] and, after few months, obliteration of the cavern with an intrathoracic transposition of extrathoracic muscle (cavernoplasty)[20] or with a tailoring thoracoplasty.[33] Cesar and colleagues[32] recently reported a large study comparing patients undergoing cavernostomy with those undergoing lung resection. However, the global results were worse in the cavernostomy group; because the cavity is not removed, relapse of *Aspergillus* infection is likely as long as the cavitation persists.

Thoracoplasty

Thoracoplasty consists of a reduction of the thoracic cavity by removing the ribs, as described

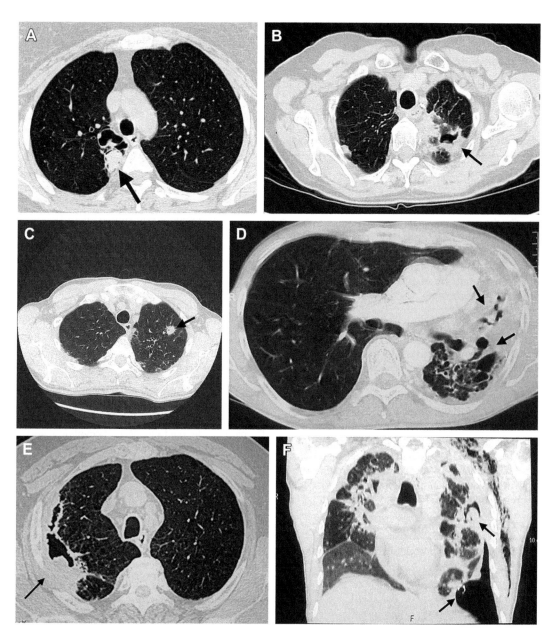

Fig. 5. Different modalities of aspergilloma presentation on CT scan. (*A*) Simple mycetoma (*arrow*) presenting a double cavitation in the right upper lobe (dorsal segment) with normal lung tissue. (*B*) Complex mycetoma: multiple cavities with a large irregular aspergilloma (*arrow*) and extensive pulmonary destruction and pleural thickening (tuberculosis sequelae). (*C*) Aspergilloma presenting as a solid nodule (*arrow*) in the left upper lobe and simulating lung cancer. (*D*) Aspergilloma (*arrow*) complicating bronchiectasis of the left lower lobe. (*E*) Pleuropulmonary aspergilloma (*arrow*) of the right upper lobe confined to the parietal pleura. (*F*) Aspergilloma (*arrow*) and aspergillus empyema with a chest drain (*arrow*) in the left pleural cavity.

by Alexander[34]; it can be limited or extended and should be offered to selected patients to obliterate the residual pleural space or pulmonary cavity (cavernostomy). Some investigators recommend immediate thoracoplasty,[35] but this mutilating procedure should be avoided at the first stage. In the specific case of cavernostomy, infection control and sealing of bronchiolar fistulas are mandatory requirements to close a cavity with a thoracoplasty. For pleural aspergillomas, the patient should be treated as for chronic empyema, and therefore a first-stage thoracoplasty or, as an alternative, an open window thoracostomy,[36] are appropriate procedures. In our patients[37] we prefer to perform an open window thoracostomy first, and a limited thoracoplasty afterward (as described by Garcia-Yuste and colleagues[33]) in combination with an intrathoracic muscle transposition, which allows obliteration of the cavity in 1 stage. This kind of operation can lead to minor side effects that we regularly find in cases of extended thoracoplasty, such as shoulder deformity, scoliosis, chronic postoperative pain, and restriction of shoulder mobility. Once the pleural or pulmonary infection has been controlled, thoracoplasty remains an option to treat the residual pleural space, and combining it with a myoplasty can improve the surgical outcomes.[38] Potential candidates for this procedure are patients affected by primary chronic empyema, postresectional empyema (postlobectomy or postpneumonectomy), or aggressive infections with consequent lung destruction (tuberculosis, fungal infections, pyogenic abscess): these conditions are all problems of residual pleural or pulmonary space in which the lung fails to reexpand.

Technical Aspects of Surgery

Pulmonary resection frequently has the following technical difficulties:

- Firm pleural adhesions: extrapleural dissection reduces the risk of disruption of the mycetoma in the pleural space with dissemination of the fungal infection, and the risk of intraoperative and early postoperative major bleeding
- Indurated hilum structures: routine taping of the main artery makes dissection of the bronchovascular hilum indurated by extrabronchial fibrosis and post–chronic infection nodes safes in case of bleeding
- Pathologic bronchial stumps: coverage of a bronchial stump with viable tissue (pericardial, omental, and muscle flap) decreases the risk of bronchopleural fistula from bronchial deficiency due to chronic inflammation, atrophy, and calcifications
- Residual pleural space: obliteration of the residual pleural cavity reduces the risk of pleural empyema from incomplete filling of the pleural space by the remaining lobes (**Fig. 10**)

Alternative Treatments

Despite high recurrence rates, direct intracavitary administration of antifungal agents should be reserved for inoperable patients.[39] Amphotericin-B, miconazole, nystatin, N-acetylcysteine, sodium iodide, and natamycin can be instilled through either percutaneous or intrabronchial catheters. Two nonprospective randomized studies[40,41] showed short-term clinical improvement.

Remy and colleagues[42] described bronchial artery embolization as effective in massive hemoptysis, either as therapy in nonsurgical patients or as a temporizing and stabilizing technique before resection.[43] The source of massive hemoptysis is

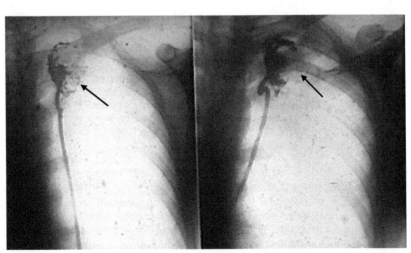

Fig. 6. Bronchography: sequential images from cavernography showing a cavity including a fungus ball (*arrow*).

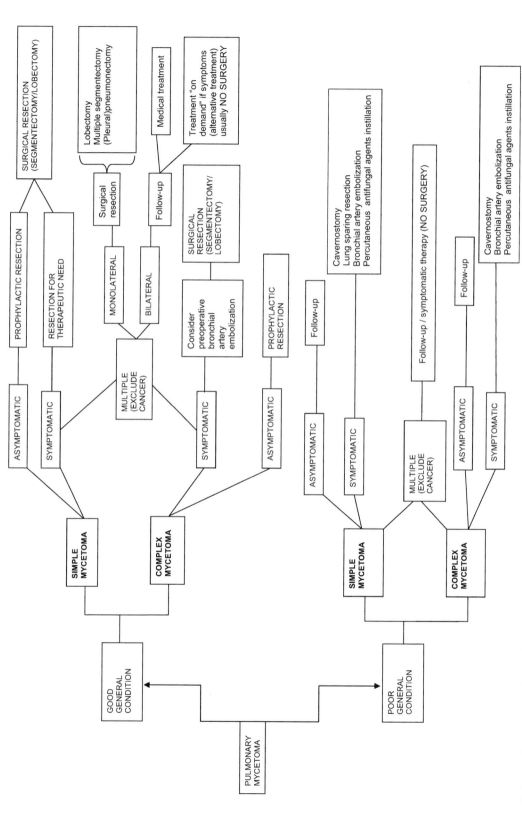

Fig. 7. Surgical management of pulmonary mycetoma.

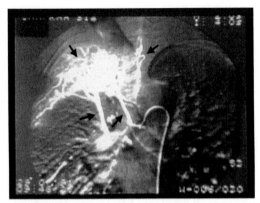

Fig. 8. Arteriography: lower arrows show a systemic vascularization of a complex aspergilloma in the right upper lobe; upper arrows reveal the classic neovascularization with an intricate tangle of vessels and neovascular anastomosis with mediastinal and pleural-chest wall vessels.

commonly the bronchial circulation (90% of cases) rather than the pulmonary circulation (5%), as in Rasmussen aneurysm, and about 5% of cases with massive hemoptysis originate from the aorta (ie, aortobronchial fistula) or nonbronchial systemic arteries.[44] However, it is often difficult to identify and control the bleeding vessel because of an undetectable vascular network in advanced disease. Furthermore, long-term results are suboptimal, with 10% to 50% recurrence within 4 years[45] caused by recanalization of the embolized vessel, or progression of disease.

Treatments in the Search for Scientific Consensus

1. Video-assisted thoracic surgery for pulmonary aspergilloma.

A recent retrospective study[46] compared video-assisted thoracic surgery (VATS) in the treatment of simple mycetoma and complex mycetoma; despite the limited number of patients, we share the investigators' wish to treat this unusual disease with a minimally invasive approach. However, we are convinced that VATS should be considered only in selected patients with small, simple, and peripheral mycetomas.

2. External beam radiotherapy

Use of radiotherapy in benign disease is not well described but it could be used when other conventional treatments have failed and the surgical option is excluded. Resolution of the hemoptysis is usually seen within 1 week of starting the radiation. The only meaningful study[47] described this procedure on 5 patients. Radiotherapy was

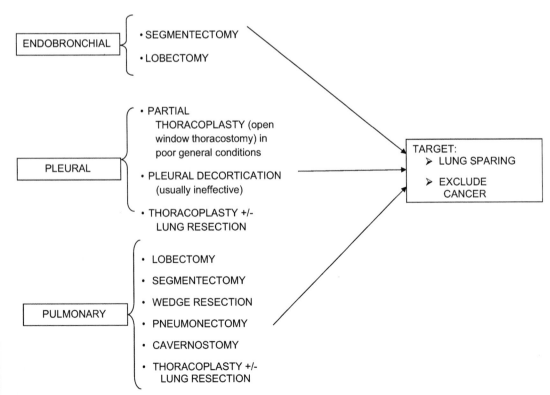

Fig. 9. Surgical options related to localization of mycetoma.

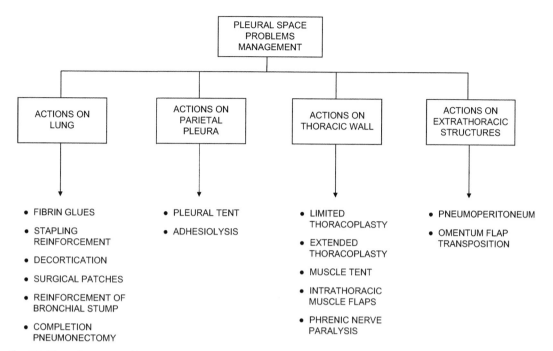

Fig. 10. Pleural space problems.

conducted with anterior-posterior parallel-opposed fields with 1-cm margins and the use of lead blocks to limit treatment margins to the cavity with the aspergilloma. A midplane dose of 3.5 Gy was administered. Three of 5 patients stopped bleeding after 2 weekly treatments (total dose 7 Gy). The other patients needed 3 (total dose 10,5 Gy) and 5 fractions (total dose 14 Gy) before bleeding cessation. No complications and no recurrences were reported after a 6-month period. The lack of an adequate follow-up (all patients were followed up for only a 6-month period) and the limited number of patients treated represent important limitations of this isolated experience.

CLINICAL OUTCOMES

Using advanced planning, appropriate preoperative management, and judicious surgical technique, surgery is the preferred treatment of pulmonary aspergilloma.[25,48]

Comparing patients without any underlying disease (simple mycetoma) with those having parenchymal sequelae (complex mycetoma), a better clinical outcome is observed in simple mycetomas.[28] Although complex mycetoma usually affects symptomatic patients with a long history of pulmonary disease and impaired functional values, they, more than others, should take advantage of surgical procedures obtaining a 79% 10-year survival rate[49]; however, patients with complex mycetoma likely to experience many

postoperative complications. Mortality ranges from 0% to 44% (**Table 1**). In high-risk patients with chronic advanced fibrosis and marked pleural-mediastinal adhesions, the average mortality may be more than 25%, and the incidence of complications related to hemorrhage, bronchopleural fistula, and empyema approaches 60%.[48] In contrast, Babatasi and colleagues[15] reported low morbidity because of selective surgical criteria in asymptomatic patients.

However, comparing surgical experience before the 1990s and after that period, it is evident that, in the last twenty years, complex mycetomas diminished due to decreasing incidence of tuberculous sequelae with the use of antitubercular drugs. With the decline of tuberculosis, surgical procedures that always presented technical difficulties[50] became less challenging; postoperative mortality and morbidity have significantly decreased since then, and postoperative outcomes have consequently improved. Furthermore, advances in surgical technique in recent years have permitted complication-free pulmonary resection for aspergilloma.

El Oakley and colleagues[30] stressed the concept of surgical assessment to optimize clinical outcomes. Patients were categorized into 4 groups: class I (fit individuals with mild or no symptoms), class II (fit individuals with severe symptoms), class III (unfit individuals with no symptoms), class IV (unfit individuals with severe symptoms). Class II was directed to traditional surgical resection; class IV was directed

Table 1
Most important publications in the English literature on surgically treated aspergillomas[a]

Author, Year	Observed Patients	Resected Patients	Year	Hemoptysis (%)	Complex Mycetoma (%)	Operative Mortality (%)	Complications (%)	Survival (%)
Karas et al,[27] 1976	41	18	1969–1974	23/41 (56)	36/41 (88)	3/15 (20)	B 2/15 (13) PSP 2/15 (13)	—
Garvey et al,[18] 1977	—	11	1972–1976	NS	NS	(8.3)	G 2/11 (18)	—
Jewkes et al,[14] 1983	85	50	1956–1980	36/49 (73.5)	80/85 (94)	C (44) LR (7) G (14)	G (15)	5 y: LR (85)
Battaglini et al,[63] 1985	—	15	1972–1983	12/15 (80)	9/15 (60)	SA (0) CA (18.1) G (13.3)	G 6/15 (40)	—
Daly et al,[28] 1986	—	53	1953–1984	—	(47)	SA (5) CA (34) G (22.6)	SA (78) CA (33)	5 y: SA (84) CA: (43)
Stamatis and Greschuchna[71] 1988	—	29	1976–1986	14/29 (48)	—	SA (0) CA (11.7) G (6.9)	6/29 (20.7)	1–10 y: 27/29 (93)
Shirakusa et al,[36] 1989	—	24	1979–1987	(58)	20/24 (83)	0	G 2/24 (8.3)	—
Al-Majed et al,[72] 1990	—	14	1985–1989	12/14 (85.7)	(100)	0	1/14 (7)	—
Massard et al,[25] 1992	77	63	1974–1991	13/63 (20.6)	51/63 (80)	SA (0) CA (10) G (9.5)	B 37/63 (59) PSP 24/63 (38)	—
Rocco et al,[16] 1994	104	77	1979–1991	(87.5)	(85.2)	(6.5)	B 0 PSP (16.9)	—
Chen et al,[48] 1997	—	67	1968–1995	(91)	66/67 (98.5)	1/67 (6.7)	G 15/67 (22.4)	—
Csekeo et al,[70] 1997	—	84	1983–1995	(48)	(50)	(9.5)	B 11/84 (13) PSP 23/84 (27.4)	—

El Oakley et al,[30] 1997	27	24	1982–1996	16/24 (66.6)	14/24 (58.3)	(28.6)	G 10/24 (41.6)	17 mo (median): 19/27 (70.4)
Chatzimichalis et al,[11] 1998	—	12	1992–1997	4/12 (33.3)	5/12 (41.6)	0	B 1/12 (8.3) PSP 2/12 (16.6)	—
Babatasi et al,[15] 2000	—	84	1959–1998	(66)	(65)	(4)	B 23/84 (27.4) PSP 31/84 (36.9)	5 y: (84) 10 y: (74)
Regnard et al,[62] 2000	—	87	1977–1997	(72)	(70)	SA 0 CA (6.2) G (5.7)	B (15.7) PSP (29.1)	5 y: (66)
Park and Jheon[69] 2002	—	110	1987–2000	(82)	81/110 (73.6)	1/110 (0.9)	G (23.6)	NS
Akbari et al,[68] 2005	—	60	1985–2003	(93.3)	(77)	SA 0 CA (4.3)	SA 0 CA (26.1)	10 y: SA (92) CA (78)
Kim et al,[49] 2005	—	88	1981–1999	40/88 (45.5)	72/88 (81.8)	(1.1)	G (27)	10 y: SA (80) CA (79.6)
Caidi et al,[66] 2006	320	278	1982–2004	(83)	TB (73)	(5.7)	B (5) PSP (24.3)	—
Demir et al,[67] 2006	—	41	1988–2003	(75.6)	(100)	(2.4)	(24.4)	—
Brik et al,[65] 2008	—	42	2001–2008	(83.3)	30/42 (71.4)	CA (3.3)	B (4.7) PSP (11.7)	5 y: SA (91.6) CA (83.3)
Lee G et al,[64] 2009	240	135	1990–2006	(61.5)	(75.6)	(4.4)	(29.6)	10 y: (84.4)
Cesar et al,[32] 2011	—	208 C 111 LR 97	1979–2010	C (95.5) LR (58.8)	(92)	C (19.5) LR (13.2)	B: C (50.5); LR (12.4) PSP: C (10.3); LR 0	—

Abbreviations: B, bleeding; C, cavernostomy; CA, complex aspergilloma; G, global; LR, lung resection; NS, not specified; PSP, pleural space problems; SA, simple mycetoma; TB, tuberculosis.

a The articles are listed in chronologic order of publication.

> **Box 5**
> **Postoperative complications**
>
> 1. Hemorrhage
> 2. Pleural space problems
>   a. Prolonged air leaks
>   b. Incomplete reexpansion
> 3. Respiratory failure
> 4. Thoracic empyema
> 5. Bronchopleural fistula
> 6. Lobar torsion

---

to a mini-invasive approach with cavernostomy. There were no operative deaths in patients treated with resection, but 2 of 7 patients in class IV died in the early postoperative period.

COMPLICATIONS AND CONCERNS

Even skillful thoracic surgeons admit that these surgical procedures can be technically arduous and have a complicated postoperative outcome. The occurrence of complications can vary from a standard procedure for a resection of a simple aspergilloma in an otherwise healthy patient[28] to a technically hazardous procedure such as a pleuropneumonectomy, which has a high rate of morbidity and mortality.[25] The most common complication is bleeding (**Box 5**). Bleeding may arise from twisted bronchial vessels, from aberrant systemic arteries growing close to the intercostals or internal mammary arteries, or from vascular adhesions resulting from chronic inflammatory pulmonary processes. Preoperative bronchial artery embolization can be attempted to reduce perioperative bleeding.[51]

Bronchopleural fistula is the most feared complication after pneumonectomy. It may lead to life-threatening complications such as respiratory insufficiency, empyema, and aspiration of purulent material to the healthy lung. Dehiscence of the bronchial suture is favored by bronchial weakness caused by chronic inflammation, atrophy, and calcification of the bronchial stump.[52] Coverage of the bronchial stump with viable tissue (pericardial, omental, and muscle flap) decreases the risk.[53]

Pleural space problems after lung resection are common, in particular in patients with a complex mycetoma, in which the lung has lost elasticity because of different underlying disease (eg, sequelae of tuberculosis or emphysema/fibrosis). To deal with such a problem, several techniques can be adopted at the time of operation or at the second stage (see **Fig. 10**).

Pleurapneumonectomies represent the most risky procedure in terms of complications and clinical outcome. This procedure should be avoided whenever possible[36]; because pleural aspergilloma is a condition that frequently produces severe symptoms, the thoracic surgeon must consider the possibility of a surgical intervention.

A local pulmonary recurrence or, worse, a pleuritic recurrence, is a dramatic event[16] and preventive adjuvant antifungal pharmacotherapy does not seem to reduce this risk of severe adverse effects.[54] A pleural empyema (pleural aspergillosis) may be clinically evident early in the postoperative period or later, even several months after resection, and it could lead to death caused by a hemorrhagic event from neoformed pleural vessels and could generate or aggravate parenchymal or bronchial fistulae. Therapeutic strategies in this situation are the same as those for chronic pleural empyema with or without bronchial fistula. In this case, an invasive approach is mandatory and this can range from a chest drain to a temporary open window thoracostomy until an extended thoracoplasty followed by a muscle flap transposition can be performed. New studies[55,56] are emerging regarding management of open window thoracostomy by vacuum-assisted closure therapy (VAC therapy), which requires careful evaluation and good experience because it can trigger clinically significant complications.[57]

WHAT LIES AHEAD FOR A MYCETOMA NOT UNDERGOING PULMONARY RESECTION?

More than half of patients develop hemoptysis, and up to 20% of these patients develop a fatal hemorrhage.[17] Some patients with aspergilloma show a progressive infective form that can vary from a CNPA to an acute aspergillosis.[58] Rupture of a pulmonary aspergilloma in the pleural space is a rare event.[25] Outcomes for these patients are mostly related to the underlying lung disease. Moreover, lung cancer is common and possibly related to tubercular sequelae (scar cancer).[59] In a few patients, aspergillomas seem to stabilize and remain asymptomatic for many years; a UK resurvey[60] reported an occasional apparent regression of aspergillomas, sometimes following a superadded bacterial infection; a spontaneous resolution has also been reported but it seems to be an anecdotal event.[61]

SUMMARY

The only effective treatment of a pulmonary mycetoma is surgery. The operative risk is low if the patient is asymptomatic and is affected by a simple mycetoma. In this case, the operation could be an anatomic resection performed on an elective basis with the same risks as a lung resection performed for cancer. Higher risk has been shown when symptoms are present and in complex mycetoma. Pleuropneumonectomy to remove a mycetoma should limited to selected patients or avoided when possible. Aspergillus empyema is a rare, often postresectional, condition usually discovered in debilitated patients: in these cases, an open window thoracostomy could be a safe and effective procedure. Even in asymptomatic patients, aggressive surgery offers 5 potential benefits: prevention of hemoptysis, eradication of the fungal and possible pyogenic component, limitation of symptoms as the result of a possible evolution to invasive aspergillosis or increased growth of the mycetoma, improvement of quality of life, and prolongation of life. Because pulmonary aspergilloma is a benign disease, the risk of early postoperative death should be avoided.

REFERENCES

1. Bonesio L, Del Curto D. Il villaggio Morelli: identità paesaggistica e patrimonio monumentale. Reggio Emilia (Italia): Edizioni Diabasis; 2011. p. 54.

2. Franquet T, Muller NL, Giménez A, et al. Spectrum of pulmonary aspergillosis: histologic, clinical, and radiologic findings. Radiographics 2001;21:825–37.

3. Pennington JE. Opportunistic fungal pneumonias: *Aspergillus, Mucor, Candida, Torulopsis.* In: Pennington JE, editor. Respiratory infections: diagnosis and management. New York: Raven Press; 1983. p. 329–39.

4. The Research Committee of the British Tuberculosis Association. *Aspergillus* in persistent lung cavities after tuberculosis. Tubercle 1968;49:1–11.

5. Young VK, Maghur HA, Luke DA, et al. Operation for cavitating invasive pulmonary aspergillosis in immunocompromised patients. Ann Thorac Surg 1992;53:621–4.

6. Degregorio MW, Lee WMF, Linker CA, et al. Fungal infections in patients with acute leukemia. Am J Med 1982;73:543–8.

7. Hinson KF, Moon AJ, Plummer NS. Bronchopulmonary aspergillosis: review and report of eight cases. Thorax 1952;7:317–33.

8. Ein ME, Wallace RJ, Williams TW. Allergic bronchopulmonary aspergillosis-like syndrome consequent to aspergilloma. Am Rev Respir Dis 1979;119:811–20.

9. Lipinski JK, Weisbrod GL, Sanders DE. Unusual manifestations of pulmonary aspergillosis. J Can Assoc Radiol 1978;29:216–20.

10. Belcher J, Plummer N. Surgery in bronchopulmonary aspergillosis. Br J Dis Chest 1960;54:335–41.

11. Chatzimichalis A, Massard G, Kessler R, et al. Bronchopulmonary aspergilloma: a reappraisal. Ann Thorac Surg 1998;65:927–96.

12. Dobbertin I, Friedel G, Jaki R, et al. [Bronchial aspergillosis]. Pneumolgie 2010;64:171–83 [in German].

13. Sharma OP, Chwogule R. Many faces of pulmonary aspergillosis. Eur Respir J 1998;12:705–15.

14. Jewkes J, Kay PH, Paneth M, et al. Pulmonary aspergilloma: analysis of prognosis in relation to haemoptysis and survey of treatment. Thorax 1983;38:572–8.

15. Babatasi G, Massetti M, Chapelier A, et al. Surgical treatment of pulmonary aspergilloma: current outcome. J Thorac Cardiovasc Surg 2000;119:906–12.

16. Rocco G, Rizzi A, Robustellini M, et al. About the surgical treatment of pulmonary mycetoma. Ann Thorac Surg 1994;57:260–2.

17. Rafferty P, Biggs BA, Crompton GK, et al. What happens to patients with pulmonary aspergilloma? Analysis of 23 cases. Thorax 1983;38:579–83.

18. Garvey J, Crastnopol P, Weisz D, et al. The surgical treatment of pulmonary aspergillomas. J Thorac Cardiovasc Surg 1977;74:542–7.

19. Pennington JE. Aspergillus. In: Sarosi GA, Davies SF, editors. Fungal Diseases of the Lung. 2nd edition. New York: Raven Press; 1993. p. 133–47.

20. Pecora DV, Toll MW. Pulmonary resection for localized aspergillosis. N Engl J Med 1960;263:785–7.

21. Breuer R, Baigelman W, Pugatch RD. Occult mycetoma. J Comput Assist Tomogr 1982;6:166–8.

22. Musher B, Fredricks D, Leisenring W, et al. *Aspergillus galactomannan* enzyme immunoassay and quantitative PCR for diagnosis of invasive aspergillosis with bronchoalveolar lavage fluid. J Clin Microbiol 2004;42:5517–22.

23. Walsh TJ, Anaissie EJ, Denning DW, et al. Treatment of aspergillosis: clinical practice guidelines of the Infectious Diseases Society of America. Clin Infect Dis 2008;46:327–60.

24. Faulkner SL, Vernon R, Brown PP, et al. Hemoptysis and pulmonary aspergilloma: operative versus nonoperative treatment. Ann Thorac Surg 1978;25:389–92.

25. Massard G, Roeslin N, Wihlm JM, et al. Pleuropulmonary aspergilloma: clinical spectrum and results of surgical treatment. Ann Thorac Surg 1992;54:1159–64.

26. Borelli D, Bran JL, Fuentes J, et al. Ketoconazole, an oral antifungal: laboratory and clinical assessment of imidazole drugs. Postgrad Med J 1979;55:657–61.

27. Karas A, Hankins JR, Attar S, et al. Pulmonary aspergilloma: an analysis of 41 patients. Ann Thorac Surg 1976;22:1–7.

28. Daly RC, Pairolero PC, Piehler JM, et al. Pulmonary aspergilloma: results of surgical treatment. J Thorac Cardiovasc Surg 1986;92:981–8.

29. Shiraishi Y, Katsuragi N, Nakajima Y, et al. Pneumonectomy for complex aspergilloma: is it still dangerous? Eur J Cardiothorac Surg 2006;29: 9–13.

30. El Oakley R, Petrori M, Goldstraw P. Indications and outcome of surgery for pulmonary aspergilloma. Thorax 1997;52:813–5.

31. Monaldi V. Endocavitary aspiration in the treatment of pathological cavities of the lung. Scand J Respir Dis Suppl 1968;65:113–21.

32. Cesar JM, Resende JS, Amaral NF, et al. Cavernostomy x resection for pulmonary aspergilloma: a 32-year history. J Cardiothorac Surg 2011;6:129.

33. Garcia-Yuste M, Ramos G, Duque JL, et al. Open window thoracostomy and thoracomioplasty to manage chronic pleural empyema. Ann Thorac Surg 1998;65:818–22.

34. Alexander J. The collapse therapy of pulmonary tuberculosis. Springfield (IL): Charles C Thomas; 1937.

35. Personne C, Toty L, Colchen A, et al. Vrais et faux problèmes de la chirurgie des aspergillomes pulmonaires. A propos de 220 cas. Rev Fr Mal Respir 1979;7:43–4.

36. Shirakusa T, Ueda H, Suito T, et al. Surgical treatment of pulmonary aspergilloma and *Aspergillus* empyema. Ann Thorac Surg 1989;48:779–82.

37. Massera F, Robustellini M, Della Pona C, et al. Open window thoracostomy for pleural empyema complicating partial lung resection. Ann Thorac Surg 2009;87:869–73.

38. Stefani A, Jouni R, Alifano M, et al. Thoracoplasty in the current practice of thoracic surgery: a single-institution 10-year experience. Ann Thorac Surg 2011;91:263–9.

39. Shapiro MJ, Albeda SM, Mayock RL, et al. Severe hemoptysis associated with pulmonary aspergilloma. Percutaneous intracavitary treatment. Chest 1988;94:1225–31.

40. Rumbak M, Kohler G, Eastrige C, et al. Topical treatment of life-threatening haemoptysis from aspergilloma. Thorax 1996;51:253–5.

41. Yamada H, Kohno S, Koga H, et al. Topical treatment of pulmonary aspergilloma by antifungals: relation between duration of the disease and efficacy of therapy. Chest 1993;103:1421–5.

42. Remy J, Voisin C, Ribet M, et al. [Treatment, by embolization, of severe or repeated hemoptysis associated with systemic hypervascularization]. Nouv Presse Med 1973;2(31):2060 [in French].

43. Uflacker R, Kaemmerer A, Neves C, et al. Management of massive hemoptysis by bronchial artery embolization. Radiology 1983;146:627–34.

44. Remy J, Remy-Jardin M, Voisin C. Endovascular management of bronchial bleeding. In: Butler J, editor. The bronchial circulation. New York: Dekker; 1992. p. 667–723.

45. Joon W, Kim JK, Kim YH, et al. Bronchial and non-bronchial systemic artery embolization for life-threatening hemoptysis: a comprehensive review. Radiographics 2002;22(6):1395–409.

46. Inchinose J, Kohno T, Fujimori S. Video-assisted thoracic surgery for pulmonary aspergilloma. Interact Cardiovasc Thorac Surg 2010;10:927–30.

47. Falkson C, Sur R, Pacella J. External beam radiotherapy: a treatment option for massive haemoptysis caused by mycetoma. Clin Oncol 2002;14: 233–5.

48. Chen J, Chang Y, Luh S, et al. Surgical treatment for pulmonary aspergilloma: a 28 year experience. Thorax 1997;52:810–3.

49. Kim YT, Kang MC, Sung SW, et al. Good long-term outcomes after surgical treatment of simple and complex pulmonary aspergilloma. Ann Thorac Surg 2005;79:294–8.

50. Lejay A, Falcoz PE, Santelmo N, et al. Surgery for aspergilloma: time trend towards improved results? Interact Cardiovasc Thorac Surg 2011;13: 392–5.

51. Hughes CF, Waugh R, Lindsay D. Surgery for pulmonary aspergilloma: preoperative embolization of the bronchial circulation. Thorax 1986;41: 324–5.

52. Massard G, Dabbagh A, Wihlm JM, et al. Pneumonectomy for chronic infection is a high-risk procedure. Ann Thorac Surg 1996;62:1033–8.

53. Shiraishi Y, Nakajima Y, Katsuragi N, et al. Pneumonectomy for non-tuberculous mycobacterial infections. Ann Thorac Surg 2004;78:399–403.

54. Sagan D, Gozdziuk K. Surgery for pulmonary aspergilloma in immunocompetent patients: no benefit from adjuvant antifungal pharmacotherapy. Ann Thorac Surg 2010;89(5):1603–10.

55. Palmen M, van Breugel HN, Geskes GG, et al. Open window thoracostomy treatment of empyema is accelerated by vacuum assisted closure. Ann Thorac Surg 2009;88:1131–6.

56. Aru GM, Jew NB, Tribble CG, et al. Intrathoracic vacuum-assisted management of persistent and infected pleural spaces. Ann Thorac Surg 2010;90: 266–70.

57. Rocco G, Cecere C, La Rocca A, et al. Caveats in using vacuum-assisted closure for post-pneumonectomy empyema. Eur J Cardiothorac Surg 2012;41:1069–71.

58. Buckingham SJ, Hansell DM. *Aspergillus* in the lung: diverse and coincident forms. Eur Radiol 2003;13: 1786–800.

59. Rizzi A, Rocco G, Robustellini M, et al. Results of surgical management of tuberculosis: experience in 206 patients undergoing operation. Ann Thorac Surg 1995;59:896–900.

60. Aspergilloma and residual tuberculous cavities: the results of a resurvey. Tubercle 1970;51:227–45.

61. Hammerman KJ, Christianson CS, Huntington I, et al. Spontaneous lysis of aspergillomata. Chest 1973;64:679.

62. Regnard JF, Icard P, Nicolosi M, et al. Aspergilloma: a series of 89 surgical cases. Ann Thorac Surg 2000;69:898–903.

63. Battaglini JW, Murray GF, Keagy BA, et al. Surgical management of symptomatic pulmonary aspergilloma. Ann Thorac Surg 1985;39: 512–6.

64. Lee JG, Lee CY, Park IK, et al. Pulmonary aspergilloma: analysis of prognosis in relation to symptoms and treatment. J Thorac Cardiovasc Surg 2009; 138(4):820–5.

65. Brik A, Salem AM, Kamal AR, et al. Surgical outcome of pulmonary aspergilloma. Eur J Cardiothorac Surg 2008;34(4):882–5.

66. Caidi M, Kabiri H, Al Aziz S, et al. [Surgical treatment of pulmonary aspergilloma. 278 cases]. Presse Med 2006;35:1819–24 [in French].

67. Demir A, Gunluoglu MZ, Turna A, et al. Analysis of surgical treatment for pulmonary aspergilloma. Asian Cardiovasc Thorac Ann 2006;14(5):407–11.

68. Akbari JG, Varma PK, Neema PK, et al. Clinical profile and surgical outcome for pulmonary aspergilloma: a single center experience. Ann Thorac Surg 2005;80(3):1067–72.

69. Park CK, Jheon S. Results of surgical treatment for pulmonary aspergilloma. Eur J Cardiothorac Surg 2002;21(5):918–23.

70. Csekeo A, Agócs L, Egerváry M. Surgery for pulmonary aspergillosis. Eur J Cardiothorac Surg 1997; 12(6):876–9.

71. Stamatis G, Greschuchna D. Surgery for pulmonary aspergilloma and pleural aspergillosis. Thorac Cardiovasc Surg 1988;36(6):356–60.

72. al-Majed SA, Ashour M, el-Kassimi FA, et al. Management of post-tuberculous complex aspergilloma of the lung: role of surgical resection. Thorax 1990;45(11):846–9.

Surgery for Other Pulmonary Fungal Infections, *Actinomyces*, and *Nocardia*

Joseph LoCicero III, MD[a],*, Jason P. Shaw, MD[b],
Richard S. Lazzaro, MD[c]

KEYWORDS

- Fungus • Infection • Lung • Abscess • Cavitary • Empyema • Chest wall

KEY POINTS

- When evaluating a patient with a pulmonary nodule, take a careful history of all previous respiratory infections and of fungal exposure.
- Use computed tomography criteria for indeterminate pulmonary nodules to avoid unnecessary operations.
- If zygomycetes infection is suspected, resect urgently to prevent extensive damage.
- Eliminate all residual spaces after resection.
- Aggressively manage fungal empyemas.

INTRODUCTION

Surgery plays a small but important niche role in modern management of fungal diseases. During the last quarter century, clinicians perfected minimally invasive biopsy procedures and techniques, researchers developed diagnostic tests that have greater accuracy, and pharmaceutical companies reformulated older antimicrobials and produced new drugs that are more effective and have fewer side effects. This article discusses the human fungal pathogens (except for *Aspergillus* species, which is discussed elsewhere in this issue). Details discussed include their behavior as pathogens, methods for their diagnosis, and the nonsurgical and surgical management (**Table 1**) of clinically significant infections and complications.

HISTOPLASMOSIS
Organism, Clinical Characteristics, and Diagnosis

Histoplasma capsulatum, the offending organism, is present in its mycelial form in soil contaminated with bird or bat droppings near large river valleys throughout the world.[1] Mammals, including humans, inhale the organism and macrophages engulf the fungus. It then transforms into the budding yeast form, causing activation of inflammatory cytokines, in particular LI-17 and tumor necrosis factor (TNF).[2] Over several months, the ongoing inflammation causes granulomas in lymph nodes, some of which become calcified.

In endemic areas, a large number of individuals have been infected with *H capsulatum*, usually as children. In those who develop symptoms, the disease may present as disseminated disease, usually only in immunocompromised patients, or may be localized in the chest.[3] Clinical symptoms may be nonexistent or mild, including fever, malaise, headache, and weakness, with substernal chest discomfort and dry cough. In cases of a large inoculum, patients present with acute fever, chills, malaise, dyspnea, cough, and chest pain. Panlobar involvement is common in this phase, but the pleura is spared. As pulmonary parenchymal involvement resolves, inflamed lymph nodes

[a] Department of Surgery, SUNY Downstate, 1158 Church Street, Mobile, AL 36604, USA; [b] Division General Thoracic Surgery, Maimonides Medical Center, 4802 Tenth Avenue, Brooklyn, NY 11218, USA; [c] Division General Thoracic Surgery, New York Methodist Hospital, 506 - Sixth Street, Brooklyn, NY 11215, USA
* Corresponding author.
E-mail address: lociceroj@comcast.net

Thorac Surg Clin 22 (2012) 363–374
doi:10.1016/j.thorsurg.2012.04.002
1547-4127/12/$ – see front matter © 2012 Elsevier Inc. All rights reserved.

Table 1
The most common surgical procedures required for different problem types, based on infecting organism

Organism	Common Problems	Common Surgical Procedures
Histoplasmosis	Broncholiths (hemoptysis/fistulas) Recurrent pericardial effusions Fibrosing mediastinitis Indeterminate nodule	Removal of broncholiths Pericardiectomy Vascular stenting Resection (obsolete)
Blastomycosis	Empyema Indeterminate nodule	Surgical management Resection (obsolete)
Coccidiodomycosis	Nonresponsive cavitary disease Indeterminate nodule	Pulmonary resection Resection
Paracoccidioidomycosis	Indeterminate nodule Airway stenosis	Resection Endobronchial management
Cryptococcosis	Empyema	Surgical management
Sporotrichosis	Cavitary disease Indeterminate nodule	Parenchymal resection Resection
Candidiasis	—	Rarely requires surgical management
Zygomycetes	Pulmonary and airway necrosis	Aggressive resection
Dematiaceous molds	Abscesses and infected cavities	Parenchyma-sparing resection Space management
Adiaspiromycosis	Parenchymal changes	Parenchyma-sparing resection
Actinomycosis	Indeterminate nodule Massive hemoptysis	Resection Resection and space management
Nocardiasis	Wound complications Draining sinuses	Debridement Resection of diseased tissue

become prominent on radiographs, looking like buckshot.

Cavitary histoplasmosis may occur in patients who have emphysema. Cavities, usually in the upper lobes, slowly enlarge compressing normal lung. Fibrosis develops in the lower lobes, possibly caused by spillage of antigen from the cavities. Without treatment, death due to diminishing pulmonary function is common.

Varying forms of mediastinitis develop in all patients with pulmonary histoplasmosis. The nodes enlarge because of granulomas with caseous necrosis. Nodes become confluent and persist for months to years. A small number of patients with smoldering mediastinitis develop broncholithiasis.

In rare instances, the inflammatory process gradually leads to scarring and fibrosing mediastinitis (**Fig. 1**). Virtually any thoracic structure may be involved, causing organ-specific obstructive symptoms. The most common sites are the airway, the pulmonary vasculature, the superior vena cava, and occasionally the aorta.

Other problems that may occur include pericarditis, rheumatologic arthritis, and, rarely, ocular histoplasmosis.

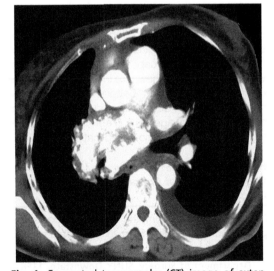

Fig. 1. Computed tomography (CT) image of extensive fibrosing mediastinitis. (*From* Hammoud ZT, Rose AS, Hage CA, et al. Surgical management of pulmonary and mediastinal sequelae of histoplasmosis: a challenging spectrum. Ann Thorac Surg 2009;88(2):399–3; with permission.)

Although index of suspicion and radiologic features of pulmonary infiltrates with massive confluent mediastinal lymph nodes are helpful, identification of the organism in tissue by biopsy and histopathologic evaluation is the best diagnostic approach. Methenamine silver or periodic acid-Schiff stains are needed to visualize the budding yeast. *Histoplasma* detection in the urine is helpful only in acute disease. *H capsulatum* may be cultured from infected body fluids and is definitive, but may take weeks. Antibody testing using immunodiffusion or complement fixation may be of use in the subacute phase of the disease, weeks after initial inhalation when the patient has had time to mount an immune response. Skin tests, which were unreliable because of cross reactivity with blastomycosis, are no longer marketed. Although polymerase chain reaction (PCR) methods are promising as the most definitive and fastest test, none are available commercially at this time.[4]

Medical Management

Guidelines published in 2007 by the Infectious Diseases Society of America[5] recommend the lipid formulation of amphotericin B for 1 to 2 weeks followed by itraconazole for moderately severe to severe acute pulmonary histoplasmosis and single-agent itraconazole for moderate disease. Cavitary disease should be treated with itraconazole for at least 1 year, but some experts prefer 18 to 24 months in view of the risk for relapse.

Itraconazole is recommended for patients with symptomatic mediastinal granulomas, but no antibiotics are recommended for mediastinal fibrosis. For patients with pericarditis or rheumatologic symptoms, itraconazole is recommended only if corticosteroids are administered.

Surgical Management

Surgeons are still called on to remove pulmonary nodules to eliminate the possibility of lung cancer in patients with a history of histoplasmosis. In many cases, operation may be avoided with careful history and radiologic evaluation, but solitary pulmonary nodules may need histopathologic evaluation. However, using strict criteria for nodules discovered on computed tomography (CT) scans in a population living in an endemic area for histoplasmosis, Stames and colleagues[6] were able to eliminate biopsies for benign disease in 132 consecutive patients followed for 5 years.

Surgery rarely plays a role in cavitary histoplasmosis in current practice. However, the Infectious Diseases Society of America[5] recommends surgical participation in the management of histoplasmosis for other specific problems. Broncholiths should be removed by the most appropriate method. Bronchoscopy is usually inadequate and removal at thoracotomy may be necessary. Both Kelly[7] and Cole and colleagues[8] suggest using the simplest method that accomplishes a good result. These patients occasionally develop massive hemoptysis or a bronchoesophageal fistula. In this author's experience, most patients with symptomatic broncholithiasis require thoracotomy with parenchyma-sparing methods and a bronchoplastic procedure. In rare instances, patients may develop recurrent broncholithiasis requiring additional surgical intervention.

The Infectious Diseases Society of America[5] also recommends pericardiectomy for recurrent effusions, but they do not recommend surgical intervention for asymptomatic mediastinal granulomas because these granulomas are self-limited and there is no evidence that mediastinal granulomas inevitably develop into mediastinal fibrosis. In cases of vascular fibrosis of the superior vena cava and pulmonary vessels, they recommend percutaneous intravascular dilation and stenting by the most appropriate interventionalist at the institution. In rare instances, surgical correction may be necessary. Hammoud and colleagues[9] presented a series of 9 patients over 17 years, and Peikert and colleagues[10] at Mayo Clinic in Arizona describe 80 patients over 9 years. Surgical management varied from simple procedures to resection in conjunction with cardiopulmonary bypass.

BLASTOMYCOSIS
Organism, Clinical Characteristics, and Diagnosis

Blastomyces dermatitidis is a dimorphic fungus living as a mold (mycelial form) in the soil of river valleys throughout the world. It releases spores (conidia) that are inhaled by humans and animals and that convert to disease, producing yeast after phagocytosis. Because alveolar macrophages inhibit the transformation of conidia into yeast, most infections are mild in immunocompetent individuals. Besides humans, blastomycosis is common in dogs, and may also be found in the horse, cow, cat, bat, and lion.[11]

Clinical presentations vary widely from virtually no pulmonary symptoms to fulminant pneumonia with acute respiratory distress syndrome.[12] Intermediate infections do occur, such as lobar pneumonia, mass lesions, single or multiple nodules, and chronic fibronodular or fibrocavitary infiltrates. Pleural effusions and empyemas are rare, but may present as empyema necessitatis.[13] The disease commonly presents with dermatologic lesions sometimes associated with thoracic disease.

Typical lesions are verrucous or ulcerative plaques but also may present as pustules.

Culture of the organism from body fluids is the usual method of diagnosis. However, identification of the yeast form may be made from histopathologic examination of surgical specimens. Patel and colleagues[14] retrospectively reviewed 53 cases and found that 79% could be diagnosed from pathologic specimens, whereas only 67% of patients whose bodily fluids were cultured were positive.

Medical Management

In 2008, the Infectious Diseases Society of America[15] recommended, for moderately severe to severe disease, initial treatment with a lipid formulation of amphotericin B for 1 to 2 weeks or until improvement is noted, followed by oral itraconazole for 6 to 12 months. For mild to moderate disease, they recommended oral itraconazole alone.

Surgical Management

Surgeons may be called on to evaluate and biopsy pulmonary nodules or hilar adenopathy months to years after resolution of an infection with B dermatitidis. The surgeon must take a careful history concerning previous infections to be aware of the possibility of residual changes and scarring caused by blastomycosis. For acute cases, the main reason for surgical involvement is for management of empyema as a complication of infection. Such empyemas should be managed aggressively in the same manner as complex bacterial empyemas. Thorough debridement leads to the best results. A case report by Wiesman and colleagues[16] outlines their experience with thoracoscopic management.

COCCIDIOIDOMYCOSIS
Organism, Clinical Characteristics, and Diagnosis

Coccidioides immitis and Coccidioides posadasii are soil-dwelling fungi found mainly in the American southwest and are the causative organisms in coccidioidomycosis. Most infections are asymptomatic and many of the remainder are associated with symptoms resembling other community-acquired pneumonia. However, acute pulmonary coccidioidomycosis is different from community-acquired pneumonia and may have hilar adenopathy, increased peripheral blood eosinophilia, severe fatigue, night sweats, and the presence of erythema multiforme or erythema nodosum. Acute cases may present with meningeal symptoms or other systemic complications, particularly in the immunocompromised host. Because of the variability of symptoms and the timing of presentation

of an infected patient, radiologic characteristics vary greatly. As the acute condition subsides, patients are left with pulmonary nodules of varying sizes.

The diagnosis may be established by immunologic testing of serum for antibodies, by the identification of coccidioidal spherules in tissue, or by culture from lesions.

Medical Management

Because coccidioidomycosis is ubiquitous and self-limited in many cases, treatment is reserved for only the symptomatic or for those with meningeal or neurologic complications. The official statement of the American Thoracic Society on the treatment of pulmonary fungal infections[12] recommends no therapy for primary pulmonary disease or for nodules, regardless of size. For diffuse pulmonary disease with symptoms, they recommend liposomal amphotericin B followed by fluconazole or itraconazole for up to a year.

Surgical Management

Surgical intervention may be indicated for only a few patients, most commonly for diagnostic dilemmas involving nodular disease, for symptomatic nonresponsive cavitary disease, or for complications of infection. Jaroszewski and colleagues[17] of the Mayo Clinic in Arizona reviewed their experience. Of the 1496 patients treated at the institution over a 10-year period, only 86 (6%) underwent operations. The most common indications were nodules in 59 patients. Eighteen had cavitary disease, 2 had infiltrates, and 7 had complications of disease such as effusion, pneumothorax, and empyema. Of the operated patients, 40% underwent resection for persistent symptoms or disease progression despite adequate antifungal therapy. Persistent air leaks were the most common morbidity, occurring in 56%, with 3 bronchopleural fistulas.

PARACOCCIDIOIDOMYCOSIS
Organism, Clinical Characteristics, and Diagnosis

Paracoccidioidomycosis, most common found in Latin America, is a systemic mycosis caused by Paracoccidioides brasiliensis that is usually acquired early in life by inhalation of conidia that convert in the lungs into yeast forms. The yeast causes an inflammatory process that may take an acute/subacute form in children or a chronic form in adults. In children and young adults, the infection frequently involves the reticuloendothelial system, including pulmonary lymph nodes. Researchers observed increased expression of CCR7 and CD103 as well as MHC-II on lung dendritic cells after infection.[18] They were able to show that bone marrow mouse dendritic cells stimulated by *P brasiliensis* migrate to the lymph nodes and activate a T helper response.

Paracoccidioidomycosis usually spares the lungs. If involved, patients show mild clinical symptoms with subtle radiological alterations. The most prominent changes are enlarged lymph nodes reminiscent of sarcoidosis.[19] High-resolution CT scanning is an important adjunct in the diagnosis of paracoccidioidomycosis. The most common CT features are parenchymal ground-glass attenuation, consolidation, varying size pulmonary nodules, cavitation, interlobular septal thickening, emphysema, and fibrotic lesions.[20] A reversed halo sign, also known as the atoll or fairy ring sign,[21] noted in cryptogenic pneumonitis may be seen in this condition (**Fig. 2**).

Medical Management

Most patients present with disseminated disease. Symptomatic or critically ill patients are treated with regimens that include 1 or more agents such as ketoconazole, itraconazole, or sulfadiazine.[12]

Surgical Management

Because the condition in adults is rarely acute, surgeons are rarely involved in the diagnosis of the infection. Surgical intervention may be needed to rule out carcinoma or to manage persistent consolidation caused by impingement of airways.

CRYPTOCOCCOSIS
Organism, Clinical Characteristics, and Diagnosis

Cryptococcus exists in nature as a minimally encapsulated yeast that rapidly synthesizes a polysaccharide capsule on entering the lungs.

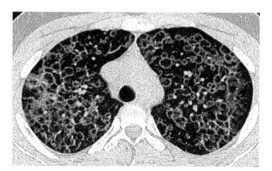

Fig. 2. CT image of ring opacities, some of which surround a center of ground-glass opacification, throughout the lung. (*From* Walsh SLF, Roberton BJ. The atoll sign. Thorax 2010;65:1029–30; with permission.)

Cryptococcus neoformans commonly produces disease in immunocompromised hosts. Patients with acquired immune deficiency syndrome are particularly susceptible. By contrast, *Cryptococcus gattii* more commonly infects immunocompetent hosts and is an emerging pathogen in the Pacific northwest and Canada as well as the Pacific Rim countries.[22]

It causes mainly pulmonary disease with pneumonialike symptoms resulting in residual nodules. Also about one-third of patients may present with cerebral cryptococcosis. The most common problem is the diagnosis of suspicious lung nodules. Characteristically, they may be solid or have a cavitating center. Diagnosis is made by identifying the fungus in tissue specimens. On microscopy, the mucinous capsules are visible and aid in the identification of the pathogen (**Fig. 3**).

Medical Management

Fluconazole or itraconazole are recommended for the treatment of mild to moderate acute disease. For patients with central nervous system involvement or disseminated disease, amphotericin is recommended.[12]

Surgical Management

Surgical intervention is rarely indicated for acute disease. However, *Cryptococcus* may cause a pleural effusion. Kurahara and colleagues[23] reported a case of fibrinopurulent cryptococcal empyema that required thoracoscopic management.

SPOROTRICHOSIS
Organism, Clinical Characteristics, and Diagnosis

The dimorphic fungus *Sporothrix schenkii* causes sporotrichosis. The organism is found throughout the world and causes disease in both canines and man. The most common form of the infection is skin or lymphocutaneous sporotrichosis. When sufficient spores are inhaled, pulmonary disease may occur and may become disseminated. Pulmonary radiologic patterns include involvement of the tracheobronchial lymph nodes, sometimes presenting with cavitary disease, predominantly involving the upper lobes (**Fig. 4**).

Medical Management

Although cutaneous disease is treatable with itraconazole, pulmonary sporotrichosis is difficult to eradicate, especially if cavitary disease is present. Conventional amphotericin B deoxycholate or a lipid formulation of amphotericin is used for

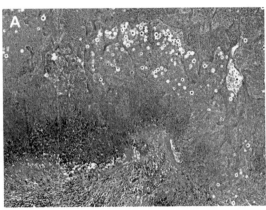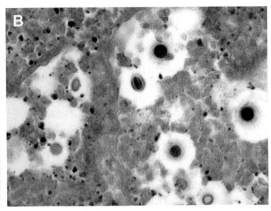

Fig. 3. (*A*) Photomicrograph of a necrotic lung nodule containing multiple cryptococci with halos in the necrotic debris. The granulomatous border of the nodule is visible on the lower left-hand side (hematoxylin and eosin stain). (*B*) Photomicrograph of cryptococci within the necrotic debris. Some organisms are round and some are oval. The mucinous capsules are seen in the organisms on the lower right-hand side of the image (hematoxylin and eosin stain, original magnification ×400). (*From* Dewar GJ, Kelly JK. *Cryptococcus gattii*: an emerging cause of pulmonary nodules. Can Respir J 2008;15(3):153–8; with permission.)

meningeal disease and may be used for severe pulmonary disease.[12]

Surgical Management

Surgical involvement may be necessary for both diagnosis and management. Surgical involvement may be necessary for both diagnosis and management. Resection for cavitary components may be necessary. Resectional therapy may be associated with air space problems.[24]

CANDIDIASIS
Organism, Clinical Characteristics, and Diagnosis

Candidiasis caused by *Candida albicans* occurs in many forms from gastrointestinal colonization to fulminant septicemia. *Candida* may colonize a cavity, but is rarely the cause of the infection. Diagnosis is based on the clinical picture and culture of the organism.

Medical Management

No treatment is required for *Candida* if it is an interloper or colonizer. Bloodstream infection is difficult to eradicate and requires aggressive treatment with amphotericin or one of the newer antifungal agents such as vorconazole, caspofungin, micafungin, or anidulafungin, sometimes combined with fluconazole. For stable disease, a regimen of fluconazole, caspofungin, micafungin, or anidulafungin is recommended.

Surgical Management

Infections involving *C albicans*, even localized ones, rarely require surgical intervention. However, recent cases of candida empyema have been reported, some of which have been fatal.[25,26]

RARE AND EMERGING FUNGI INCLUDING ZYGOMYCOSES, HYALOHYPHOMYCOSES, PHAEOHYPHOMYCOSES, TRICHOSPOROSIS, AND ADIASPIROMYCOSIS
Organism, Clinical Characteristics, and Diagnosis

Although the fungi of this group may be rare or only recently been proved to be human pathogens, zygomycetes (ie, *Rhizopus*, mucormycosis, *Cunninghamella*, and other species), hyaline molds or hyalohyphomycoses (ie, *Paecilomyces*, *Fusarium*, and *Scedosporium*), dematiaceous (black) molds or phaeohyphomycoses (ie, *Curvularia*, *Bipolaris*, *Exophiala*, and *Alternaria*), *Trichosporon*, and adiaspiromycosis caused by *Emmonsia crescens* cause significant and fulminant, often fatal, disease. Although most of the initial cases are identified among immunodepressed patients or patients with poorly controlled diabetes, many of these species now cause life-threatening infections in immunocompetent patients as well.

Although some species may produce disseminated disease, the most significant problems are related to the lungs. Zygomycetes that is angioinvasive produces pulmonary infiltrates that become necrotic, sometimes including the airway itself. Others such as the dematiaceous molds produce abscesses and infected cavities that are difficult to eradicate with antimicrobials alone. *E crescens* produces a diffuse pulmonary picture resembling tuberculosis or histoplasmosis and is diagnosed using PCR methods.[27]

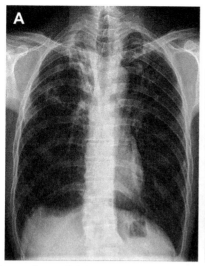
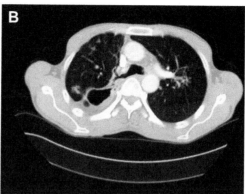

Fig. 4. Chest radiograph (*A*) and CT image (*B*) of a patient with sporotrichosis. (*From* Palomino J, Saeed O, Daroca P, et al. 47-year-old man with cough, dyspnea, and an abnormal chest radiograph. Chest 2009;135;872–5; with permission.)

Diagnosis is confirmed by culture or by identification of fungi invading tissue. Because many of these patients are critically ill and are intubated and ventilated for long periods, airway cultures showing exotic fungi must be correlated with the patients' radiographic findings and clinical course.

Medical Management

Amphotericin B in both standard and lyposomal forms, as well as vorconazole and posaconazole, are the mainstays of treatment of these serious pathogens. In some cases in which persistently infected cavities are present and cannot be resected, or in cases of residual spaces after resectional therapy, local irrigation has been used.[12]

Surgical Management

In general, rare and newly discovered fungal infections require more surgical involvement than common well-known fungal infections because there are fewer effective antimicrobials available. However, angioinvasive fungi such as zygomycetes (eg, *Rhizopus*, mucormycosis, *Cunninghamella*) cause necrosis and may move rapidly, leading to extensive destruction and death in a short period of time. These patients require urgent surgical intervention with complete removal of all devitalized tissue, even if it requires a pneumonectomy. Coverage of the stump with a vascularized pedicle of muscle, pericardium, or omentum is advisable with interval bronchoscopic surveillance during the early postoperative period. **Figs. 5–7**

show such a patient. A 32-year-old uncontrolled diabetic Hispanic man presented to the emergency room with severe sepsis and right upper lobe pneumonia and a large cavity. After initial resuscitation, he stabilized. Bronchoscopy showed purulent material draining from the right upper lobe orifice. Images of the parenchyma obtained with probe-based confocal laser endomicroscopy (Mauna Kea Technologies, Inc. Newtown, PA, USA) showed little normal parenchyma in the right upper lobe. Overnight, he became critically ill. He was taken to the operating room where repeat bronchoscopy showed necrosis of the posterior wall

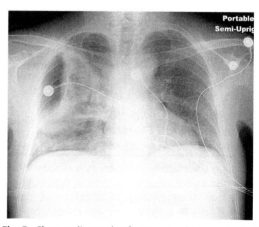

Fig. 5. Chest radiograph of a 32-year-old uncontrolled diabetic Hispanic man with a cavitary right upper lobe pneumonia and sepsis. Subsequent cultures proved mucor infection.

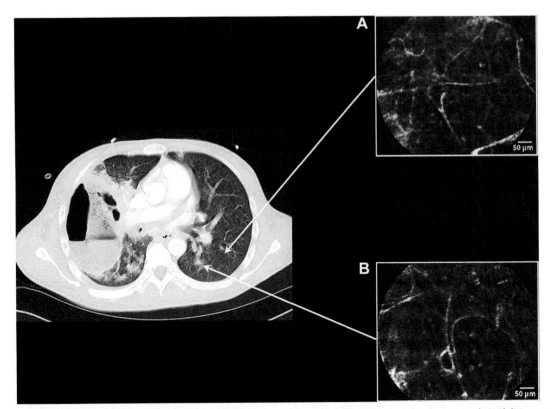

Fig. 6. CT image of patient in **Fig. 5** with images from probe-based confocal laser endomicroscopy (pCLE) (Mauna Kea Technologies, Inc. Newtown, PA, USA) performed at the time of bronchoscopy of the left lower lobe. (*A*) Normal alveolar architecture. (*B*) Aspirated material, possibly from cavity in right upper lobe.

of the right upper lobe bronchus. He underwent immediate right upper lobectomy with a serratus muscle flap patch and subsequently recovered completely.

In cases in which the culprit fungi are not angioinvasive, the goal of resective therapy is similar to tuberculosis operations: remove as much of the diseased parenchyma as possible while still using parenchyma-sparing techniques such as segmentectomy. Residual spaces should be avoided with tenting or thoracoplasty techniques. All of these patients require perioperative and long-term postoperative antimicrobials.

ACTINOMYCOSIS AND *NOCARDIA*
Organism, Clinical Characteristics, and Diagnosis

Although traditionally included in a discussion of fungal infections, *Actinomyces* and *Nocardia* are not fungi. They belong to a group of gram-positive bacteria that cause infections that resemble fungal infections. For classification purposes, the biological order Actinomycetales includes both aerobic species (*Nocardia*, *Gordona*, *Tsukamurella*,

Streptomyces, *Rhodococcus*, *Streptomyces*, and *Corynebacterium*) and anaerobic species (*Actinomyces*, *Arachnia*, *Rothia*, and *Bifidobacterium*), all of which cause veterinary and human disease.[28]

According to a review by Mabeza and Macfarlane,[29] pulmonary *Actinomyces* species is only the third most common form of human infection. Cervicofacial infections are most common (50%–60%), followed by abdominopelvic (20%) and thoracic (15%) infections. Pulmonary infections result from aspiration of contaminated oral microflora or by extension from complicated cervical infections. In the chest, *Actinomyces* species cause an initial acute pneumonitis producing chronic inflammation, fibrosis, and cavitation that may invade and destroy surrounding structures. Invasion into major blood vessels may cause life-threatening hemorrhage.

Nocardia can cause acute pulmonary infection with pneumonia, as well as chronic disease with nodules, cavities, or empyema.[30] In many cases, it has an indolent course mimicking tuberculosis with fever, chills, productive cough, sweats, weight loss, anorexia, dyspnea, and hemoptysis. Left untreated, the infection may burrow into thoracic structures including the mediastinum

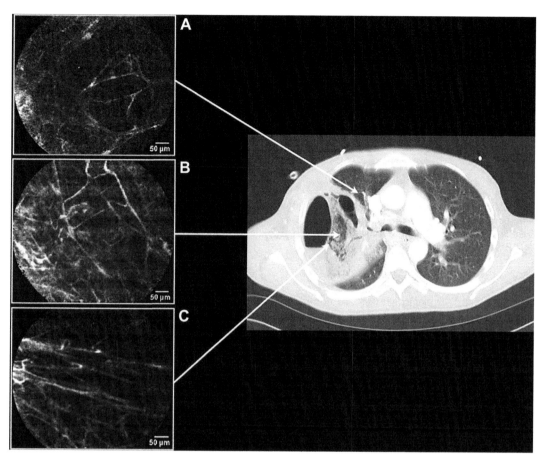

Fig. 7. CT image of patient in **Figs. 5** and **6** with images from pCLE performed at the time of bronchoscopy of the right upper lobe. Normal alveolar structure (*A*), fluid-filled alveoli next to destroyed alveoli (*B*), and compressed and broken alveolar walls (*C*) are seen next to the cavity with evidence of ischemia.

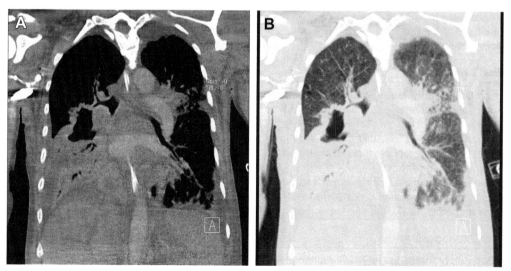

Fig. 8. Images from mediastinal (*A*) and lung (*B*) windows of a reformatted chest CT with contrast of a man presenting with massive hemoptysis. Note that the cavitary lesion communicates with the bronchus intermedius. Subsequent cultures of the resected lobectomy specimen grew *Actinomyces*.

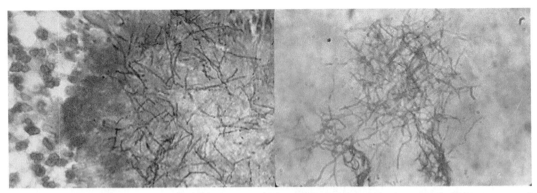

Fig. 9. Filamentous actinomycetes. Anaerobic gram-positive *Actinomyces* species have a beaded appearance in tissue (*left panel*), whereas the aerobic *Nocardia* species (*right panel*) stain acid fast in this sputum specimen. (*From* Sullivan DC, Chapman SW. Bacteria that masquerade as fungi: actinomycosis/Nocardia. Proc Am Thorac Soc 2010;7(3):216–21; with permission.)

and chest wall.[31] Draining sinuses are common. *Nocardia* infections in lung transplant recipients is an increasing problem[32] and an outbreak of sternal wound infections occurred among open heart surgical patients, which was transmitted by a team member.[33]

Because these organisms mimic both tuberculosis and other chronic fungal infections, a combination of microbiologic, pathologic, and molecular studies may be required for definitive diagnosis, best done by isolation and identification of the organism from the patient's tissue. The presence of sulfur granules in cavities is characteristic but not sufficient for absolute diagnosis of actinomycosis. Clinical suspicion for *Actinomyces* species or *Nocardia* should be raised by the identification of gram-positive beaded branching bacilli, but a Ziehl Neelsen stain (**Fig. 8**) distinguishes between acid-fast *Nocardia* species from non–acid-fast *Actinomyces* species.[30]

Medical Management

Antimicrobial therapy is necessary for infections involving both bacteria. *Actinomyces* species, except for rare isolates of *Actinomyces israelii*, remain susceptible to penicillins and extended spectrum penicillins, cephalosporins, clindamycin, carbapenems, and tetracycline. *Nocardia* species are generally susceptible to trimethoprim sulfamethoxazole, but resistance is reported in *Nocardia farcinica* and other newly identified species.[30]

Surgical Management

In both types of infections, surgical management may be necessary. In a recent study of 40 patients with actinomycosis, more than 40% required surgical resection.[34] However, the indication for resection is changing. In 1996, Rizzi and colleagues[35] reported of 13 patients who required resection. Among the indications, 46% were for hemoptysis, 15% for drug resistance, 23% for an undefined mass, and 15% for a combination of hemoptysis and resistance. In 2010, Song and colleagues[34] reported on 40 patients with actinomycosis; 23 underwent operation. Among these patients, 45% had a lung lesion. Hemoptysis was the second most common indication, followed by failure of antimicrobial therapy. In both series, results were excellent for the surgically treated group. Although some patients were not treated with antibiotics before surgery because the establishment of the diagnosis of actinomycosis was not made before surgery, all patients were treated after surgery with antibiotics.

An illustrative case of a 53-year-old smoker who presented with massive hemoptysis and a large lower lobe cavity is shown in **Fig. 9**. After stabilization, he underwent a bilobectomy with reinforcement of the resected bronchus. Pathologic evaluation showed *Actinomyces*.

The need for surgical intervention in nocardiasis is less common but the conditions requiring operative intervention are more complex. Some of the cases begin as complications of surgical site infections that require further surgical debridement. In a case of mediastinitis with superior vena cava syndrome, pericardiectomy was required.[36]

SUMMARY

Fungal organisms remain important human and veterinary pathogens causing a wide variety of chest problems. Although some fungal infections are best managed with antimicrobials, other infections and their complications also require surgical management. One of the main problems is the indeterminate nodule. Using a combination of careful history and radiologic guidelines, this problem now requires less surgical participation. Certain fungal infections produce life-threatening complications and advanced disease may require surgical management. These operations may be among the most challenging a thoracic surgeon may face.

REFERENCES

1. Kauffman CA. Histoplasmosis. Clin Chest Med 2009; 30(2):217–25, v.

2. Deppe GS, Gibbons RS. Interleukins 17 and 23 Influence the host response to *Histoplasma capsulatum*. J Infect Dis 2009;200(1):142–51.

3. Kauffman CA. Histoplasmosis: a clinical and laboratory update. Clin Microbiol Rev 2007;20(1):115–32.

4. Bracca A, Tosello ME, Girardini JE, et al. Molecular detection of *Histoplasma capsulatum* var. *capsulatum* in human clinical samples. J Clin Microbiol 2003;41:1753–5.

5. Wheat LJ, Freifeld AG, Kleiman MB, et al. Clinical practice guidelines for the management of patients with histoplasmosis: 2007 update by the Infectious Diseases Society of America. Clin Infect Dis 2007; 45(7):807–25.

6. Starnes SL, Reed MF, Meyer CA, et al. Can lung cancer screening by computed tomography be effective in areas with endemic histoplasmosis? J Thorac Cardiovasc Surg 2011;141(3):688–93.

7. Kelley WA. Broncholithiasis: current concepts of an ancient disease. Postgrad Med 1979;66(3):81–6, 88, 90.

8. Cole FH, Cole FH Jr, Khandekar A, et al. Management of broncholithiasis: is thoracotomy necessary? Ann Thorac Surg 1986;42(3):255–7.

9. Hammoud ZT, Rose AS, Hage CA, et al. Surgical management of pulmonary and mediastinal sequelae of histoplasmosis: a challenging spectrum. Ann Thorac Surg 2009;88(2):399–403.

10. Peikert T, Colby TV, Midthun DE, et al. Fibrosing mediastinitis: clinical presentation, therapeutic outcomes, and adaptive immune response. Medicine (Baltimore) 2011;90(6):412–23.

11. Chapman SW, Lin AC, Hendricks KA, et al. Endemic blastomycosis in Mississippi: epidemiological and clinical studies. Semin Respir Infect 1997;12(3): 219–28.

12. Limper AH, Knox KS, Sarosi GA, et al. American Thoracic Society Fungal Working Group. An official American Thoracic Society statement: treatment of fungal infections in adult pulmonary and critical care patients. Am J Respir Crit Care Med 2011; 183(1):96–128.

13. Reyes CV. Cutaneous tumefaction in empyema necessitatis. Int J Dermatol 2007;46(12):1294–7.

14. Patel AJ, Gattuso P, Reddy VB. Diagnosis of blastomycosis in surgical pathology and cytopathology: correlation with microbiologic culture. Am J Surg Pathol 2010;34(2):256–61.

15. Chapman SW, Dismukes WE, Proia LA, et al. Infectious Diseases Society of America. Clinical practice guidelines for the management of blastomycosis: 2008 update by the Infectious Diseases Society of America. Clin Infect Dis 2008;46(12): 1801–12.

16. Wiesman IM, Podbielski FJ, Hernan MJ, et al. Thoracic blastomycosis and empyema. JSLS 1999; 3(1):75–8.

17. Jaroszewski DE, Halabi WJ, Blair JE, et al. Surgery for pulmonary coccidioidomycosis: a 10-year experience. Ann Thorac Surg 2009;88(6):1765–72.

18. Silvana dos Santos S, Ferreira KS, Almeida SR. *Paracoccidioides brasilinsis*-induced migration of dendritic cells and subsequent T-cell activation in the lung-draining lymph nodes. PLoS One 2011; 6(5):e19690.

19. Simon CY, Castro CN, Romero GA. Thoracic adenomegaly as the predominant manifestation of paracoccidioidomycosis. Rev Soc Bras Med Trop 2005; 38(5):448–9.

20. Barreto MM, Marchiori E, Amorim VB, et al. Thoracic paracoccidioidomycosis: radiographic and CT findings. Radiographics 2012;32(1):71–84.

21. Walsh SLF, Roberton BJ. The atoll sign. Thorax 2010;65:1029–30.

22. Dewar GJ, Kelly JK. *Cryptococcus gattii*: an emerging cause of pulmonary nodules. Can Respir J 2008;15(3):153–8.

23. Kurahara Y, Tachibana K, Katsura H, et al. [A case of cryptococcal empyema successfully treated by debridement by medical thoracoscopy with local anesthesia]. Nihon Kokyuki Gakkai Zasshi 2011; 49(2):142–7 [in Japanese].

24. Palomino J, Saeed O, Daroca P, et al. 47-year-old man with cough, dyspnea, and an abnormal chest radiograph. Chest 2009;135:872–5.

25. Baradkar VP, Mathur M, Kulkarni SD, et al. Thoracic empyema due to *Candida albicans*. Indian J Pathol Microbiol 2008;51(2):286–8.

26. Chuang TY, Yeh CY, Ko SW, et al. Fatal case of community-acquired empyema thoracis and candidemia caused by *Candida albicans*. Diagn Microbiol Infect Dis 2011;71(2):156–8.

27. Dot JM, Debourgogne A, Champigneulle J, et al. Molecular diagnosis of disseminated adiaspiromycosis due to *Emmonsia crescens*. J Clin Microbiol 2009;47(4):1269–73.

28. Sullivan DC, Chapman SW. Bacteria that masquerade as fungi: actinomycosis/*Nocardia*. Proc Am Thorac Soc 2010;7(3):216–21.

29. Mabeza GF, Macfarlane J. Pulmonary actinomycosis. Eur Respir J 2003;21:545–51.

30. Yildiz O, Doganay M. Actinomycoses and *Nocardia* pulmonary infections. Curr Opin Pulm Med 2006;12: 228–34.

31. Kroe DM, Shulman N, Kirsch CM, et al. An anterior mediastinal mass with draining sternal sinus tracts due to *Nocardia braziliensis*. West J Med 1997;167(1):47–9.

32. Poonyagariyagorn HK, Gershman A, Avery R, et al. Challenges in the diagnosis and management of *Nocardia* infections in lung transplant recipients. Transpl Infect Dis 2008;10(6):403–8.

33. Wenger PN, Brown JM, McNeil MM, et al. *Nocardia farcinica* sternotomy site infections in patients following open heart surgery. J Infect Dis 1998; 178:1539–43.

34. Song JU, Park HY, Jeon K, et al. Treatment of thoracic actinomycosis: a retrospective analysis of 40 patients. Ann Thorac Med 2010;5(2):80–5.

35. Rizzi A, Rocco G, Della Pona C, et al. Pulmonary actinomycosis: surgical considerations. Monaldi Arch Chest Dis 1996;51(5):369–72.

36. Abdelkafi S, Dubail D, Bosschaerts T, et al. Superior vena cava syndrome associated with *Nocardia farcinica* infection. Thorax 1997;52(5): 492–3.

Surgical Management for Hydatid Disease

Semih Halezeroglu, MD, FETCS[a],*, Erdal Okur, MD[b],
M. Ozan Tanyü, MD[c]

KEYWORDS

- Hydatid disease • Echinococcosis • Lung • Treatment • Surgery • VATS

KEY POINTS

- Hydatid disease is a parasitic infection caused by the *Echinococcus* family. It characterizes with cystic lesions located mainly in liver and the lungs.
- Diagnosis of a pulmonary cystic lesion in a patient who is living or has lived in an endemic area where hydatid disease is relatively common can be done by radiological findings and serologic tests.
- Although medical treatment with albendazole has promising results, surgical excision of the cyst by a parenchyma-saving operation remains the method of choice for most patients.
- Postoperative mortality can be related to an unrecognized cyst located in the brain or major vessels instead of the operation itself. For this reason, brain and mediastinal contrast-enhanced CT scans should be done in all patients with multiple hydatid cysts.

Hydatid disease is a parasitic infection caused by *Echinococcus*, a cestode of the Taeniidae family. It is characterized by cystic lesions occurring in different parts of the human body. The lung is second only to the liver as the main affected organ. Although not frequently, cysts can also be detected in the kidneys, brain, heart, soft tissues, and bones, along with intravascular lodgment. The disease is common in animal-raising regions and poses a significant public health problem in many areas worldwide.

THE PARASITE

Echinococcus is made up of a specialized attachment structure, the scolex, which contains a hook and several suckers, a neck, and two to six reproductive segments. The parasite is only a few millimeters long, rarely more than 7 mm. Among the four types of *Echinococcus*, *E granulosus* is the most common in humans. In addition, the rarely found *E multilocularis (alveolaris)* is responsible for the more disseminated form named alveolar hydatid disease. *E vogeli* and *E oligharthrus*, the causes of polycystic echinococcosis, are rare pathogens found only in Central and South America.[1]

In this article, only hydatid disease caused by *E granulosus* is discussed.

EPIDEMIOLOGY

The World Health Organization reports that *E granulosus* has a worldwide geographic distribution and it may occur in countries all over the world.[2] A high parasite prevalence is found in areas of Europe and Asia, including the Balkan and Mediterranean

All the authors of this paper declare no conflict of interest.
[a] Thoracic Surgery Department, Faculty of Medicine, Acibadem University, Acibadem Maslak Hospital, Buyukdere Cad, 34457 Istanbul, Turkey; [b] Thoracic Surgery Department, Faculty of Medicine, Acibadem University, Acibadem Bakirkoy Hospital, Halit Ziya Uşaklıgil Cad. 1 Bakırköy, 34140 Istanbul, Turkey; [c] Radiology Department, Acik MR Radiology Center, Abdi İpekci Cad. 40/1, Nisantasi, 34367 Istanbul, Turkey
* Corresponding author.
E-mail address: semihh@atlas.net.tr

regions, the Russian Federation and adjacent independent states, and in China. Also, the disease is observed in Australia and South America; whereas prevalence in up to 3% of the population has been reported in northern and eastern Africa where *E granulosus* is highly endemic.[2] Occurrence is sporadic in other regions including northern and central Europe and North America.

PATHOGENESIS

Echinococcosis is a cyclozoonosis, which means that it requires two vertebrate hosts to support its life cycle. The primary host is generally a dog, wolf, or other carnivore (except for cat). The parasite lives in the intestines of the primary host. After a disruption in the intestines, parasitic eggs are released into the environment via feces. The egg-carrying embryos can survive 1 week in water or up to 1 year in soil. The intermediate hosts, which are sheep, cattle, horses, goats, deer, pigs, elks, and so forth, ingest infected grass or vegetables or drink infected water and become infested. Embryos are released from the eggs and, by their hooklets, attach to and penetrate the duodenal or jejunal wall of the intermediate host. They are then brought to the liver via portal circulation. Most of the parasitic embryos are embedded in liver sinusoids but some can bypass them and, through the hepatic vein and inferior vena cava, enter the right heart and, finally, the lungs. Others enter the systemic circulation and disseminate to other organs such as spleen, brain, kidneys, and so forth.

Another pathway to the lung is also thought to exist. Embryos can proceed through the intestinal lymphatics into the thoracic duct and then to the right heart, finally reaching the lung. If a primary host eats infected viscera of the intermediate host, the cycle continues.

DISEASE IN HUMANS

Humans can be infested accidentally and become intermediate hosts as well. Because most of the embryos were captured in its sinusoids, the liver is the organ most commonly infected—between two to eight times more often than the lung.[3,4] An asymptomatic cyst is more commonly found in the liver than in the lung. In most reported series, the lower lobes of both lungs are affected more often than the upper lobes.[5–7]

In general, the cysts are solitary (**Fig. 1**), but some may be bilateral (**Fig. 2**), concomitantly locating in the lung and liver (**Fig. 3**), or multiple (**Fig. 4**). When the embryo has settled into an organ, the second larval stage begins. The natural

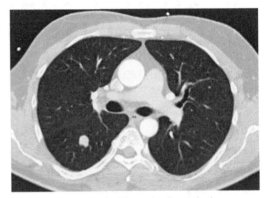

Fig. 1. A solitary hydatid cyst in the right lung.

course is the progressive growth of the cyst over a long period of time, but sometimes it may remain static.[8,9]

The growth rate of the hydatid cyst varies in different organs. Tissue elasticity probably plays a major role in limiting the growth rate. Growth in soft organs is faster than in dense organs. There is evidence that liver cysts grow at a lower rate than lung cysts.[10,11] Negative intrathoracic pressure may result in rapid growth of a lung cyst, whereas the compact tissue and hepatobiliary capsules in the liver probably limit its growth.[12] In a child's lung, the hydatid cyst can probably develop more rapidly than in an adult's lung and grow to unusual size.[11]

THE CYST

A hydatid cyst (**Fig. 5A, B**) consists of a three-layered wall and fluid inside. The cyst fluid is clear, colorless, odorless, and sterile. Electrolyte level and pH are similar to that of the host's serum. The germinal membrane, also called the endocyst, is the innermost layer. It is the living part of the parasite and produces scolices and daughter

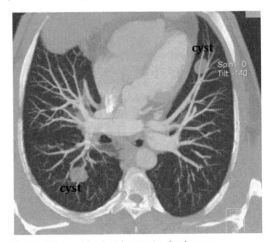

Fig. 2. Bilateral hydatid cysts in the lungs.

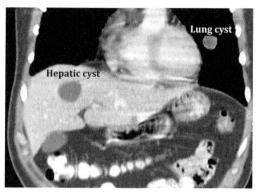

Fig. 3. Concomitant hydatid cysts in the liver and the left lung.

vesicles by budding through its inner surface. They may be a few millimeters to centimeters in size and may be multiple.

The germinal membrane is responsible for production of the outer layer, the laminated membrane. The laminated membrane, also called the ectocyst, is a protective barrier for the cyst. It is a thin (1–3 mm), relatively transparent, acellular membrane. When the laminated membrane is disrupted, the osmotic balance within the cyst is disturbed and the cyst ruptures. The laminated membrane has no adhesion to the outer layer, the adventitia, and can easily be separated during surgery.

The adventitia, also called the pericyst, is not a component of the parasite, but represents the host's reaction to the parasite. When the parasite is settled in the viscera, because of a local immune reaction, inflammatory cells are collected. Fibroblasts later replace these inflammatory cells and the host's viscera form a fibrinous layer around the cyst.

Signs and Symptoms

There are no symptoms indicating the presence of a small, intact cyst. Clinical symptoms are related

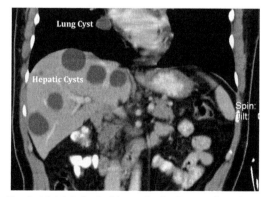

Fig. 4. Multiple hydatid cysts in the liver and a solitary hydatid cyst in the right lung.

mostly either to the increasing size of the cyst and its pressure over the lung, bronchus, or (rarely) major vessels, or to the occurrence of complications such as infection or rupture.

Cough is the major symptom (52%–62%)[6,11] and may be due to irritation of the bronchus by the enlarging cyst or rupture of the cyst into the bronchus. A giant cyst (diameter >10 cm) may cause dyspnea or even chest wall asymmetry in a child.

In most patients the clinical course is mild and patients present with symptoms such as fever, malaise, pruritus, and urticaria. Empyema and pneumothorax may also be seen. Aribas and colleagues[13] reported hepatopleural and hepatobronchial fistulas as late sequelae of cyst ruptures. Balci and colleagues[14] reported a 4.7% mortality rate after rupture. Rupture of the cyst into a pulmonary vessel and pulmonary embolism are rare but devastating complications and may lead to death or severe chronic pulmonary hypertension.[15,16] Rupture of a hydatid cyst, into bronchus, pleura, or vessel, may result in dissemination of the disease. In cases of involvement of other organs (eg, brain, liver, bone), symptoms specific to these organs (convulsions, increased intracranial pressure, pathologic bone fracture, and jaundice) can also be seen.

Rupture of the cyst is reported to occur in 34% to 64% of the patients.[17,18] Rupture may occur spontaneously or during coughing, sneezing, or because of a blunt chest trauma. Iatrogenic rupture during needle aspiration may also occur. A giant cyst is expected to rupture more easily. The rupture may be contained within the pericyst or drained into a bronchus. Massive drainage of cyst fluid into the bronchus may cause severe anaphylaxis, aspiration, suffocation, or even death.[19,20] Pieces of cyst membrane may be expectorated (hydatoptysis). Spontaneous healing is theoretically possible if one expectorates the whole cyst membrane. Hemoptysis may occur owing to rupture of the cyst, but massive bleeding is very rare. Suppuration of the cyst after rupture may also occur. In this situation, the patient expectorates purulent sputum and may have fever and leukocytosis.

A lung abscess can develop in the cyst cavity. The cyst may rupture into the pleural space leading to severe chest pain, dyspnea, cough, and cyanosis in acute cases. A tension pneumothorax maybe seen when an air leak occurs in the lung.[21]

Diagnosis

History of animal contact (especially dogs) and living in a sheep-raising or cattle-raising rural area is generally present. History of travel to an

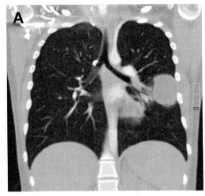
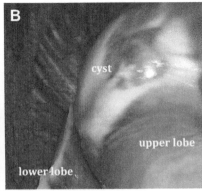

Fig. 5. (*A*) A hydatid cyst in the left upper lobe. (*B*) Intraoperative appearance of a hydatid cyst in the left upper lobe.

endemic region should also be considered in a patient with cystic lesions. Expectoration of a bolus of fluid together with a membrane is very specific for hydatid disease. Patient may not report this symptom unless asked specifically. Physical examination generally does not show any specific sign of the disease.

Imaging

Chest radiograph

A plain radiograph of the chest usually shows pathologic findings (**Fig. 6**). An unruptured cyst appears as a spherical, well-circumscribed, homogenous opacity. Its size may vary from a few centimeters to 20 cm. The shape of the lesion changes from spherical to oval during forced deep inhalation and exhalation (Escudero-Nemerow sign).

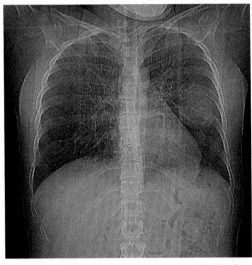

Fig. 6. A chest radiograph of a patient with a hydatid cyst in the left upper lobe.

The cyst may compress hilar bronchovascular structures, presenting radiologically as a depression or indentation, known as a notch sign, at the site of bronchovascular compression. However, presence of atelectasis or obstructive pneumonitis is rare. A small amount of air may enter the zone between the pericyst and ectocyst layers due to increased intrathoracic pressure (eg, coughing, trauma). In a radiograph, it looks like an air shadow at the top of the cyst and is known as a crescent sign, moon sign, or meniscus sign.[22] This is probably the first sign before rupture of the cyst. When air freely enters the cyst and displaces the cystic fluid after complete rupture of the laminated membrane, an air-fluid level is formed.

A cyst membrane floating on cystic water with free air above yields a classic radiologic finding known as the water-lily sign or Camelot sign. These classic radiologic signs are not always present. Actually, a complicated hydatid cyst may mimic the signs of a wide variety of pulmonary diseases, including intrathoracic tumors. Radiologically, signs of cyst complications, such as empyema, pneumothorax, lung abscess, pneumonia, and bronchial obstruction, may be observed. Numerous unusual radiologic findings have been reviewed by Turgut and colleagues[23] and by Kilic and colleagues.[24]

Ultrasound scanning helps to differentiate the cystic nature of the lesion from solid masses and represents a useful tool to diagnose a coexisting liver cyst.

CT scan

This is the mainstay of diagnosis in a patient with an appropriate history. If the cyst is intact, a CT scan with contrast enhancement may demonstrate a thin enhancing rim. It can also elucidate the cystic nature of the lung mass. Classically, an intact cyst is a round, small opacity (**Fig. 7**). However, a different

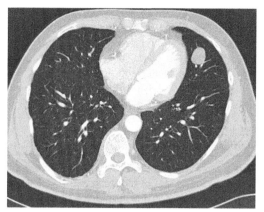

Fig. 7. A CT scan of a round, small, intact hydatid cyst in the lingual segment of left upper lobe.

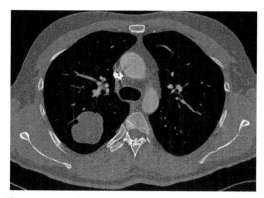

Fig. 9. An indentation is seen in the margin of hydatid cyst in the right upper lobe.

contour of a pulmonary cystic lesion does not rule out a hydatid cyst (**Figs. 8** and **9**). The content of intact cysts is homogenous, with a density close to that of water (**Fig. 10**).[25]

A ruptured cyst in the lung may mimic lung abscess; however, lacking of adjacent pulmonary infiltration in hydatid cyst differentiates it from an abscess (**Fig. 11**). CT is able to show additional small ipsilateral or contralateral cysts, often not visible on plain radiographs. The daughter cysts attached to the endocyst or lying free within the main cyst may also be noticed. In addition, an increase in the CT density of the lung mass and/or a thick wall should not negate a diagnosis of hydatid disease.[26]

MRI

On MRI, cysts show low-signal intensity on T1-weighted images and high-signal intensity on T2-weighted images.[27] The magnetic resonance signal characteristics of a hydatid cyst may differ depending on the developmental phase, that is, whether it is unilocular or multilocular, and whether the cyst is viable, infected, or dead. Information regarding reactive changes in the host tissue, capsule, and signal intensity of parent and daughter cysts is also obtained.[28]

In general, MRI is not used in defining a lung hydatid cyst. However, fistulization of a hydatid cyst located on the liver dome through the transdiaphragmatic way to the pleural cavity can be visualized perfectly by MRI view (**Fig. 12**A, B).

Laboratory tests

Blood eosinophilia is reported to occur in 20% to 34% of patients.[4] It is a nonspecific sign because it may be seen in numerous other pathologies. A higher rate of eosinophilia was found in patients with a ruptured cyst.[8]

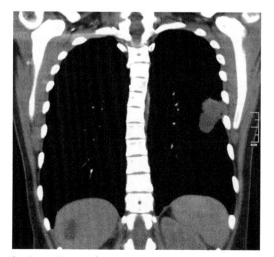

Fig. 8. A CT scan of an intact, cylindrical cyst in the left upper lobe.

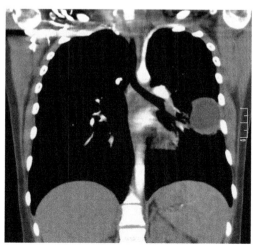

Fig. 10. The fluid density is recognized within the cyst in the left upper lobe.

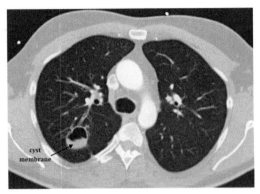

Fig. 11. A ruptured hydatid cyst in the right upper lobe. The cyst membrane is floating in the fluid.

The Casoni intradermal skin test, Weinberg complement fixation (CF) test, indirect hemagglutination (IHA) test, ELISA, and Western blot (WB) are the commonly used laboratory tests for diagnosis of hydatid disease. Akisu and colleagues[29] reported the overall sensitivity of the IHA, ELISA and WB tests used for the serodiagnosis of pulmonary hydatid disease as 96.7%, 87.1%, and 100%, respectively, and the specificities were 82.2%, 89.2%, and 85.7%, respectively. Wattal and colleagues[30] compared the results of the Casoni, IHA, and ELISA tests in 46 patients with surgically proved hydatid disease. Positive test results were found in 29 (63%), 32 (70%), and 46 (100%) patients. They concluded that the ELISA is highly sensitive and specific in detecting anti-Echinococcus antibodies in the serum of patients with hydatidosis. Chemtai and colleagues[31] analyzed 141 surgically proven cases in Africa and found an overall sensitivity of 86% for IHA and 63% for the CF test. Another study by Sbihi and colleagues[32] reported high sensitivity (93.5%), specificity (89.7%), and diagnostic efficacy (92.3%) for a specific ELISA test.

Patients with a liver cyst are reported to have a higher rate of serologic test sensitivity than those with lung cysts.[30,33] Among the several laboratory tests, ELISA and IHA seem most valuable, but a negative test should never preclude the possibility of a hydatid cyst. These tests are complementary to clinical and radiologic findings. Serologic tests can also be used in the follow-up of patients after surgical resection.[34,35]

TREATMENT
Medical Treatment

Medical treatment with benzimidazole compound, either mebendazole or albendazole, certainly has an important role in the treatment of pulmonary hydatid disease. Albendazole is known to be more effective than mebendazole.[36] Saimot[37] studied the pharmacokinetics of albendazole and reported good penetration of the drug into the liver cyst. Keshmiri and colleagues[38] reported good therapeutic results in pulmonary hydatidosis (57.7%–91% cure rate) by albendazole treatment. Dogru and colleagues[39] suggested that selected pediatric patients with uncomplicated pulmonary cysts smaller than 5 cm should have a trial of medical treatment with close follow-up. A standard dose of albendazole is 10 to 15 mg/kg/d (taken twice daily). Owing to its hepatotoxicity, a 1-week to 2-week interval should be given between 3-week and 4-week cycles and treatment may last 3 to 6 months.

The cyst may be disrupted by medical therapy, but the remaining membranes in the cavity may cause infection.[40,41] More severe complications were reported to have occurred during medical treatment, including perforation, anaphylactic shock, and expectoration of the cyst membrane.[42]

Surgical Treatment

General principles of the operation
The aim of surgery in pulmonary hydatid cyst is to remove the cyst completely while preserving the lung tissue as much as possible.[6,7,11,12,43] Lung

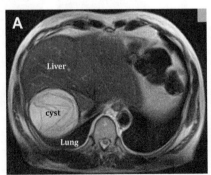
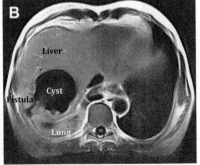

Fig. 12. (A) MRI of a hydatid cyst in the subdiaphragmatic area. (B) This MRI shows the fistulization of a subdiaphragmatic hydatid cyst into the right pleural cavity by perforating the diaphragm.

resection is performed only if there is an irreversible and disseminated pulmonary destruction. Careful manipulation of the cyst and adherence to the precaution to avoid the contamination of the operative field with the cyst content is the imperative part of the operation. The cysts located on the liver dome are easily accessible and resected via right thoracotomy with the transdiaphragmatic approach.

The surgical approach is determined depending on whether

- the cyst is intact or ruptured
- the cyst is single or multiple
- the cyst is unilateral or bilateral or together with a liver dome cyst
- the size of the cyst
- associated destruction of lung parenchyma.

Rupture of a cyst and aspiration of cyst fluid and membrane during operation may cause severe problems, such as obstruction of the contralateral bronchus, anaphylaxis, or parasitic dissemination. Intubation with a double-lumen tube is vitally important to protect the contralateral lung. For this reason, the anesthesiologists should be informed preoperatively about the possibility of such a complication.

Pulmonary hydatid cyst surgery can be performed by an open technique, such as thoracotomy or median sternotomy (for bilateral cases), or an endoscopic technique with videothoracoscopy.

Operative steps that were prepared by the first author (SH) of this paper can be watched on *Multimedia Manual of Cardiothoracic Surgery* (www.mmcts.org).[43]

Open Technique

Surgical technique for intact cyst: needle aspiration

The needle aspiration method entails no risk of cyst rupture or contamination of pleura. However, a small leak may occur when the needle punctures the cyst. On opening of the chest, the hydatid cyst is generally easily noticed with its white-gray pericystic extension to the visceral pleural surface of the lung. Rarely, the cyst is located entirely within the lung parenchyma and cannot be seen but only felt by light palpation. To prevent contamination of the pleura, a few towels soaked in povidone-iodine solution are placed around the cyst.[43] The authors have developed an apparatus consisting of a medium-sized needle placed on a 40 to 50 cm catheter that is connected to a three-way stopcock.[43] A 20 mL or 50 mL syringe is connected to one end and a 20 cm catheter connected to the other end of the stopcock. One or two well-

functioning suction devices should be prepared and directed toward the cyst surface near the puncture site. After puncturing the cyst with the needle, cyst fluid is aspirated into the syringe in a controlled way and then directed to the other catheter with the help of the three-way stopcock. Because the syringe and catheters are outside the chest cavity, there is no risk of contamination. After most of the cyst fluid is aspirated, the free end of the short catheter is immersed in povidone-iodine solution and aspirated povidone-iodine is directed to the cyst cavity exactly the inverse of aspiration procedure. After the cyst is almost filled with povidone-iodine solution, there is a wait of a few minutes to allow the scolicidal agent to take effect. Then the pericyst is incised with scissors and the fluid within the cyst is aspirated. If daughter cysts are present, they are also aspirated completely and the whole cyst membrane is taken out after being grasped with 1 or 2 ringed forceps (**Fig. 13**). The remaining cavity is irrigated with an isotonic saline solution to locate bronchial air leaks.[43] The air leaks, if present, are obliterated with absorbable sutures. To create a wide opening, a partial pericystectomy is performed by resecting the white, avascular, pericystic area on the visceral pleural surface. Either electrocautery or a tissue-sealing instrument may be used for this purpose. After checking for bronchial and parenchymal air leaks once more, the cyst cavity is either left open or closed by approximating sutures within the cavity (capitonnage) is performed (see later discussion).[11,43] Scolicidal solutions other than povidone-iodine, such as formaldehyde or hypertonic saline, may be used.[21] All preparations may have similar side effects, such as irritation of lung parenchyma and pulmonary edema. The ideal scolicidal agent has not yet been, and needs to be, ascertained.

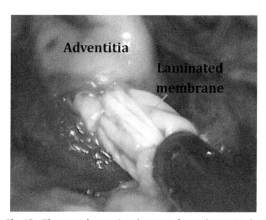

Fig 13. The membrane is taken out from the cavity by an aspirator.

Surgical technique for intact cyst: enucleation

In this method, the intact cyst is delivered without being punctured. It is technically a demanding procedure and suitable only for relatively small cysts because larger cysts have a higher risk of rupture during delivery. The patient is prepared in the manner described above. Povidone-iodine–soaked towels are placed at the periphery of the cyst surface. An incision is carefully made over the adventitial layer of the cyst and the underlying white-colored laminated membrane is observed.[43] The laminated membrane is totally free of adhesions to the adventitia and the plane in between is easily dissected. The lung is inflated minimally in order not to increase the pressure exerted on the cyst. Forceps grasp both edges of the adventitial layer and the incision on the adventitial layer is extended in four directions so as to be almost equal to the cyst diameter. The anesthesiologist is then asked to forcefully inflate the lung. The inflated lung pushes the cyst out of its adventitial covering and the cyst is delivered. During the procedure the laminated membrane is not grasped with any kind of forceps and should be manipulated gently to avoid rupture. The remaining cyst cavity (**Fig. 14**) is irrigated with isotonic saline solutions and air leaks are obliterated as described above. The remaining cyst cavity is either obliterated with capitonnage or left as it is. In this context, the authors prefer the enucleation method for small cysts.

Obliteration of the cyst cavity: capitonnage

The term capitonnage is used for a method of obliterating the remaining cyst cavity (**Fig. 15**).

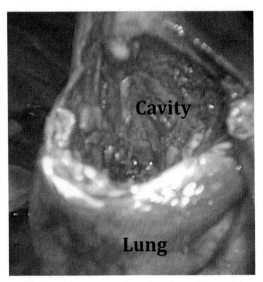

Fig 14. The cyst cavity after cleaning with povidone iodine.

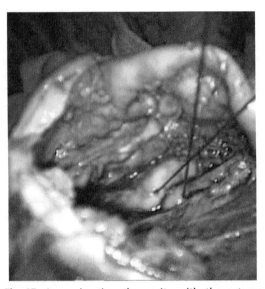

Fig 15. Approximating the cavity with the sutures from within the cavity. This closes the bronchial openings and obliterates the space.

After checking for air leaks in the cyst cavity, apposition of cyst walls is done by direct suturing. As already described, separate absorbable sutures are used and a few rows of sutures may be needed, depending on the size of the cavity.[43] The need for obliteration of the remaining cyst cavity is debatable. Some investigators suggest that the capitonnage of pulmonary hydatid cysts is necessary because it reduces morbidity (especially prolonged air leakage) and hospital length-of-stay.[44,45] Conversely, some investigators claim that capitonnage provides no advantage in operations for pulmonary hydatid cysts.[46] In most large series in the literature, the capitonnage method was used and suggested for most resected hydatid cysts.[11,43,47,48]

Resection of a complicated cyst

A hydatid cyst may rupture into a bronchus or into the pleural cavity. Infection may develop within the remaining cyst cavity owing to contamination through bronchial orifices. When a cyst cavity is infected, parasites within the cavity die, but an abscess may develop within the cavity. The cyst membrane, however, may cause obstruction of the bronchus and obstructive pneumonia may develop. Parenchymal destruction and fibrosis of neighboring lung tissue may be observed in chronic cases.

When destruction and fibrosis are not severe, simple cystectomy, obliteration of the bronchial opening by sutures, and irrigation of the cyst cavity are enough to treat a ruptured cyst. In cases of lung destruction, a wide-wedge resection or a lobectomy may be needed.[17] An attempt should be made to preserve as much lung parenchyma as possible; this endeavor is successful in most cases, as reported in the literature.[47,48] The lobectomy rate in complicated hydatid cysts is reported to be much higher than for uncomplicated ones.[21] Rupture of the cyst into the pleura may lead to hydrothorax or sometimes to hydropneumothorax. An empyema may develop because of contamination of the pleural space, which leads to pleural thickening and lung entrapment. In such a case, decortication may be needed in addition to cystectomy and capitonnage.

Resection of multiple hydatid cysts

There may be unilateral or bilateral multiple hydatid cysts. A patient with a bilateral pulmonary hydatid cyst may undergo a median sternotomy or staged thoracotomies.[49] If the bilateral approach is chosen, the side on which to operate first must be considered. If there is an intact cyst on one side, and a ruptured cyst on the other, the side of the intact cyst should be operated on first to prevent its rupture. In cases of an intact cyst on both sides, the side having a bigger cyst or having more cysts is done first. In cases when there is, simultaneously, a cyst in the right lung and in the upper dome of the liver, a one-stage operation by right thoracotomy and phrenicotomy and resection of the cysts in both organs may be a good approach.[40]

Video-Assisted Thoracic Surgery for Pulmonary Hydatid Cyst

Videothoracoscopic resection of a hydatid cyst was reported to have been safely performed in selected patients.[50,51] A ruptured cyst, as it poses no risk of contamination, may be a good candidate for video-assisted thoracic surgery (VATS) resection. An intact pulmonary hydatid cyst can also be resected by a VATS approach; however, a certain level of experience with thoracoscopic procedures is necessary to avoid postoperative complications such as prolonged air leak or recurrence.

Percutaneous therapy, which was used for selected liver hydatid cysts, is not advised for pulmonary hydatid disease because of the high risk of rupture and contamination.

Transthoracic-Transdiaphragmatic Approach to the Subdiaphragmatic Hydatid Cysts

Not infrequently, thoracic surgeons are asked for the management of hydatid cysts located at the upper part (subdiaphragmatic location) of the liver. A thoracotomy provides better exploration and access to the cyst located in this area when compared with the laparotomy.

The principal of the resection of liver cyst is similar to that of the pulmonary cyst; however, there are important technical differences between the two operations. The hepatic cysts contain daughter vesicles more commonly than the pulmonary cysts.[43] For this reason, a scolicidal agent (to kill the parasite) such as hypertonic saline solution or 10% povidone iodine must be injected through the diaphragm into the cyst to prevent the spreading of the living vesicles in the abdomen or thorax before the opening and removal of the cyst. The diaphragm is cut using a scissors and its muscle is separated from the cyst by blunt and sharp dissections with no pressure over the cyst. When the intracystic pressure has been lowered, the cyst is opened from the uppermost part of the cyst and its content is aspirated by a large-holed suction device.

Technique

Povidone iodine is injected into the cyst through the diaphragm located on the liver dome. Diaphragm muscle is cut by a scissors and the muscle is dissected from the cyst. Then the cyst is opened, a suction device aspirates the content and a grasper takes out the membranes from the cavity. Because the cyst contains numerous daughter vesicles that are not technically possible to aspirate with a suction device or take out by a grasper, a spoon is used to completely evacuate the cavity.

After the diaphragm is incised enough to evacuate the cyst completely, the content that contains daughter vesicles is removed with a sterile spoon. The cavity remaining between the upper surface of the liver and the fibrous pericyst is cleaned with the gauze steeped in povidone iodine. A rubber tube is inserted into the cavity and taken out from the skin under the diaphragm. Finally, the edges of the fibrous capsule of the cyst are closed with mattress sutures.

SUMMARY

The prognosis after resection of hydatid cysts is excellent:

- Postoperative complication rate is 0.8% to 4% for the intact cysts and 4% to 6% for the ruptured cysts.[5–7,11,12] The most common postoperative complications are prolonged air leak, empyema, and pneumonia due to the aspiration of cystic content or washing solution through an open bronchus adjacent to the cyst.
- The overall mortality rate is lower than 1% for intact cysts and about 2% for complicated cysts. The mortality rate is closely related to the presence of unrecognized

cysts in the central nervous system or in the proximal part of the pulmonary artery. The size of the cyst is another factor that may be associated with an increased complication rate.

- The CNS and the pulmonary arteries must be evaluated before surgical attempt is made in every case with disseminated hydatidosis.
- Recurrence rate is between 1% and 6%. Adherence to the precaution to avoid spreading of the cystic material and the use of albendazole in selected patients decreases the recurrence rate. Recurrence may be seen 15 to 18 years after first resection.[7,51] Arinc and colleagues[52] reported that 7 of 10 recurrences were in a different location in the lung and one patient needed a pneumonectomy and another needed a lobectomy. Two recurrences were observed out of 10 patients (20%) in their series.
- Pulmonary resection (ie, lobectomy) is necessary in less than 10% of the patients.[11,17,43]

REFERENCES

1. D'Alessandro A. Polycystic echinococcosis in tropical America: *Echinococcus vogeli* and *E. oligarthrus*. Acta Trop 1997;67(1-2):43–65.
2. Eckert J, Schantz PM, Gasser RB, et al. Geographic distribution and prevalence. In: Eckert J, Gemmell MA, Meslin FX, et al, editors. World Health Organization (WHO)/World Organization for Animal Health (Office International des Epizooties) (OIE) Manual on Echinococcosis in Humans and Animals: a Public Health Problem of Global Concern. Paris: World Organisation for Animal Health; 2002. p. 101–43.
3. Ahmadi NA, Hamidi M. A retrospective analysis of human cystic echinococcosis in Hamedan province, an endemic region of Iran. Ann Trop Med Parasitol 2008;102(7):603–9.
4. Eckert J, Deplazes P. Biological, epidemiological, and clinical aspects of echinococcosis, a zoonosis of increasing concern. Clin Microbiol Rev 2004;17:107–35.
5. Dakak M, Genç O, Gurkok S, et al. Surgical treatment for pulmonary hydatidosis (a review of 422 cases). J R Coll Surg Edinb 2002;47:689–92.
6. Dogan R, Yuksel M, Cetin G, et al. Surgical treatment of hydatid cysts of the lung: report on 1055 patients. Thorax 1989;44:192–9.
7. Burgos R, Varela A, Castedo E, et al. Pulmonary hydatidosis: surgical treatment and follow-up of 240 cases. Eur J Cardiothorac Surg 1999;16:628–34.
8. Schantz P. Echinococcosis. In: Guerrant R, Walker DH, Weller PF, editors. Tropical infectious disease. Philadelphia: WB Saunders Company; 1999. p. 1005–25.
9. Blanton R. Pulmonary echinococcosis. Lung Biol Health Dis 1997;101:171–89.
10. Larrieu EJ, Frider B. Human cystic echinococcosis: contributions to the natural history of the disease. Ann Trop Med Parasitol 2001;95:679–87.
11. Halezeroglu S, Celik M, Uysal A, et al. Giant hydatid cysts of the lung. J Thorac Cardiovasc Surg 1997; 113:712–7.
12. Dincer SI, Demir A, Sayar A, et al. Surgical treatment of pulmonary hydatid disease: a comparison of children and adults. J Pediatr Surg 2006;41(7):1230–6.
13. Aribas OK, Kanat F, Gormus N, et al. Pleural complications of hydatid disease. J Thorac Cardiovasc Surg 2002;123:492–7.
14. Balci AE, Eren N, Eren S, et al. Ruptured hydatid cysts of the lung in children: clinical review and results of surgery. Ann Thorac Surg 2002;74:889–92.
15. Bus S, Knosalla C, Mulahasanovic S, et al. Severe chronic pulmonary hypertension caused by pulmonary embolism of hydatid cysts. Ann Thorac Surg 2007;84:2108–10.
16. Koksal C, Baysungur V, Okur E, et al. A two-stage approach to a patient with hydatid cysts inside the right pulmonary artery and multiple right lung involvement. Ann Thorac Cardiovasc Surg 2006; 12:349–51.
17. Vasquez JC, Montesinos E, Peralta J, et al. Need for lung resection in patients with ruptured hydatid cysts. Thorac Cardiovasc Surg 2009;57:295–302.
18. Topcu S, Kurul IC, Tastepe I, et al. Surgical treatment of pulmonary hydatid cysts in children. J Thorac Cardiovasc Surg 2000;120:1097–101.
19. Boots RJ. "Near drowning" due to hydatid disease. Anaesth Intensive Care 1998;26(6):680–1.
20. Fanne RA, Khamasi M, Mevorach D, et al. Spontaneous rupture of lung echinococcal cyst causing anaphylactic shock and respiratory distress syndrome. Thorax 2006;61:550.
21. Kuzucu A, Soysal O, Ozgel M, et al. Complicated hydatid diseases of the lung: clinical and therapeutic issues. Ann Thorac Surg 2004;77:1200–4.
22. Barret NR, Thomas D. Pulmonary hydatid disease. Br J Surg 1952;40:222.
23. Turgut AT, Altinok T, Topçu S, et al. Local complications of hydatid disease involving thoracic cavity: imaging findings. Eur J Radiol 2009;70(1):49–56.
24. Kilic D, Tercan F, Sahin E, et al. Unusual radiologic manifestations of the echinococcus infection in the thorax. J Thorac Imaging 2006;21(1):32–6.
25. Saksouk FA, Fahl MH, Rizk GK. Computed tomography of pulmonary hydatid disease. J Comput Assist Tomogr 1986;10:226–32.
26. Koul PA, Koul AN, Wahid A, et al. CT in pulmonary hydatid disease: unusual appearances. Chest 2000;118:1645–7.
27. Morar R, Feldman C. Pulmonary echinococcosis. Eur Resp J 2003;21:1069–77.

28. Singh S, Gibikote SV. Magnetic resonance imaging signal characteristics in hydatid cysts. Australas Radiol 2001;45:128–33.

29. Akisu C, Bayram Delibas S, Yuncu G, et al. [Evaluation of IHA, ELISA and western blot tests in diagnosis of pulmonary cystic hidatidosis]. Tuberk Toraks 2005;53(2):156–60 [in Turkish].

30. Wattal C, Malla N, Khan IA, et al. Comparative evaluation of enzyme-linked immunosorbent assay for the diagnosis of pulmonary echinococcosis. J Clin Microbiol 1986;24(1):41–6.

31. Chemtai AK, Bowry TR, Ahmad Z. Evaluation of five immunodiagnostic techniques in echinococcosis patients. Bull World Health Organ 1981;59(5):767–72.

32. Sbihi Y, Rmiqui A, Rodriguez-Cabezas MN, et al. Comparative sensitivity of six serological tests and diagnostic value of ELISA using purified antigen in hydatidosis. J Clin Lab Anal 2001;15(1):14–8.

33. Babba H, Messedi A, Masmoudi S, et al. Diagnosis of human hydatidosis: comparison between imagery and six serologic techniques. Am J Trop Med Hyg 1994;50(1):64–8.

34. Gonzalez AN, Muro A, Barrera I, et al. Usefulness of four different echinococcus granulosus recombinant antigens for serodiagnosis of unilocular hydatid disease (UHD) and postsurgical follow-up of patients treated for UHD. Clin Vaccine Immunol 2008;15:147–53.

35. Nouir NB, Nunez S, Gianiazzi C, et al. Assessment of echinococcus granulosus somatic protoscolex antigens for serological follow-up of young patients surgically treated for cystic echinococcosis. J Clin Microbiol 2008;46:1631–40.

36. Anadol D, Ozcelik U, Kiper N, et al. Treatment of hydatid disease. Paediatr Drugs 2001;3:123–35.

37. Saimot AG. Medical treatment of liver hydatidosis. World J Surg 2001;25:15.

38. Keshmiri M, Baharvahdat H, Fattahi SH, et al. A placebo controlled study of albendazole in the treatment of pulmonary echinococcosis. Eur Respir J 1999;14:503–7.

39. Dogru D, Kiper N, Ozcelik U, et al. Medical treatment of pulmonary hydatid disease: for which child? Parasitol Int 2005;54:135–8.

40. Keramidas D, Mavridis G, Soutis M, et al. Medical treatment of pulmonary hydatidosis: complications and surgical management. Pediatr Surg Int 2004; 19:774.

41. Kurul IC, Topcu S, Altinok T, et al. One stage operation for hydatid disease of the lung and liver: principles of treatment. J Thorac Cardiovasc Surg 2002; 124:1212.

42. Kurkcuoglu IC, Eroglu A, Karaoglanoglu N, et al. Complications of albendazole treatment in hydatid disease of the lung. Eur J Cardiothorac Surg 2002; 22:649–50.

43. Halezeroglu S. Resection of intrathoracic and subdiapragmatic hydatid cysts. Multimed Man Cardiothorac Surg Available at: http://mmcts.ctsnetjournals.org/. Accessed 2004. DOI: 10.1510/mmcts.2004.000307.

44. Turna A, Yilmaz MA, Haciibrahimolu G, et al. Surgical treatment of pulmonary hydatid cysts: is capitonnage necessary? Ann Thorac Surg 2002;74(1):191–5.

45. Kosar A, Orki A, Haciibrahimoglu G, et al. Effect of capitonnage and cystotomy on outcome of childhood pulmonary hydatid cysts. J Thorac Cardiovasc Surg 2006;132:560–4.

46. Bilgin M, Oguzkaya F, Akcali Y. Is capitonnage unnecessary in the surgery of intact pulmonary hydatic cyst? ANZ J Surg 2004;74:40–2.

47. Dakak M, Caylak H, Kavakli K, et al. Parenchyma-saving surgical treatment of giant pulmonary hydatid cysts. Thorac Cardiovasc Surg 2009;57(3): 165–8.

48. Kavukcu S, Kilic D, Tokat AO, et al. Parenchyma-preserving surgery in the management of pulmonary hydatid cysts. J Invest Surg 2006;19(1):61–8.

49. Petrov DB, Terzinacheva PP, Djambazov VI, et al. Surgical treatment of bilateral hydatid disease of the lung. Eur J Cardiothorac Surg 2001;19:918–23.

50. Chowbey PK, Shah S, Khullar R, et al. Minimal access surgery for hydatid cyst disease: laparoscopic, thoracoscopic, and retroperitoneoscopic approach. J Laparoendosc Adv Surg Tech A 2003;13:159–65.

51. Parelkar SV, Gupta RK, Shah H, et al. Experience with video-assisted thoracoscopic removal of pulmonary hydatid cysts in children. J Pediatr Surg 2009;44(4):836–41.

52. Arinc S, Alpay L, Okur E, et al. Recurrent pulmonary hydatid disease: analysis of ten cases. Surg Today 2008;38(11):983–6.

Pulmonary Infections of Surgical Interest in Childhood

Michele Loizzi, MD[a],*, Angela De Palma, MD, PhD[a],
Vincenzo Pagliarulo, MD[a], Domenico Loizzi, MD[b],
Francesco Sollitto, MD[b]

KEYWORDS

- Childhood • Pulmonary infections • Pleural empyema • Lung abscess • Thoracic surgery

KEY POINTS

- Pneumonia is one of the most common infection in childhood and represents an important global health problem, affecting about 150 million children of all ages each year.
- The most common complication of pneumonia are parapneumonic effusion, pleural empyema, pulmonary necrosis and lung abscess, which may require thoracic surgical procedures.
- In childhood, other pulmonary fungal and parasite infectious diseases and post-infectious pulmonary disorders or chronic pulmonary infections secondary to other pathologic conditions may need surgical treatment.
- Accurate knowledge of causes, pathophysiology, clinical aspects, diagnosis and management of pleuropulmonary infections in children is recommended to correctly select patients for thoracic surgery.

INTRODUCTION

Pneumonia is one of the most common infections in the pediatric population and represents an important global health problem, affecting about 150 million children of all ages each year.[1,2] In addition, pneumonia represents the leading cause of mortality (more than 2 million deaths per year) in children less than 5 years of age worldwide.[3,4] Although most cases of pneumonia occur in developing countries, about 3% to 4% of children are affected in high-income areas.[1,5] Causes are variable, with viral pneumonia being more common in younger children and *Streptococcus pneumoniae* the most common bacterial agent in children older than 5 years.[6] The causes of pneumonia in childhood by age groups are reported in **Table 1**.[1,4,6] The cornerstones of modern treatment are supportive care (adequate analgesia, oxygen if saturation falls below 92%, fluid balance control[4]) and adequate antibiotics.[1,4]

Although pneumonia is effectively treated and prevented with antibiotics and vaccines on an outpatient basis in most cases,[1] some children still require hospitalization, especially in immunocompromised patients. Pneumonia complicated by pulmonary necrosis, lung abscess, parapneumonic effusion, and empyema may need more invasive treatment, including interventional radiology and thoracic surgical procedures.

Moreover, in childhood there are other pulmonary infectious diseases (fungal and parasitic infections) that primarily require a surgical approach, and postinfectious pulmonary disorders (pneumatoceles, acquired bronchiectasis, posttuberculosis sequelae) or chronic pulmonary infections secondary to other pathologic conditions (congenital bronchiectasis, retained endobronchial foreign body, pulmonary sequestration, mycetoma) that may necessitate a surgical treatment (**Table 2**).

[a] Department of Thoracic Surgery, University of Bari "Aldo Moro", Piazza Giulio Cesare 11, Bari 70124, Italy;
[b] Department of Thoracic Surgery, University of Foggia, Viale Pinto 1, Foggia 71100, Italy
* Corresponding author. Corso Alcide De Gasperi 513/B, 70124 Bari, Italy.
E-mail address: mloizzi@chirtor.uniba.it

Thorac Surg Clin 22 (2012) 387–401
doi:10.1016/j.thorsurg.2012.04.005
1547-4127/12/$ - see front matter © 2012 Elsevier Inc. All rights reserved.

thoracic.theclinics.com

Table 1
Causes of pneumonia in childhood distinguished by age

Neonatal period	*Streptococcus agalactiae* (group B streptococcus) *Escherichia coli* Cytomegalovirus *Listeria monocytogenes*
1–12 mo	Respiratory syncytial virus Parainfluenza viruses *Chlamydia trachomatis* *Staphylococcus aureus* *S pneumoniae* *Bordetella pertussis*
1–4 y	Respiratory syncytial virus Parainfluenza viruses Adenovirus *S pneumoniae* *Haemophilus influenzae* *Mycoplasma pneumoniae* *Mycobacterium tuberculosis*
5–16 y	Human metapneumovirus *S pneumoniae* *Mycoplasma pneumoniae* *C pneumoniae* *M tuberculosis*

This article reviews the causes, pathophysiology, clinical aspects, diagnosis, and management of pleuropulmonary infections of surgical interest in childhood.

COMPLICATIONS OF PNEUMONIA

The most common complications of pneumonia are parapneumonic effusion, pleural empyema, pulmonary necrosis, and lung abscess. The management of these complications has changed in recent years and remains controversial.

PARAPNEUMONIC EFFUSION AND PLEURAL EMPYEMA

Pleural effusion (fluid into the chest cavity) can be classified according to the type, mechanisms and causes (**Table 3**).

Parapneumonic pleural effusion (PPE) is an exudate within the pleural space associated with underlying pneumonia. Complicated effusion refers to secondary contamination of the pleural fluid by an infectious agent. In particular, empyema is defined by the presence of a purulent collection in the pleural cavity and by inflammatory pleural changes that can lead to impairment, sometimes irreversible, of the thoracopulmonary function. The incidence of empyema in childhood is increasing. It affects almost 1 in 150 children with pneumonia,[7] possibly due to recent changes in health politics. It is more frequent in immuno-compromised (HIV-infection, immunosuppressive therapy, chemotherapy) and in malnourished patients. Empyema in children is a very different condition from that in adults because it is almost never fatal, probably due to the higher incidence of comorbidities in the adult empyema population.

Causes and Pathophysiology of Empyema

Currently, streptococci and *Staphylococcus aureus* are the most frequent causes of empyema.[1,6] *Staphylococcus* spp are the main cause of pediatric pulmonary infections in children under 2 years of

Table 2
Pleuropulmonary infections of surgical interest in childhood

Complications of pneumonia	Parapneumonic effusion Pleural empyema Pulmonary necrosis Lung abscess
Other pulmonary infectious diseases	Parasites infections (hydatidosis, amebiasis) Fungal infections (aspergillosis, candidiasis, mucormycosis)
Postinfectious pulmonary disorders	Pneumatocele Acquired bronchiectasis Posttuberculosis sequelae
Chronic pulmonary infections secondary to other pathologic conditions	Congenital bronchiectasis Retained endobronchial foreign body Pulmonary sequestration Mycetoma

Table 3
Classification of pleural effusions

Type of Effusion	Mechanism	Causes
Transudate	Increased vascular pressure	Congestive heart failure
		Mitral valve disease
	Reduced capillary oncotic force	Nephrotic syndrome
		Liver disease
Exudate	Pleural inflammation leading to an increase of pleural capillary permeability and reduced lymphatic absorption	Parapneumonic effusion
		Empyema
		Connective tissue disease
		Malignancy (eg, lymphoma)
		Direct extension of abdominal inflammation (eg, pancreatitis, hepatic abscess)
	Malignant pleural infiltration	Thoracic malignancies (eg, lymphoma, chest wall sarcoma)
Hemorrhagic effusion	Bleeding	Chest trauma
		Vessel infiltration (eg, inflammation, neoplasms)
Chyle	Structural defect of pleural lymphatic system or thoracic duct	Pulmonary lymphangiectasia or pulmonary lymphangiomatosis
	Disruption of pleural lymphatic system or thoracic duct	Extrinsic compression (eg, lymphoma, postcardiac surgery)
		Chest trauma

age and produce parenchymal microabscesses, sometimes emptying in the pleural cavity, and pneumatoceles during the healing phase.[1,6] Aerobic gram-negative bacteria (*Klebsiella*, *Haemophilus influenzae*, *Escherichia coli*, *Pseudomonas aeruginosa*) and anaerobic organisms (*Peptostreptococcus*, *Peptococcus*, *Fusobacterium*, *Bacteroides*, *Clostridium*, *Lactobacillus* spp) are more frequently causes of empyema in children with neurodevelopmental disorders and immunodeficiency. Worldwide, tuberculosis accounts for approximately 6% of all empyema cases, but this is rare in the developed world where effective antituberculosis therapy is aggressively administered.[8,9]

Pathophysiologic mechanisms of infection of the pleural cavity can be various (**Table 4**).[10] More than 50% of cases are related to a pulmonary infection, because of the common visceral pleural and pulmonary lymphatic and hematic circulation. Sometimes infectious processes of the abdominal cavity (subdiaphragmatic abscesses, suppurative appendicitis) can extend to the pleural cavity, because of the presence of little diaphragmatic lacunae with direct contact zones between pleura and peritoneum and the contiguity of the peritoneal and pleural lymphatic and hematic circulation.[10]

Stages

Pleural empyema can involve the entire pleural cavity or be confined to a part of it depending on the quantity of pus and the causing pathogen (*S pneumoniae*

Table 4
Pathophysiologic mechanisms of infection of the pleural cavity in children

Contiguity or continuity	From inflammatory or suppurative process of adjacent organs (bronchopneumonia, lung abscess, specific or aspecific pulmonary infiltrates, suppurated bronchiectasis, lymphadenitis, mediastinal cellulitis, esophagitis, pericarditis, chest wall phlegmon, vertebral abscess, subdiaphragmatic suppurative processes)
Hematic or lymphatic spread	From extrathoracic infectious foci or pleural localization of a bacteremia (polytraumatized, immunocompromised children undergoing cardiac surgery with septicemia)
Direct contamination	By penetrating wounds or surgical procedures

usually produce tenacious pleural-pulmonary adhesions yielding a plurilocular empyema, whereas *Streptococcus* spp generate an all cavity empyema by the production of fibrinolytic enzymes).[10]

In 1962, the American Thoracic Society described three stages (not rigidly defined) in the natural course of the disease, recently summarized by Hamm and Light[11] and termed Light's stages with an initial precollection stage (pleuritis sicca) when the underlying lung inflammation extends to the pleura causing pleural rub and pleuritic chest pain. The typical three stages (**Table 5**) are (1) exudative, (2) fibrinopurulent or transitional, and (3) organization or chronic (producing an inelastic membrane, the pleural peel, limiting lung expansion). The organization process starts 7 to 10 days after the onset of the disease, but the chronic stage occurs 4 to 6 weeks after the initial development of the empyema.[10]

Factors promoting chronicization of empyema include delayed diagnosis, inadequate antibiotic therapy, loculation, bronchopleural fistula, pleural foreign bodies, chronic pulmonary infection unresponsive to antibiotics, lung trapping by a thick pleural peel, and inadequate drainage or its premature removal.[10] Recognized complications of empyema include pneumothorax, bronchopleural or cutaneous fistula, lung necrosis, purulent pericarditis, and spread of infection to other sites.[4]

Clinical Presentation

PPE and empyema should be considered in children with pneumonia and persisting fever, despite treatment with appropriate antibiotics for 48 hours. Symptoms are similar to those of pneumonia but more prominent. The patient appears suffering, tired, lacking appetite, and pale. Fever is irregular and recedes when a spontaneous (necessitatis) or surgical pleural drainage of pus occurs. Chest pain may be less severe but persistent at the onset of the disease. Subsequently, it becomes pulsating due to the parietal retraction caused by peel organization. Cough is related to concomitant bronchopulmonary lesions and to pleural irritation. Dyspnea can be present.[10]

Physical examination may reveal limited respiratory excursions, dullness on percussion, and decreased breath sounds on the affected side. Pain on percussion as well as a friction rub over the involved chest wall may be evident.

Diagnostic Procedures

Differential diagnosis includes all other causes of pleural effusion (see **Table 3**).

Imaging in the form of chest radiographs (x-rays) (CXR) and ultrasound (US) is recommended for the diagnosis and to identify and guide drainage of the PPE or empyema. Computed tomography (CT) is recommended in special circumstances only.

CXR is frequently the first investigation to suggest the presence of pleural effusion. CXR in two views, when feasible, can show a more or less extended and homogeneous opacity, defining a curve line with internal and upwards concavity (meniscus sign). "White hemithorax" occurs when a pleural cavity collects a very large effusion, causing contralateral mediastinal displacement. CXR cannot distinguish between fluid and extensive consolidation, and US is usually required (**Fig. 1**, Appendix 1).[12] CXR may also show a scoliosis concave to the side of fluid collection, reflecting splinting of the chest wall to reduce pain.[9]

Table 5 Stages of empyema	
Exudative stage	Accumulation in the pleural cavity of a sterile pleural fluid, with few cells and leukocytes Low lactate dehydrogenase and normal glucose and pH levels
Fibrinopurulent stage	Invasion of the pleural fluid by bacteria Increase of neutrophil granulocytes and fluid Fibrin deposit on the parietal-visceral pleura as a continuous sheet or membrane, preventing extension of the empyema but trapping the lung Loculation, making tube thoracostomy drainage difficult Increase of lactate dehydrogenase and reduction of pH and glucose levels
Organization or chronic stage	Organization of the deposited fibrin, with ingrowth of fibroblasts and capillaries from both the parietal and visceral pleural surfaces Formation of the pleural peel, an inelastic membrane, severely limiting lung expansion

A   B   C

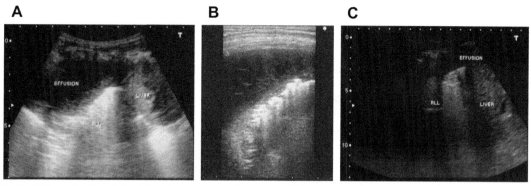

Fig. 1. (*A*) Longitudinal lateral basal sonograms of a 4-year-old boy with respiratory distress and fever of unclear cause showing a large pleural effusion and consolidated right lower lobe of the lung. (*B*) Linear probe scansion reveals a pleural empyema with formation of fibrinous septations (echoic material). Pleural decortication through a right anterolateral thoracotomy was successfully accomplished. (*C*) Postoperative sonogram at 1 week from surgery showing almost complete resolution of pleural effusion and right lower lobe reexpansion.

Chest computed tomography (CT) should not be considered a routine investigation and pediatric dose optimization should be used.[9] CT contributes to identify the site and extension of empyema and the characteristics of surrounding structures but is generally unable to visualize pleural septation or fibrin stranding because septations are too thin. The authors usually do not use chest CT for radio-protective reasons, limiting its use to selected cases because CXR and, especially, chest US allow us to obtain a lot of information that does not require further imaging investigations.

In this setting, several studies have tried to use a US-based staging system correlating with Light's empyema stages and found a US capacity to predict outcome.[13]

Bronchoscopy is a valid option in case of clinical-suspicion of endobronchial obstruction (eg, foreign body, tumors) or structural bronchial disease as causes of bronchopneumonia and empyema.[10]

Thoracentesis is the mainstay of the diagnostic process, allowing physicochemical and microbiological pleural fluid examination. In the initial stage, glucose, lactate dehydrogenase and pH levels can suggest the diagnosis. Advanced molecular biology techniques (eg, polymerase chain reaction [PCR]) are increasingly used to identify causative organisms. Immunologic, genetic, and advanced laboratory investigations should be considered in case of atypical clinical presentations, history of previous recurrent infections, or identification of unusual pathogens.

Treatment

The optimal treatment modality for children with PPE or empyema is significantly debated. In fact, regardless of treatment options, the outcome in children is generally better than adults.[14]

Supportive care (adequate analgesia and intravenous fluids) and appropriate systemic antibiotics are cardinal principles of PPE or empyema medical treatment.

The primary aims of treatment are clearance of pleural cavity and complete lung reexpansion. Time to defervescence and length of hospital stay are also important outcomes. Some investigators favor early surgical intervention and drainage of the pleural cavity,[14] as in the authors' center. Other institutions prefer the instillation of fibrinolytics via an intrapleural chest drain, reserving definitive surgery for failures.[14]

Because empyema is a dynamic process that progresses through different stages, a stepwise algorithm has been suggested for its treatment.[15–17] During the first and second Light's stages or US evidence of anechoic or not loculated pleural effusion, the first therapeutic procedure is pleural aspiration, by repeated thoracentesis or thoracostomic pleural drainage.[10] Repeated aspiration is not a satisfactory option in children because it is painful and requires considerable cooperation from the patient. At the authors' institution, US-guided chest tube drainage, adequate in size and fenestrations, is preferred. Smaller-bore tubes or Seldinger-technique pigtail catheters can be adopted.[9] The use of intrapleural fibrinolytics is debated.[18] It can be effective to improve drainage, but should not change the underlying principles of PPE or empyema management. Adequate antibiotics, optimal nutritional status, effective immunity response, complete control of infection cause, and appropriate pleural drainage can lead to clinical recovery. Effective drainage with lung reexpansion is imperative to reduce morbidity and progression of the disease to the chronic phase.

Persistent sepsis with a pleural collection after a maximum of 7 days conservative management is an absolute indication for surgical referral.[9] Seven days is an arbitrary period chosen to acknowledge different rates of disease progression, yet provides a clear limit on the duration of medical therapy. Failure of chest tube drainage with fibrinolytics and antibiotics should refer the patient to surgical procedures that, according to the evolution of the pleural disease, should be debridement and/or decortication.

There are different surgical approaches, varying from the less invasive (video-assisted thoracic surgery [VATS]) to the more invasive (thoracotomy), with the intermediate one represented by minithoracotomy. Early surgery and debridement produces good postoperative lung expansion in almost all cases.[19,20] The authors support that, if the child is undergoing general anesthesia for simple drain insertion, the procedure should be combined with early VATS or minithoracotomy for debridement.[19,20] Selective endobronchial intubation or bronchial blockers in young children when double-lumen tubes are not available may be useful to avoid contamination of the contralateral lung and comfortably perform surgical procedures with a deflated lung. VATS, through three small thoracostomic accesses and, eventually, an auxiliary minithoracotomy, achieves debridement of the fibrinous pyogenic material, breakdown of loculation, and pus drainage from the pleural cavity under direct vision. There is no trial evidence comparing VATS to minithoracotomy in children, and it is currently not possible to determine whether one technique is superior to another.[9] Although early VATS is safe and effective, the failure rate is higher in late-presenting cases and it is not suitable for advanced organized empyema.

Minithoracotomy and thoracotomy are open procedures that achieve complete debridement and decortication of the thick fibrous pleural rind with evacuation of pyogenic material. The anesthetized child is placed in lateral decubitus and incision is made in the fifth or sixth intercostal space as an anterolateral or standard posterolateral incision (preferably muscle-sparing). Decortication (removal of the parietal and visceral pleural peel) involves sharp dissection to excise the thickened pleura and carries a significant morbidity from bleeding and air leaks. With adequate pleural drainage, it allows recuperation of the normal chest wall mobility and complete lung reexpansion. This surgical procedure should be performed neither too early nor too late.[10] The best interval is 4 to 6 weeks after the initial development of the empyema when a well-defined peel has constituted, not yet conglomerated with the pulmonary parenchyma and the endothoracic fascia (**Fig. 2**).

Between January 1993 and December 2011, the authors treated 648 children (ages 0–16 years) for the following indications: malformation (95), infectious-inflammation (98), trauma (63), dystrophy (109), neoplasia (46), foreign body aspiration (201), and miscellaneous (36). Of 98 children affected by infectious-inflammatory diseases, 33 had pleural effusion or empyema, which were treated with pleural drainage only in 12 cases and with VATS or minithoracotomy pleural debridement and decortication in 21 cases. In six of the latter group, an atypical lung resection was also performed and, in one case, a left lower lobectomy for a lung abscess was required (**Fig. 3**). No postoperative morbidity and mortality was observed.

Chest physiotherapy is not recommended, but the authors usually suggest early mobilization, even with a drain in situ, keeping the child comfortable with adequate analgesia, to allow a complete and faster recovery.

Clinical Outcomes

Child overall mortality in the developed world is very low.[14]

A repeat CXR should be performed at approximately 1 month from discharge to confirm radiological resolution of consolidation and scoliosis. Children usually show a complete clinical recovery and CXR can be expected to return to almost normal by 3 to 6 months.[9]

Long-term follow-up with pulmonary function tests have not been routinely assessed in children because of age limitations associated with these investigations.[14]

PULMONARY NECROSIS

Pulmonary necrosis is an area of infected, consolidated parenchyma characterized by formation of necrotic cavities.

Causes and Pathophysiology

S pneumoniae and S aureus are the most common causes. Pulmonary necrosis is primarily a vascular phenomenon related to the infectious process, leading to thrombotic occlusion of intrapulmonary vessels associated with adjacent inflammation, resulting in ischemia and, eventually, necrotic parenchymal lesions.[4,6] PPE or empyema are frequently associated. Lung necrosis results in cavity formation, often with associated abscesses.[4]

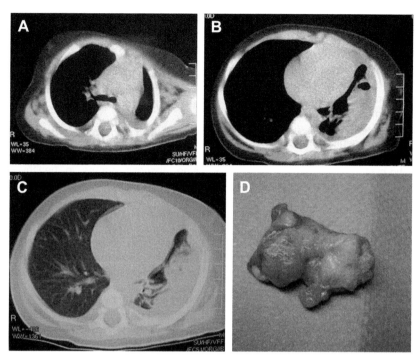

Fig. 2. (*A–C*) Chest CT scans of a 4-month-old infant boy showing a left pleural empyema in the organization stage. Left hemithorax asymmetry due to retraction by the pleural peel and lung parenchyma trapping are evident. (*D*) Pleural decortication through minithoracotomy, resecting the entire empyematic sac, was successfully performed.

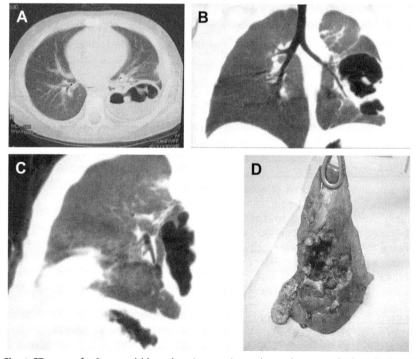

Fig. 3. (*A–C*) Chest CT scans of a 3-year-old boy showing a primary lung abscess, a thick-walled cavity containing an air-fluid level, of the apical segment of the left lower lobe. The causing pathogen was *S pneumoniae*. Due to the severity of infection, unresponsive to systemic antibiotics, a lung lobectomy through anterolateral thoracotomy was successfully performed. (*D*) The necrotic abscess cavity within the left lower lobe is clearly evident.

Clinical Presentation

Signs and symptoms are the same of pneumonia. However, patients are often disproportionately sick with persistent fever, respiratory distress, and chest pain, and they respond poorly to standard antibiotic therapy. Clotting indices may be deranged with thrombocytosis or, less frequently, thrombocytopenia.[4] Differential diagnosis may include infection in congenital lung diseases or in immunocompromised children, traumatic pseudocyst, and hydatid cyst.[4]

Diagnostic Procedures

Necrotizing pneumonia cannot normally be diagnosed on CXR. US may detect lung consolidation. However, chest CT is superior to both CXR and US for detecting necrotic lung disease, showing cystic heterogeneous areas of necrosis and air-filled cavities within solid consolidation and nonenhancing lung parenchyma.[6,21] CT is also useful to confirm or exclude congenital lung malformations.[4]

Treatment

Prolonged systemic antibiotic therapy is required. Some investigators suggest that surgery should be avoided in pulmonary necrosis because bronchopleural fistulae may occur.[4] Nevertheless, this is usually not practicable because necrotizing pneumonia is often associated with empyema, requiring surgery, and concomitant lung necrosis is frequently discovered only at the time of operation. The authors recommend being particularly careful in the surgical maneuvers, eventually suturing or resecting the coexisting necrotic lung area by stapler and reinforcing the suture or staple line with thrombin glue or fibrinogen patch to prevent postoperative air leaks. Some investigators have also proposed the interposition of muscle flaps.[4]

Clinical Outcomes

The long-term outcome for children affected by necrotic pneumonia is generally good, although recovery is usually more prolonged than in children with less complicated disease. A follow-up CXR is required to ensure resolution of the process and to detect possible long-term complications, such as bronchiectasis and persistent pulmonary consolidation.[4]

LUNG ABSCESS

A lung abscess is a thick-walled parenchymal cavity containing purulent material, resulting from a necrotizing pulmonary infection.[10,22] It has progressively become less frequent owing to improvements in antibiotic therapy. It is less frequent in children than adults and is an uncommon pediatric problem, with a paucity of quality data on this subject in the literature.[10,22] Some investigators impose a minimum size of 2 cm as a diagnostic criterion.[22] If left untreated, a lung abscess may be complicated by significant morbidity, such as pleural empyema and fistula formation.[22]

Causes and Pathophysiology

There are two types of lung abscess: a primary lung abscess occurs in healthy children with normal lungs, a secondary lung abscess in children with an underlying congenital or acquired lung disease (**Table 6**).[22,23]

Numerous pathogens can cause a lung abscess: species of Streptococci, Staphylococci, Klebsiella, and other gram-negative bacteria and anaerobic organisms.[1,10,22,23] These pathogens can reach the pulmonary site of infection in different ways (**Table 7**).[10]

Pulmonary aspiration is considered to be a central factor in the development and evolution of lung abscess in children, especially in those with neurodevelopmental delay or immunodeficiency.[1,22] Indeed, people of any age may present daily microaspirations. However, what is determinant is the number of episodes, the volume of aspirated material, and the presence of an impairment of mucociliary clearance mechanisms.[22,24] Supporting this concept is that lung abscesses occur more commonly in the most dependant parts of the lung for the supine patient (upper lobes and apical segments of lower lobes).[22,24]

Clinical Presentation

Clinical findings can vary from severe and acute symptoms to insidious or asymptomatic situations, in relationship to the pathogenesis, the stage of the disease, and its extension.[10]

The evolution of a lung abscess may be surprisingly indolent, lasting several weeks, with tachypnea, cough, and fever being the most common symptoms. The main clinical signs are a dull percussion note or reduced air entry locally and localized crepitations.[1,22,24] In severe and acute forms (nowadays extremely rare in children owing to early antibiotic therapy), the main symptoms resemble a bacterial pneumonia: high fever, sweats, chest pain, dyspnea, persistent cough that becomes productive, and severe prostration. Chest physical examination can be negative and blood examination can reveal neutrophil leukocytosis. Some days later, cough with putrid purulent secretions may appear due to the opening and total or partial emptying of the abscess cavity. Clinical examination reveals a typical amphoric

Table 6
Etiologic classification of lung abscess in children

Primary lung abscess (healthy children, normal lung)	Anaerobic aspiration (*Bacteroides, Fusobacterium*) Specific pneumonia (*S pneumoniae, S aureus, K pneumoniae*)

Secondary lung abscess (underlying lung disease)	Congenital
	  Cystic fibrosis
	  Immunodeficiency
	  Cyst adenomatoid malformation
	  Bronchogenic cyst
	  Pulmonary sequestration
	Acquired
	  Achalasia, other esophageal motility problems
	  Neurodevelopmental abnormality (eg, cerebral palsy)
	  Immunodeficiency (chemo-immunosuppressive therapy, HIV)
	  Nutritional deficiency
	  Bronchial obstruction (foreign body, lymphadenopathy)
	  Bronchiectasis

breath sound and a rapid improvement of general conditions occurs.[10]

Diagnostic Procedures

The basic diagnostic test for a lung abscess is CXR, but US and CT are useful adjuncts to confirm the diagnosis.[1,22]

In the initial stage, CXR can show a more or less homogeneous consolidation, with definite margins, similar to a bronchopneumonic process: after the lung abscess empties, a cavity containing an air-fluid level and with thick wall appears.[4,10,22]

US may better define a lung abscess. The optimal roles of US may be in the initial evaluation of a critical child at the bedside and the ability to detect peripheral abscesses, adjacent to the pleura or the hemidiaphragm.[22] Before cavitation, a lung abscess may appear as an avascular, hypoechoic mass. Some interventional radiologists prefer to use US guidance under general anesthesia to aspirate or place drainage into peripheral lung abscesses. When CT is not available, US is a safe noninvasive test useful to monitor recovery.[22]

Contrast-enhanced chest CT is usually considered to be the investigation of choice for lung abscess because it allows definition of the extension of the lesion and its characteristics and differentiation of an abscess from empyema, necrotizing pneumonia, pulmonary sequestration, pneumatoceles, or other cystic congenital diseases.[10,22] It

Table 7
Pathophysiology of lung abscess in children

Descending respiratory way	Infectious foci of the rhinopharyngeal or oral cavity (sinusitis, tonsillar, dental abscesses)
Aspiration of oral secretion	Impaired consciousness, immunocompromised patients (neurologic diseases, anesthesia, comatose state)
Hematic spread	From extrapulmonary infectious foci (thrombophlebitis, endocarditis)
Contiguity	From mediastinal, pleural, or subdiaphragmatic suppurative processes
Suppurative complication	Of preexisting pulmonary diseases (bronchopneumonia, bronchiectasis, pulmonary sequestration)
Transthoracic way	By penetrating wounds (posttraumatic)

can also guide the interventional radiologist during diagnostic aspiration or therapeutic drainage of the abscess.[22] The typical CT finding is a thick-walled cavity containing mobile, central fluid, within an area of consolidated lung. An air-fluid level is often present.[22]

Sputum examination and cultures of the material aspirated from the lung abscess are fundamental to identify the responsible pathogens and to start an adequate antibiotic therapy.[10]

In some cases, bronchoscopy is useful to assess bronchi status and it can reveal the presence of retained foreign bodies.[10]

Treatment

The mainstay of treatment of lung abscess is hospital admission and intravenous antibiotic therapy, which may lead to recovery up to 90% of patients.[1,22] The duration of systemic antibiotics varies with investigators' experience from 5 days to 3 weeks.[1,22,25] However, 4 weeks oral antibiotic therapy is always required after intravenous medications have been stopped.[1,22,25] With the aim of tailoring antibiotics to the causing pathogen, aspiration of the lung abscess and placement of pigtail catheters play a significant role in the treatment algorithm.[1,25] About 60 years ago, Monaldi[26] described the first percutaneous drainage of a lung abscess under fluoroscopic control.[26] Recently, the rediscovery of interventional radiology has led to a renewed use of CT-guided aspiration and pigtail drainage for peripheral lung abscesses in children, with reports of a higher proportion of positive cultures overall, improved success rates, reduced morbidity and mortality, and a shorter hospital stay.[22] However, outcome data are limited. Owing to these improvements, nowadays chronicization is rare and most lung abscesses have an attenuate clinical course and usually recover with minimal radiological scar.

Surgical resection of lung abscesses is rarely required.[1,23] A pulmonary lobectomy or segmental or atypical resection can become mandatory in some cases, including abscess worsening (despite adequate medical therapy, see **Fig. 3**), complications (endobronchial pus diffusion with pulmonary spread, bronchopleural fistula with pyopneumothorax, massive hemoptysis not responsive to embolization, embolic infection diffusion to other organs), or chronicization (formation of empty residual cavities at risk of colonization such as mycetomas).[10]

Moreover, indications to surgery may be the treatment of underlying diseases in secondary lung abscess (**Fig. 4**): resection of bronchogenic cyst, removal of bronchial obstruction (foreign body, lymphadenopathy), resection of localized bronchiectasis, or pulmonary sequestration. Bilateral lung transplantation may be required for cystic fibrosis.

This kind of surgery in children can be challenging. Indeed, surgery for lung abscess in adult and pediatric patients has been associated with significant morbidity, such as empyema, bronchoalveolar air leaks, and a mortality rate of 5% to 10%.[22] Some investigators have compared surgical management with medical therapy alone or medical therapy coupled with interventional radiology. However, most studies are retrospective.[22,25,27] In these patients, the authors recommend extreme caution in all surgical maneuvers, reducing lung manipulation to a minimum, and favoring a delicate dissection. After suturing the bronchus or the parenchyma, or after resection of the lung abscess by stapler, it is advisable to reinforce the suture. Usually, a child's postoperative course is faster and characterized by lower morbidity than adults. The authors have never had significant morbidity after this type of surgery.

Clinical Outcomes

A follow-up CXR about 1 month after hospital discharge may be useful to confirm the resolution of the abscess or to monitor children who underwent surgery. Where available, US is a safe, noninvasive test to check recovery.[22]

In the literature, prognosis and overall outcome are extremely good, especially for immunocompetent children with primary lung abscesses. Morbidity and mortality rates are lower than those of adults. Mortality is in the order of less than 5% and occurs mostly in children with secondary lung abscesses[1,22,27] because their prognosis is influenced by the predisposing disease.[22,25]

Very few long-term follow-up data in children are available. Some investigators have reported a normal lung function after primary lung abscesses[22,28] and in children who underwent surgical management.[22,29]

OTHER PULMONARY INFECTIOUS DISEASES

Children may be affected by other pulmonary infectious diseases, caused by fungi or parasites, which primarily require a surgical treatment. This article particularly focuses on aspergillosis and pulmonary hydatidosis.

Aspergillosis is one of the most common fungal pneumonias in children, especially in the immunocompromised group. It refers to any infection caused by several species of Aspergillus (A fumigatus, A flavus, A niger, A terreus). The fungus is ubiquitous and asymptomatic colonization is common.

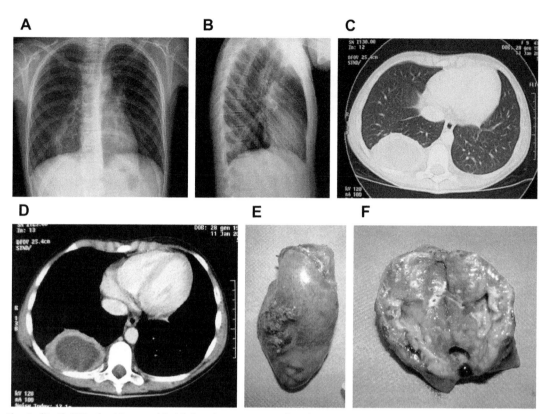

Fig. 4. (*A, B*) CXR of a 10-year-old girl showing a posterior-basal opacity of the right hemithorax. (*C, D*) Contrast-enhanced chest CT revealed a secondary lung abscess in a congenital bronchogenic cyst of the right lower lobe, which was resected by stapler (*E*) through anterolateral thoracotomy. (*F*) Section of the resected specimen showing the thick-walled infected cystic cavity with epithelial lining.

Three factors are important in the development of active infection: the virulence of the fungus, the type and amount of exposure, and the immune status of the child.[6] The spectrum of lung diseases ranges from allergic reactions and colonization of preexisting lung cavities (aspergilloma) to progressive vascular invasion and destruction of lung tissue (angioinvasive aspergillosis).[6,30] Clinical presentation may be characterized by cough with bloody or blood-streaked sputum.[30] Allergic bronchopulmonary aspergillosis is usually treated with steroids, with or without association of itraconazole.[30] Aspergilloma usually occurs in individuals with preexisting lung cavities resulting from chronic lung diseases and pulmonary sequelae (tuberculosis, bronchiectasis, chronic lung abscess) or congenital malformations (pulmonary sequestration, bronchogenic cyst).[6,30] Invasion to lung parenchyma and pleura is minimal, and a fungus ball consisting of fungal hyphae, mucus, and cellular debris may be present. The disease can persist for months or years. Chest CT usually reveals a consolidation with an interposed cavitation and an ovoid intracavitary mass (fungus ball

or mycetoma).[6] Angioinvasive aspergillosis is one of the most common forms of fungal infection among immunocompromised, neutropenic children. Chest CT in the initial phase may show a characteristic halo sign (edema or hemorrhage around a solid nodule) and, in the later stage, the air crescent sign (areas of necrotic tissue and pulmonary sequestration within the surrounding parenchyma).[6] In these patients, resection of aspergilloma or lung involved by angioinvasive aspergillosis is recommended principally to avoid extension of the fungal infectious process in an already immunocompromised host (**Fig. 5**). Hemorrhage, empyema, and bronchopleural fistula are the main postoperative complications. Some investigators have suggested intrathoracic transposition of chest wall muscles in patients with large residual pleural space.[30]

Pulmonary hydatidosis is a parasitic disease usually caused by *Echinococcus granulosus*, which affects children who have direct contact with infected domestic animals or accidentally ingest parasite eggs released in the feces of definitive hosts, such as dogs, foxes, and so forth. The eggs

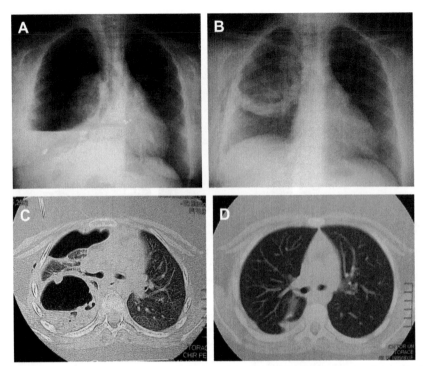

Fig. 5. (A) CXR of an 8-year-old obese girl, with high fever, showing a right hydropneumothorax that was drained (B) revealing a pyopneumothorax. (C) Chest CT at 5 days from drainage, performed due to symptoms worsening despite antibiotics, revealed persistent right pneumothorax with lung abscess. A lateral thoracotomy was performed and the necrotic lung resected by stapler, protecting the suture by intrathoracic transposition of intercostal muscle. Specimen culture was positive for *Aspergillus fumigatus* and systemic antifungine drugs were postoperatively administered. (D) Chest CT at 3 months from surgery shows recovery and the intercostal muscle is evident as an area of calcification.

hatch into larvae in the duodenum and then migrate through the portal system to the liver and to alveolar lung capillaries, where they develop into spherical or oval cysts (hydatid). Hydatidosis is more frequent in developing countries. CT may show single or multiple cysts (which may present daughter and nephew cysts) and ruptured cysts with internal floating membranes (water lily sign).[6] When pulmonary hydatidosis in children is diagnosed, it is recommended to surgically eliminate the disease because of the possibility of progressive enlargement of the cyst (causing compression of the surrounding healthy thoracic structures, **Fig. 6**) and its infection or rupture, which is a dramatically dangerous situation, called vomica. The patient eliminates the hydatid liquid, which is extremely allergenic, in the tracheobronchial tree and may die of anaphylactic shock. Different surgical techniques (Posadas, Ugon-Dubau, Perez-Fontana) have been described to resect the hydatid cysts. Whatever the procedure, the main aims of the operation are to avoid contamination and dissemination of the disease in the healthy lung and pleural cavity, to elide the residual cavity, and to close properly all

potential sources of postoperative air leaks. A typical lung resection is rarely required. For peripheral cysts, an atypical lung resection by stapler may be performed. Antiparasitic drugs should be administered postoperatively, to prevent recurrences.

POSTINFECTIOUS PULMONARY DISORDERS AND CHRONIC PULMONARY INFECTIONS SECONDARY TO OTHER PATHOLOGIC CONDITIONS

A surgical approach may be necessary to eradicate some postinfectious pulmonary disorders or chronic pulmonary infections secondary to other pathologic conditions.

Among postinfectious pulmonary disorders, pneumatoceles and bronchiectasis are the most common **postinfectious sequelae of bacterial pneumonia**.

Pneumatocele is a thin-walled cyst, with or without septations, that develops within the lung parenchyma, occurring after an acute pneumonia, most often caused by *S aureus*.[6] If big or increasing in size, or when it becomes symptomatic because

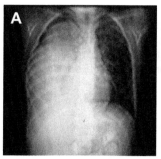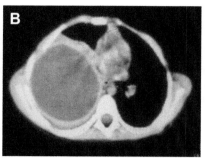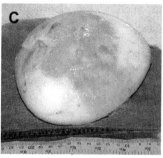

Fig. 6. (A) CXR of a 4-year-old boy showing a subtotal opacity of the right hemithorax. (B) Chest CT showed a huge cystic lesion almost occupying the entire right hemithorax, compressing the surrounding healthy thoracic structures. An anterolateral thoracotomy was performed, revealing a giant hydatid cyst, about 15 cm in maximum diameter (C) that was successfully removed using the Ugon-Dubau technique.

of recurrent infections, pneumatocele should be resected, usually by atypical resection with stapler through VATS or minithoracotomy. A lobectomy is seldom necessary.

Bronchiectasis is an abnormal irreversible dilatation of subsegmental bronchi caused by weakening or destruction of the muscular and elastic components of the bronchial walls.[6,23]

Bronchiectasis can be distinguished in congenital and acquired forms. Congenital bronchiectasis is caused by congenital disorders of the mucociliary or humoral defense mechanisms, or of the bronchial wall structure, leading to recurrent suppurative infections that permanently impair subsegmental bronchi.[23] Acquired bronchiectasis is generally secondary to an infectious pulmonary process or to persistent bronchial obstruction (foreign body, lymphadenopathy with middle lobe syndrome). It usually occurs in older children after destructive pulmonary infections that cause impaired clearance of bronchial secretions, leading to chronic infection. Both CXR and CT may show the thickening of the bronchial walls and a marked enlargement of the bronchial channel. Although bronchiectasis can be managed by medical treatment associated with respiratory physiotherapy, surgical lung resection may be indicated in cases of acquired localized bronchiectasis and its complications (recurrent suppurative infections, hemoptysis, if interventional radiology is unsuccessful). A complete resection of all disease should be performed, to prevent recurrence, preserving nonsuppurative areas. Lung transplantation may be indicated for children with congenital bronchiectasis and cystic fibrosis.

Posttuberculosis Sequelae

The incidence of tuberculosis, caused by *Mycobacterium tuberculosis*, is increasing worldwide.

Sixty percent of new childhood infections occur in children younger than 5 years old.[6,31] Childhood tuberculosis generally results from infection spread by an adult with active pulmonary disease.[1,32] Children are most severely affected by this infection and positive skin tests are an effective means of identifying children with the disease.[1] Primary pulmonary tuberculosis especially involves the lymphatic system (primary complex). Infection of the mediastinal or hilar lymph nodes can result in bronchial damage or obstruction, leading to atelectasis, chronic infection, and bronchiectasis.[1] Most primary infections heal, with deposition of calcium within mediastinal or hilar lymph nodes (Ghon complex). If the host response is depressed, the inoculating dose large, and the pathogen particularly virulent, the primary infection may not be adequately controlled, causing symptoms such as fever, dyspnea, and cough. CXR may reveal lung opacities ranging from consolidation to cavitary lesions and/or pleural effusions.[1] Thus, tubercular infection must be suspected in any child with a chronic cough, unwell status, or recent contact with an adult with active tuberculosis.[1] The diagnosis may be confirmed by sputum, bronchial washings, gastric aspirate and urine bacterioscopy, culture, and PCR.[1,33]

Indications for surgery include all the conditions that do not recover with specific medical therapy (rarely) and posttuberculosis sequelae, such as pulmonary cavity, pulmonary consolidation or destruction, bronchial extrinsic obstruction by lymph nodes (middle lobe syndrome), and bronchial stenosis.

Pulmonary cavity is an evolution of tuberculosis infection, characterized by a progressive colliquation leading to formation of a persistent primary cavity. Chest CT may show a lung cavity lesion associated with important hilar and mediastinal lymphadenopathy with aspects of colliquation or calcification in relationship to the earlier or later phase of the disease.[6] Surgical resection of post-tubercular cavity is recommended when recurrent infections and/or hemoptysis occur and to prevent or eradicate fungal colonization (mycetoma).

Pulmonary consolidation and destruction are possible evolutions of tuberculosis infection, characterized by parenchymal carnification and necrosis, respectively. These conditions can favor recurrent suppurative infections, thus surgical resection may be indicated to remove the damaged tissue.

Middle lobe syndrome is caused by the involvement of lymph nodes and the middle lobe bronchus from the tuberculosis process. A progressive bronchial extrinsic obstruction occurs, which may favor retention of secretions with recurrent infections leading to bronchiectasis, requiring surgery.

Bronchial stenosis is very rare in children. It may require an endoscopic treatment (dilatation, stent) and, in some cases when this is unsuccessful, a typical resection to remove the infected lung below the stenosis.

Pediatric thoracic surgery in tuberculosis patients can be particularly difficult owing to chronic infection. All surgical procedures—especially the dissection, identification, and isolation of hilar structures in cases of typical lung resection—should be made with maximal caution. Preventive measures to reduce the potential risk of postoperative air leaks, bronchopleural fistula, and hemorrhage are recommended.

Finally, there are **chronic pulmonary infections secondary to other pathologic conditions** (congenital bronchiectasis, retained endobronchial foreign body, pulmonary sequestration, and mycetoma) that may require surgical treatment.

Concerning retained endobronchial foreign body, the mechanism causing persistent infection is bronchial obstruction with consequent retention of secretions that may lead to bronchiectasis and, eventually, suppuration and lung abscess.

Pulmonary sequestration (intralobar or extralobar) is a congenital malformation consisting of the presence of an anomalous lung segment, variable in size, without connection to the tracheobronchial tree and the pulmonary arteries. Over the years, stasis of secretions inside the unconnected lung segment leads to recurrent infections, bronchiectasis, suppuration, and lung abscess. Usually a lobectomy is required, using extreme caution in the isolation of the systemic arterial supply coming from a thoracic or subdiaphragmatic vessel.

Mycetoma is a fungal colonization of a preexisting lung cavity, mainly a sequela of tuberculosis, but it can also be found in congenital malformations (pulmonary sequestrations). The main colonizing fungus in children are *Aspergillus* spp (see previous discussion). Resection of mycetomas is advisable for both a diagnostic and a therapeutic aim, especially in immunocompromised children.

SUMMARY

Although effectively treated and prevented with antibiotics and vaccines, in some children pneumonia still requires hospitalization and its complications involving the lung and the adjacent pleura (pulmonary necrosis, lung abscess, parapneumonic effusion, and empyema) may need more invasive treatment, including interventional radiology and thoracic surgical procedures. Moreover, in childhood there are other pulmonary fungal and parasite infectious diseases and post-infectious pulmonary disorders or chronic pulmonary infections secondary to other pathologic conditions that may necessitate surgical treatment. Accurate knowledge of the causes, pathophysiology, clinical aspects, diagnosis, and management of pleuropulmonary infections in children is recommended to correctly select patients for whom thoracic surgery is indicated.

APPENDIX1: CHEST SONOGRAPHY IN THE MANAGEMENT OF EMPYEMA IN CHILDREN

US can detect even very small effusions and is capable of distinguishing between pleural fluid and underlying lung consolidation. Occasionally, a highly organized empyema may appear solid and difficult to distinguish from the underlying lung on gray-scale imaging. In this scenario, color Doppler is useful because the pleural collection will be avascular, clearly visible, separately from the highly vascular consolidated lung. A recommendation of the British Thoracic Society guidelines[9] is that US should be used in all cases to confirm the presence of pleural fluid before attempt aspiration. The authors consider the placement of chest tubes using the ultrasound assistance safer and more effective. The operator should never use superficial markers as reference (the usual fifth intercostal space between the anterior and midaxillary lines or the safe triangle) because these reference points do not correspond to the exact pleural effusion position. This is particularly important when a "White hemithorax" is present. The US technique should comprise as complete an evaluation of pleural space as possible. The authors use a combination of a convex probe with frequency of 3.5 MHz to identify a collection, with supplemental scans with a linear probe at high frequency (8 MHz) to further characterize an effusion so identified (see **Fig. 1**). US appearances reflect the presence of cellularity, hemorrhage, and fibrin deposits within a pleural collection. Effusion may appear entirely anechoic or be echoic with floating pinpoints echoes. Fibrin deposition produces a variety of appearances: fibrinous strands floating, fibrinous septations, and pleural thickening. Loculation, in the sense of fluid that does not move freely, can also be identified by scanning the patient supine and sitting if the effusion does not move with this change of posture.

REFERENCES

1. Puligandla PS, Laberge JM. Respiratory infections: pneumonia, lung abscess, and empyema. Semin Pediatr Surg 2008;17:42–52.
2. Bhutta ZA. Dealing with childhood pneumonia in developing countries: how can we make a difference? Arch Dis Child 2007;92:286–8.
3. Wardlaw T, Salama P, Johansson EW, et al. Pneumonia: the leading killer of children. Lancet 2006; 368:1048–50.
4. Thomas MF, Spencer DA. Management and complications of pneumonia. Pediatr Child Health 2011; 21(5):207–12.
5. Colin AA. Pneumonia in the developed world. Pediatr Respir Rev 2006;7(Suppl 1):S138–40.
6. Daltro P, Santos EN, Gasparetto TD, et al. Pulmonary infections. Pediatr Radiol 2011;41(Suppl 1):S69–82.
7. Avasino JR, Goldman B, Sawis RS, et al. Primary operative versus nonoperative therapy for pediatric empyema: a meta-analysis. Pediatrics 2005;115: 1652–9.
8. Jaffè A, Balfour-Lynn IM. Management of empyema in children. Pediatr Pulmonol 2005;40:148–56.
9. Balfour-Lynn IM, Abrahamson E, Cohen G, et al. BTS guidelines for the management of pleural infection in children. Thorax 2005;60(Suppl 1):i1–21.
10. De Palma A, Loizzi D, Sollitto F. Lung abscess and pleural empyema. In: Sartelli M, Catena F, editors. Emergency surgery manual. Rome (Italy): Alpes Italia Editions; 2008. p. 333–9.
11. Hamm H, Light RW. Parapneumonic effusion and empyema. Eur Respir J 1997;10:1150–6.
12. Coley BD. Chest sonography in children: current indications, technique, and imaging findings. Radiol Clin North Am 2011;49:825–46.
13. Yang PC, Luh KT, Chang DB, et al. Value of sonography in determining the nature of pleural effusion: analysis of 320 cases. AJR Am J Roentgenol 1992; 159:29–33.
14. Sonnappa S, Jaffè A. Treatment approaches for empyema in children. Pediatr Respir Rev 2007;8: 164–70.
15. Puligandla PS, Laberge JM. Infections and diseases of the lungs, pleura, and mediastinum. In: Grosfeld JL,

O'Neill JA, Coran AG, et al, editors. Pediatric surgery. Philadelphia: Mosby; 2006. p. 1001–37.
16. Finck C, Wagner C, Jackson R, et al. Empyema: development of a critical pathway. Semin Pediatr Surg 2002;11:25–8.
17. Fuller NMK, Helmarth MA. Thoracic empyema, application of video-assisted thoracic surgery and its current management. Curr Opin Pediatr 2007; 19:328–32.
18. Thomson AH, Hull J, Kumar MR, et al. Randomised trial of intrapleural urokinase in the treatment of childhood empyema. Thorax 2002;57:343–7.
19. Kosloske AM, Cartwright KC. The controversial role of decortication in the management of pediatric empyema. J Thorac Cardiovasc Surg 1988;96(1): 166–70.
20. Gofrit ON, Engelhard D, Abu-Dalu K. Post-pneumonic thoracic empyema in children: a continued surgical challenge. Eur J Pediatr Surg 1999;9:4–7.
21. Calder A, Owens CM. Imaging of parapneumonic pleural effusion and empyema in children. Pediatr Radiol 2009;39:527–37.
22. Patradoon-Ho P, Fitzgerald DA. Lung abscess in children. Paediatr Respir Rev 2007;8:77–84.
23. Miller JI. Bacterial infections of the lungs and bronchial compressive disorders. Chapter 86. In: Shields TW, LoCicero J III, Ponn RB, et al, editors. General Thoracic Surgery. 6th edition. Philadelphia: Lippincott Williams & Wilkins; 2005. p. 1219–32.
24. Brook I. Anaerobic pulmonary infections in children. Pediatr Emerg Care 2004;20:636–40.
25. Tan TQ, Seilheimer DK, Kaplan SL. Pediatric lung abscess: clinical management and outcome. Pediatr Infect Dis J 1995;14:51–5.
26. Monaldi V. Endocavitary aspiration in the treatment of lung abscess. Chest 1956;29:193–201.
27. Yen CC, Tang RB, Chen SJ, et al. Pediatric lung abscess: a retrospective review of 23 cases. J Microbiol Immunol Infect 2004;37:45–9.
28. Asher MI, Spier S, Beland M, et al. Primary lung abscess in childhood. Am J Dis Child 1982;136:491–4.
29. Nonoyama A, Tanaka K, Osako T, et al. Surgical treatment of pulmonary abscess in children under ten years of age. Chest 1984;85:358–62.
30. Lucke JC. Thoracic mycotic and actinomycotic infections of the lung. In: Shields TW, LoCicero J III, Ponn RB, et al, editors. General thoracic surgery. 6th edition. Philadelphia: Lippincott Williams & Wilkins; 2005. p. 1262–89.
31. Adler B, Effmann E. Pneumonia and pulmonary infection. In: Slovis TL, editor. Caffey's pediatric diagnostic imaging. 11th edition. Philadelphia: Mosby; 2008. p. 1184–228.
32. Donald PR. Childhood tuberculosis. Curr Opin Pulm Med 2000;6:187–92.
33. Lodha R, Kabra SK. Newer diagnostic modalities for tuberculosis. Indian J Pediatr 2004;71:221–7.

Pulmonary Infections Following Lung Transplantation

Chad A. Witt, MD[a],*, Bryan F. Meyers, MD, MPH[b],
Ramsey R. Hachem, MD[a]

KEYWORDS

- Lung transplantation • Immunocompromised • Infectious complications • Cytomegalovirus
- Aspergillosis • Prophylaxis

KEY POINTS

- Lung transplant recipients are at a higher risk of infectious complications than recipients of other solid organs.
- The major cause of mortality beyond 1 year after lung transplantation is bronchiolitis obliterans syndrome (chronic allograft rejection).
- Infections with cytomegalovirus (CMV), *Pseudomonas aeruginosa*, and *Aspergillus* species have been associated with the development of bronchiolitis obliterans syndrome.
- CMV and fungal prophylaxis regimens vary by transplant center.
- *Pneuomcystis jiroveci* pneumonia is rare in the era of prophylaxis.

INTRODUCTION

In 2009, 3272 lung transplant procedures were reported to the International Society for Heart and Lung Transplantation for end-stage lung disease, the highest annual number to date. Survival for lung transplant recipients continues to lag behind that of other solid organ transplant recipients, with a median survival ("half-life") of 5.5 years.[1] Graft failure and non-cytomegalovirus (non-CMV) infection remain the major reported causes of postoperative mortality in the first year after transplantation. After the first year, the most common identifiable causes for mortality are bronchiolitis obliterans syndrome (BOS) and non-CMV infection. Immunosuppression contributes significantly to posttransplant infections in all recipients; however, lung transplant recipients are generally more intensively immunosuppressed than other solid organ recipients and have more frequent and more severe infectious complications. In addition, factors such as preoperative microorganism colonization, transmission of infectious agents from the donor organs, blunted cough mechanism due to denervation, impaired mucociliary clearance, poor lymphatic drainage, ischemic large airways in the immediate postoperative period, and constant exposure to the environment uniquely place lung transplant recipients at higher risk for infections than other organ recipients.[2]

Chronic allograft rejection, in the form of BOS, is the major life-limiting complication after lung transplantation. Pulmonary infections with viruses, including CMV; gram-negative bacilli, especially *Pseudomonas aeruginosa*; and *Aspergillus* species have all been associated with an increased risk of BOS.[3–7] These findings underscore the importance of prevention, diagnosis, and treatment of infections in the population that has undergone lung transplantation.

[a] Department of Internal Medicine, Washington University School of Medicine in St Louis, 660 South Euclid Avenue Campus Box 8052, St Louis, MO 63110, USA; [b] Department of Surgery, Washington University School of Medicine in St Louis, 660 South Euclid Avenue Campus Box 8234, St Louis, MO 63110, USA
* Corresponding author.
E-mail address: cwitt@dom.wustl.edu

Thorac Surg Clin 22 (2012) 403–412
doi:10.1016/j.thorsurg.2012.04.006
1547-4127/12/$ – see front matter © 2012 Elsevier Inc. All rights reserved.

PERIOPERATIVE PERIOD

During the perioperative period, lung transplant recipients are at increased risk for bacterial, fungal, and viral infections. In this patient population, gram-negative organisms, including *P aeruginosa*, and methicillin-resistant *Staphylococcus aureus* (MRSA) are often encountered.[8] Infections can result from chronic preoperative recipient colonization, as is common in suppurative conditions such as cystic fibrosis (CF). Other mechanisms include acute perioperative donor colonization or infection and postoperative infection in early recipients via mechanical ventilation or through other means throughout the initial hospital stay.

Donor airway sputum specimens are typically obtained for culture in patients before implantation. The results of Gram stain and culture from the donor sputum are followed up to ensure that the initial antibiotic regimen appropriately covers organisms identified in the donor airway specimens. In transplant recipients colonized with known organisms, perioperative antibiotic prophylaxis is based on the results of prior cultures and sensitivity data. This is especially important in patients with CF or non-CF bronchiectasis because these patients are often chronically infected with multidrug-resistant organisms. When such patients are placed on the waiting list for lung transplantation, the perioperative antibiotic regimen is usually planned ahead of time. In addition to results of bacterial cultures, any recent positive cultures for *Aspergillus* species or nontuberculous mycobacteria are considered when selecting the perioperative antimicrobial regimen.

For patients without previous airway cultures, prophylactic perioperative antibiotic therapy must provide coverage against multidrug-resistant gram-negative organisms and MRSA. At our center, patients are initiated on an antipseudomonal β-lactam (eg, cefepime [Maxipime], meropenem [Merrem] or piperacillin/tazobactam [Zosyn]) and vancomycin perioperatively.[9] The choice of antipseudomonal agent should be based on the local sensitivities for each institution. This antibiotic combination is continued for 7 days unless an indication for a longer course of therapy arises in the postoperative period.

Surgical site infections in the postoperative period are most commonly caused by skin flora, the most frequent organism being *Staphylococcus aureus*. Patients colonized with gram-negative organisms preoperatively and those with surgical complications can develop pleural, and less commonly mediastinal, infectious complications in the postoperative period. Ischemic airway injury is the major risk factor for the development of *Aspergillus* tracheobronchitis. Rare occurrences of challenging surgical site infections have been observed in recipients with multidrug-resistant organisms present preoperatively. It seems logical, although largely not supported by evidence, that such patients should undergo longer and more vigorous infectious prophylaxis.

Fungal colonization and infections, most commonly *Candida* species or *Aspergillus* species, can occur in the perioperative period. *Candida albicans* remains the most common *Candida* species to be isolated from lung transplant recipients, although there has been a recent rise in non-*albicans* species. It is sometimes difficult to distinguish an invasive candidal infection from airway colonization. At our center, we usually treat patients with either fluconazole (Diflucan) or an echinocandin if they have ischemic airway injury or copious secretions and *Candida* species are the only organisms that are cultured. The major risk factors for *Aspergillus* infections are previous colonization and ischemic airway injury.[10] **Table 1** outlines some common prophylaxis regimens for viral, fungal, and *Pneumocystis jiroveci* infections.

BACTERIAL INFECTIONS

In contrast to nontransplant hosts, patients who have undergone lung transplantation are at much higher risk of becoming colonized and infected with drug-resistant organisms. Gram-negative organisms are the most frequent cause of bacterial pneumonia, with *P aeruginosa* being the most common. Other gram-negative organisms identified less frequently include, but are not limited to, *Acinetobacter baumannii*, *Escherichia coli*, *Klebsiella pneumoniae*, *Stenotrophomonas maltophilia*, *Burkholderia cepacia*, and *Serratia marcescens*. De novo colonization of the airways with *P aeruginosa* after transplantation has been demonstrated to be an independent risk factor for the development of BOS.[6] *Staphylococcus aureus* is the most common gram-positive organism causing pneumonia and the second most common specific organism causing bacterial pneumonia among lung transplant recipients.[10,11]

Infection with *B cepacia* has historically been associated with poor outcomes after transplantation, and many centers consider chronic infection with *B cepacia* an absolute contraindication to lung transplantion.[12,13] However, it has since been recognized that organisms formally classified as *B cepacia* represent a group complex (*B cepacia* complex, BCC) comprising several distinct species (genomovars). *Burkholderia cenocepacia* (genomovar III) and *Burkholderia multivorans* (genomovar II) account for the majority of infections.[14] *B cenocepacia* is associated with a much higher risk of

Table 1
Some common prophylaxis regimens in the lung transplant recipient

Infection	Viruses/Organisms	Common Prophylaxis Regimens
Viral	Herpes simplex virus CMV	Acyclovir, 200 mg, po twice daily indefinitely High risk (D$^+$/R$^-$) Valganciclovir, 900 mg, po daily for 6–12 mo Medium Risk (D$^+$/R$^+$, D$^-$/R$^+$) 1. Weekly CMV polymerase chain reaction, treat when test result is positive 2. Valganciclovir, 900 mg, po daily for 3–12 mo
Pneumocystis jiroveci pneumonia	Pneumocystis jiroveci	Trimethoprim/sulfamethoxazole, 160/800 mg, po 3 times weekly indefinitely Alternatives for sulfa intolerant, all continued indefinitely 1. Atovaquone, 1500 mg, po daily 2. Pentamidine, 300 mg, inhaled monthly 3. Dapsone, 100 mg, po daily
Fungal	C albicans	Until corticosteroid dose weaned postoperatively or 3 mo 1. Nystatin, 5 mL, po 4 times daily 2. Fluconazole, 100 mg, po daily
	Aspergillus species	When colonized preoperatively or immediately postoperatively, continued until cultures negative 1. Voriconazole, 200 mg, po twice daily 2. Itraconazole, 200 mg, po twice daily 3. Amphotericin, 20–40 mg, inhaled daily

Abbreviation: po, by mouth (oral).

posttransplant mortality, including a 6-fold higher risk of death at 1 year compared with patients infected with BCC organisms other than B cenocepacia and an 8-fold higher risk of death at 1 year compared with patients not infected with any BCC organism.[15] In that series, BCC infection with organisms other than B cenocepacia did not increase the risk of death after transplantation in comparison with patients not infected with BCC. B cenocepacia can cause pneumonia, locally invasive disease with empyema, and disseminated infection. Although not a member of the BCC, Burkholderia gladioli has also been associated with an increased mortality.[16] Transplant centers have to consider the specific species of Burkholderia and the risk of B cenocepacia infection when evaluating patients with CF infected with these organisms.

Because lung transplant recipients are immunocompromised lifelong, empiric antibiotic treatment in lung recipients for pneumonia should include coverage for MRSA, P aeruginosa, and atypical organisms (Listeria, Mycoplasma, Chlamydia). Based on the patient's clinical status, bronchoscopy with bronchoalveolar lavage, with or without transbronchial biopsies, should be considered. In addition to culture data, bronchoscopy helps to evaluate for noninfectious causes of shortness of breath and abnormal chest radiography, including airway complications and acute or chronic rejection. Lung transplant recipients often require up to 14 days of antibiotic therapy or longer if recovery is slow or airway cultures remain positive. As with any patient with pneumonia, the spectrum of the antibiotic therapy should be narrowed based on culture results when possible.

VIRAL INFECTIONS
CMV

CMV infection is a significant cause of morbidity in all transplant recipients. Among lung recipients, CMV is the most common opportunistic infection.[17] The major risk factor for the development of CMV disease is the interaction of the CMV status of the recipient and the CMV status of the donor. Patients who are CMV negative receiving CMV-negative donor organs (D$^-$/R$^-$) are at very low risk for CMV infection. CMV-positive recipients receiving either a CMV-positive or CMV-negative allograft (D$^-$/R$^+$ or D$^+$/R$^+$) are at medium risk, and CMV-negative recipients receiving a CMV-positive allograft (D$^+$/R$^-$) are at the highest risk of developing CMV disease. CMV infection most commonly occurs within the first 3 to 6 months after transplantation, and the risk wanes after the first year in most recipients unless the immunosuppressive regimen is augmented. However, a minority of recipients have recurrent CMV infections beyond the first year after transplantation, and this can result in increased morbidity and mortality.

CMV prophylaxis may delay the onset of invasive disease. In general, there are 2 main prophylactic strategies, but practices in specific centers are highly variable. Most centers advocate valganciclovir (Valcyte) or intravenous ganciclovir (Cytovene) for 6 to 12 months in high-risk recipients (D+/R−), and some encourage lifelong prophylaxis. In contrast, controversy exists on the optimal approach for recipients at medium risk (D−/R+ or D+/R+) for CMV disease. One strategy involves universal prophylaxis for all at-risk patients. The second strategy is based on monitoring and preemptive therapy at the time of identification of active viral replication, ideally before symptomatic infection. Using this strategy, medium-risk patients are monitored frequently (once to twice weekly), screening either for viral pp65 antigenemia or with a plasma polymerase chain reaction (PCR) for CMV. Assays vary, and different virology laboratory tests have different thresholds of positivity. At present, fewer centers rely on testing for pp65 antigenemia because the PCR assay has become more widely available and is less prone to technical errors. Treatment of CMV infection is started at the first sign of viral replication.

Concerning prophylactic therapy, most centers either start with intravenous ganciclovir and then transition to oral valganciclovir or administer oral valganciclovir from the outset. Valganciclovir is typically administered at a dose of 900 mg orally daily for prophylaxis in patients with normal renal function, but the dose may need to be adjusted in the setting of low body mass or leukopenia.[18] The most frequent adverse effects from ganciclovir or valganciclovir therapy are leukopenia and thrombocytopenia. There is also a small risk of ganciclovir resistance in patients on prophylaxis, especially if treatment is periodically interrupted. In addition, a limitation of prophylaxis for a given time course is shifting the timeline of CMV disease to a later time point after transplantation. CMV-specific immunoglobulin (Cytogam) is used at few centers as part of the prophylactic regimen for high-risk patients.[19] No randomized controlled trials have demonstrated the superiority of universal prophylaxis over a preemptive strategy. However, one large multicenter trial demonstrated that in at-risk patients, 12 months of prophylaxis with valganciclovir was superior to 3 months after 13 months of follow-up with respect to CMV infection, with no change in acute rejection, CMV UL97 ganciclovir resistance mutations, or laboratory abnormalities.[20]

The term CMV infection applies to any situation in which viral replication is identified. CMV disease indicates CMV infection with symptoms, including mononucleosis-like syndrome with fever, malaise, and fatigue, or organ-specific invasion involving the lung (Fig. 1), liver, gastrointestinal tract, central nervous system, or retina.[21] As discussed earlier, there is no universal standard of the viral load cutoff that represents a positive blood PCR result. However, if symptoms are present, the general consensus is to initiate treatment of CMV infection. Standard therapy includes intravenous ganciclovir, 5 mg/kg twice daily, or oral valganciclovir, 900 mg twice daily, with dose adjustments for renal function and leukocyte count. Oral valganciclovir has been shown to be noninferior to intravenous ganciclovir in a mixed population of transplant recipients and can be considered as initial therapy, especially in patients with subclinical CMV infection and mild disease.[22,23] Antiviral therapy is generally continued for at least 1 week after viral replication is no longer detectable. CMV-specific immunoglobulin can be

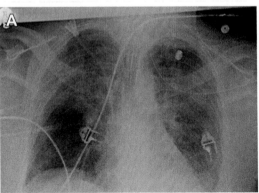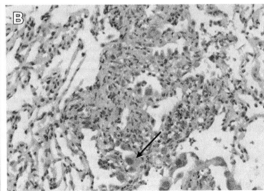

Fig. 1. (*A*) A bilateral lung recipient who CMV seropositive developed severe CMV pneumonia and respiratory failure. (*B*) Pathologic examination of CMV pneumonia with characteristic inclusion bodies (*black arrow*).

used as add-on therapy in severe cases or in patients not responding to initial therapy, especially in seronegative recipients. In patients not responding to conventional therapy, resistance to ganciclovir must be evaluated. The UL 97 gene encodes a protein kinase involved in the phosphorylation and activation of ganciclovir, and mutations within this gene are the most common mechanisms of ganciclovir resistance. Mutations within the UL54 region, which encodes for CMV DNA polymerase, also confer ganciclovir resistance and are more likely to result in resistance to cidofovir and foscarnet. Many patients with UL 97 mutations, and some with UL54 mutations, respond to therapy with cidofovir or foscarnet; however, drug toxicity is the major obstacle to treatment.

Community-Acquired Respiratory Viruses

Community-acquired respiratory virus (CARV) infections, including respiratory syncytial virus (RSV), influenza, parainfluenza, rhinovirus, and adenovirus, have been associated with increased risk of BOS and death.[24] Other CARVs have been identified, including human metapneumovirus, coronavirus, and bocavirus, but the role of these viruses in the development of BOS is not yet established.

Given that influenza infection is treatable, it is important to evaluate patients with clinical symptoms during the typical influenza season and treat them accordingly. As in nontransplant recipients, the first-line therapy for influenza in lung transplant recipients is the neuraminidase inhibitor oseltamivir (Tamiflu). When the severity of illness is high, the duration of therapy is often extended beyond the conventional 5 days to 7 to 14 days.

The decision to treat RSV with ribavirin, either inhaled or systemic, varies from center to center and between individual patients. The RSV season overlaps with the influenza season and may extend later into the spring. In patients with RSV, the goal is to reduce the progression from upper respiratory tract infection to lower respiratory tract infection and thus the risk of BOS.[25] Given this risk, in addition to high clinical suspicion for influenza, patients with upper respiratory tract symptoms during the winter and early spring should be tested for RSV as well. At our center, patients with a positive result for nasopharyngeal viral swab for RSV are treated with 3 days of inhaled ribavirin therapy. Intravenous ribavirin therapy is limited by drug toxicity, especially hemolytic anemia. Other treatment modalities, including palivizumab, an immunomodulating RSV-specific monoclonal antibody; intravenous immunoglobulin (IVIG); and RSV-IVIG (no longer commercially available), have been evaluated in children and in hematopoietic stem cell transplant

recipients. These agents seem to decrease viral loads in animal studies and have shown trends toward efficacy in clinical trials in the stem cell transplant population; however, few data exist in lung transplant recipients.[26]

Epstein-Barr Virus and Posttransplant Lymphoproliferative Disorder

The Epstein-Barr virus (EBV) is the agent that most commonly causes infectious mononucleosis. In transplant recipients, the major morbidity of EBV is posttransplant lymphoproliferative disorder (PTLD). There are 2 major subtypes of PTLD. Polymorphic PTLD is characterized by a monoclonal B-cell population in various stages of maturation and reactive T cells. Monomorphic PTLD is characterized by homogenous sheets of transformed monoclonal B cells, frequently with cytogenetic abnormalities. Monomorphic PTLD is a subtype of non-Hodgkin lymphoma.[27]

PTLD occurs in the setting of immunosuppression, and evidence of EBV infection has been identified in as many as 80% to 90% of patients with PTLD.[28,29] PTLD frequently occurs in the first year after transplantation but can present years later. Among transplant recipients, those who have undergone heart and lung transplants are at the highest risk of developing PTLD, which is likely related to the higher intensity of immunosuppression maintained in these patients.[30] The reported incidence of PTLD after lung transplantation varies between 2.5% and 8%, with a recent series identifying 34 cases in 705 patients (4.8%) who had undergone lung transplantation at a single center.[31] PTLD frequently occurs in the transplanted organ, and, in lung recipients, this neoplasm can present as solitary or multiple pulmonary nodules or masses, hilar or mediastinal lymphadenopathy, or a pleural effusion. In general, cases of PTLD that develop in the first year after lung transplantation tend to be isolated to the chest, but cases that develop beyond the first year after transplantation tend to be extrathoracic, often involving the abdomen and pelvis.[32,33] It is noteworthy that late extrathoracic cases tend to have a worse prognosis and are less likely to respond to de-escalation of immunosuppression.

The diagnosis of PTLD requires tissue examination, and, similar to the evaluation for lymphoma, excisional biopsies are ideal. Serum PCR testing for EBV has been evaluated as a tool to aid in the diagnosis and follow-up of patients with PTLD. While the specificity of a positive test in patients with PTLD is near 100%, the sensitivity has been reported to be as low as 40% because many patients with pathologically confirmed PTLD will have negative serum EBV PCR results.[34]

The initial treatment of PTLD is generally a deescalation of immunosuppression.[35] There is an increased risk of allograft rejection with this approach. The anti-CD20 monoclonal antibody rituximab (Rituxan) is the next line of therapy for PTLD. Rituximab is used when remission is not achieved with reduced immunosuppression. In addition, recent studies suggest that administering rituximab earlier in the course of PTLD improves the response and duration of remission.[36,37] If reducing immunosuppression and administration of rituximab does not induce remission of PTLD, systemic chemotherapy with CHOP (cyclophosphamide, doxorubicin, vincristine, and prednisone) is usually administered. Surgical resection can be curative in cases of PTLD with localized disease. Radiation therapy can also be considered in cases of local diseases that are not amenable to surgical resection. When performed, both surgery and radiation should be combined with a reduction in immunosuppression with or without rituximab.

FUNGAL INFECTIONS
Prophylaxis

Antifungal prophylaxis in the immediate posttransplant period varies widely from center to center. This variation is demonstrated in a survey of 50 lung transplant centers published in 2006.[38] Universal prophylaxis and targeted prophylaxis (patients colonized with Aspergillus species before transplantation or becoming colonized after transplantation) were the 2 most common approaches in the survey. Regimens used by different centers included inhaled amphotericin B with or without an azole (usually itraconazole [Sporanox]), itraconazole alone, and fluconazole alone. Universal voriconazole (Vfend) prophylaxis has been shown to decrease the incidence of invasive aspergillosis at 1 year in comparison with targeted prophylaxis with itraconazole with or without inhaled amphotericin B; however, there were increased adverse events in the treatment group, predominantly an elevation of serum liver enzyme levels suggestive of hepatic toxicity.[39] At our center, we practice a targeted approach using itraconazole or voriconazole in patients colonized with Aspergillus before transplantation or immediately after transplantation. In addition, patients are administered prophylaxis with nystatin or fluconazole for oropharyngeal thrush until the corticosteroid doses have been tapered.

Aspergillus Species Infections

Aspergillus fumigatus causes most fungal infections in lung transplant recipients. However, other species, including Aspergillus flavus, Aspergillus niger, Aspergillus terreus, and Aspergillus ustus, have been increasingly reported as causes of invasive fungal infection.[40] Aspergillus infections can be classified as localized airway infection or invasive disease. Invasive diseases include Aspergillus tracheobronchitis, invasive pulmonary aspergillosis, and disseminated aspergillosis.[41]

Aspergillus tracheobronchitis is characterized by the involvement of anastomotic sites and distal airways, especially areas of ischemic injury without extension into the lung parenchyma. Necrosis, ulceration, and pseudomembrane formation are the characteristic features of Aspergillus tracheobronchitis, and the diagnosis is made using bronchoscopy.[42] The risk of developing Aspergillus tracheobronchitis is highest in the first 3 months after transplantation. Progression of the infection is possible if treatment is delayed.

In contrast to the stem cell transplant population, patients who have undergone any solid organ transplant and develop invasive pulmonary aspergillosis do not regularly demonstrate the characteristic halo sign radiologic finding on computed tomography of the chest.[43,44] The most common radiologic findings are nonspecific, including focal or multifocal consolidation, infiltration, or nodular lesions with or without cavitation (**Fig. 2**).

The diagnosis of invasive Aspergillus infections is based on appropriate clinical signs and symptoms combined with pathologic and microbiological confirmation. The Aspergillus galactomannan antigen assay has been used as a marker of angioinvasive disease, especially in the stem cell recipient population, but the sensitivity of the assay for the diagnosis of invasive disease in lung transplant recipients has been reported to be only 30% and is especially poor in patients with

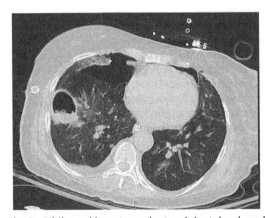

Fig. 2. A bilateral lung transplant recipient developed a thick-walled right lower lobe cavity, which was confirmed to be due to invasive aspergillosis histologically. The recipient developed respiratory failure and pneumothorax and did not respond to therapy.

tracheobronchitis.[45] Testing the bronchoalveolar fluid for the presence of the galactomannan antigen appears to be more sensitive than testing the serum when looking for tracheobronchitis or invasive pulmonary aspergillosis; however, the overall clinical condition of the patient must be considered before deciding on any one diagnostic test to make the diagnosis of invasive aspergillosis.[46] False-positive results of the serum galactomannan assay can occur in the presence of certain antibiotics, especially piperacillin/tazobactam.

The treatment of *Aspergillus* infections involves the use of azoles, echinocandins, and amphotericin B and generally depends on the severity of illness, with the lipid formulation of amphotericin B remaining the first line of treatment in severe disease. There is emerging data that echinocandins, (caspofungin [Cancidas], micafungin [Mycamine], and anidulafungin [Eraxis]), alone or in combination with voriconazole may be an effective first-line treatment of pulmonary aspergillosis, with significantly less toxicity.[47,48] Voriconazole is generally preferred over itraconazole, given the more predicable bioavailability of voriconazole over itraconazole. Posaconazole (Noxafil) also has activity against *Aspergillus* species, but there is not as much experience with this agent, and it is not available in an intravenous formulation. In addition, azoles have a potent interaction with calcineurin inhibitors, and the cyclosporine (Neoral) or tacrolimus (Prograf) doses need to be significantly reduced when itraconazole or voriconazole are inititated.[41]

Candida Species Infections

C albicans remains the most common *Candida* species causing fungal infections in lung transplant recipients but a shift toward non-albicans species has been observed.[10] Clinical patterns of candidiasis in lung transplantation recipients range from mucocutaneous to invasive disease, with candidemia and multiorgan involvement. Although *C albicans* is generally sensitive to azole agents, including fluconazole, some non-albicans *Candida* species are resistant to fluconazole. Several recent studies have demonstrated the effectiveness of echinocandins in invasive candidiasis and should be considered as a first-line treatment pending identification and speciation of the *Candida* species in culture.[49–51] Amphotericin B is effective for invasive candidiasis; however, given its toxicity and the effectiveness of safer echinocandins and azoles, it should be reserved for treatment failures or patients who are intolerant of echinocandins and are infected by organisms that are resistant to azole agents.

P jiroveci

P jiroveci (formerly *Pneumocystis carinii*) is an organism that is ubiquitous in the environment and can cause pneumonia in any immunosuppressed patient. In the era of prophylaxis, it is rare for patients to develop *P jiroveci* pneumonia.[52] The first-line prophylactic is trimethoprim/sulfamethoxazole (Bactrim, Septra), although in patients who are allergic to sulfa drugs alternative options include inhaled pentamidine (Pentam), atovaquone (Mepron), and dapsone. This infection is treated with high doses of trimethoprim/sulfamethoxazole, often with an increase in the corticosteroid dose, especially when complicated by hypoxemia.[53] In patients who are allergic to sulfa drugs, desensitization can be considered in order to use trimethoprim/sulfamethoxazole for either prophylaxis or treatment in the event of *Pneumocystis* pneumonia.

Other Fungi

Many other fungal pathogens have been associated with clinical disease in lung transplant recipients. *Cryptococcus neoformans* can infect the lung itself, in addition to causing disseminated multisystem disease. Depending on the geography, endemic fungi can cause disease in lung transplant recipients (eg, histoplasmosis, coccidioidomycosis, and blastomycosis). In addition, several non-*Aspergillus* mycelial fungi, including zygomycetes (eg, mucormycosis) and *Scedosporium* species, have more recently been recognized as important pathogens in the transplant recipient population and are generally associated with worsened outcomes compared with *Aspergillus* species.[54]

MYCOBACTERIA
Nontuberculosis Mycobacteria

Nontuberculosis mycobacterial infection before lung transplantation is generally observed in patients with bronchiectasis, especially CF. The prevalence of these organisms has been reported as 3% to 10% in patients with adult onset bronchiectasis and 13% to 28% in patients with CF.[55,56] The risk of recurrence of nontuberculosis mycobacterial infection and significant clinical disease seems to be the highest with *Mycobacterium abscessus*, although in one study the posttransplant course was not affected by *M abscessus* infection.[57] Although difficult to manage, it is possible to successfully treat infections caused by *Mycobacterium avium-intracellulare* (**Fig. 3**) and *M abscessus* in lung transplant recipients.[58] Treatment is guided by the American Thoracic Society (ATS)/Infectious Diseases Society of America (IDSA) statement regarding nontuberculous mycobacterial disease

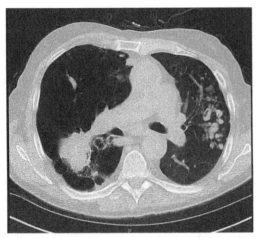

Fig. 3. A left single lung transplant recipient developed a masslike infiltrate in the native emphysematous lung and multiple nodules in the allograft. Pathologic conditions were consistent with granulomatous inflammation and cultures showed positive results for *Mycobacterium avium-intracellulare*. The recipient responded well to treatment.

and is the same as in the nontransplant immunocompetent host.[59]

Mycobacterium tuberculosis

Transplant recipients should be evaluated for latent infection with *Mycobacterium tuberculosis* using the tuberculin skin test. In the event of a positive test result and no evidence of active tuberculosis on chest radiograph, INH therapy should be administered for 6 to 9 months.[60] Active tuberculosis should be treated according to ATS/Centers for Disease Control/IDSA guidelines and is the same as in the nontransplant host.[61]

SUMMARY

Throughout their lives lung transplant recipients are at an increased risk of infectious complications from the immediate postoperative period. Appropriate antimicrobial prophylaxis, knowledge of the timing of risk of infectious complications, and aggressive appropriate treatment of the infections decrease morbidity and mortality in this population. Many infectious complications, including bacterial, viral, and fungal infections, confer an increased risk for BOS, the leading cause of death in lung recipients after more than 1 year after transplantation. Continued investigations regarding the ideal antimicrobial prophylaxis and immunosuppressive regimens will allow clinicians caring for lung transplant recipients to minimize the risks of infection, maximize allograft function by limiting rejection,

and minimize the adverse effects that are associated with prolonged antimicrobial therapy.

REFERENCES

1. Christie JD, Edwards LB, Kucheryavaya AY, et al. The registry of the International Society for Heart and Lung Transplantation: twenty-eighth adult lung and heart-lung transplant report—2011. J Heart Lung Transplant 2011;30(10):1104–22.
2. Alexander BD, Tapson VF. Infectious complications of lung transplantation. Transpl Infect Dis 2001;3(3): 128–37.
3. Snyder LD, Finlen-Copeland A, Jackson W, et al. Cytomegalovirus pneumonitis is a risk for bronchiolitis obliterans syndrome in lung transplantation. Am J Respir Crit Care Med 2010;181:1391–6.
4. Vos R, Vanaudenaerde BM, Geudens N, et al. Pseudomonal airway colonization: risk factor for bronchiolitis obliterans syndrome after lung transplantation? Eur Respir J 2008;31:1037–45.
5. Gottlieb J, Mattner F, Weissbrodt H, et al. Impact of graft colonization with gram-negative bacteria after lung transplantation on the development of bronchiolitis obliterans syndrome in recipients with cystic fibrosis. Respir Med 2009;103:743–9.
6. Botha P, Archer L, Anderson RL, et al. Pseudomonas aeruginosa colonization of the allograft after lung transplantation and the risk of bronchiolitis obliterans syndrome. Transplantation 2008;85:771–4.
7. Weigt SS, Elashoff RM, Huang C, et al. Aspergillus colonization of the lung allograft is a risk factor for bronchiolitis obliterans syndrome. Am J Transplant 2009;9:1903–11.
8. Campos S, Caramori M, Teizeira R, et al. Bacterial and fungal pneumonias after lung transplantation. Transplant Proc 2008;27:528–35.
9. Chang ST, Krupnick AS. Perioperative antibiotics in thoracic surgery. Thorac Surg Clin 2012;22:35–45.
10. Solé A, Salavert M. Fungal infections after lung transplantation. Curr Opin Pulm Med 2009;15: 243–53.
11. Aguilar-Guisado M, Givalda J, Ussetti P, et al. Pneumonia after lung transplantation in the RESITRA Cohort: a multicenter prospective study. Am J Transplant 2007;7:1989–96.
12. Chaparro C, Maurer J, Gutierrez C, et al. Infection with Burkholderia cepacia in cystic fibrosis: outcome following lung transplantation. Am J Respir Crit Care Med 2001;163:43–8.
13. Meachery G, De Soyza A, Nicholson A, et al. Outcomes of lung transplantation for cystic fibrosis in a large UK cohort. Thorax 2008;63:725–31.
14. Luong M, Morrissey O, Husain S. Assessment of infection risks prior to lung transplantation. Curr Opin Infect Dis 2010;23:578–83.

15. Alexander BD, Petzold EW, Reller LB, et al. Survival after lung transplantation of cystic fibrosis patients infected with Burkholderia cepacia complex. Am J Transplant 2008;8:1025–30.

16. Murray S, Charbeneau J, Marshall BC, et al. Impact of Burkholderia infection on lung transplantation in cystic fibrosis. Am J Respir Crit Care Med 2008; 178:363–71.

17. Zamora MR. Cytomegalovirus and lung transplantation. Am J Transplant 2004;4:1219–26.

18. Kotton CN, Kumar D, Caliendo AM, et al. International consensus guidelines on the management of cytomegalovirus in solid organ transplantation. Transplantation 2010;89:779–95.

19. Zuk DM, Humar A, Weinkauf JG, et al. An international survey of cytomegalovirus management practices in lung transplantation. Transplantation 2010; 90:672–6.

20. Palmer SM, Limaye AP, Banks M, et al. Extended valganciclovir prophylaxis to prevent cytomegalovirus after lung transplantation. Ann Intern Med 2010;152:761–9.

21. Kotloff RM, Ahya VN. Medical complications of lung transplantation. Eur Respir J 2004;23:334–42.

22. Asberg A, Humar A, Rollag H, et al. Oral valganciclovir is noninferior to intravenous ganciclovir for the treatment of cytomegalovirus disease in solid organ transplant recipients. Am J Transplant 2007;7:2106–13.

23. Snydman DR, Limaye AP, Potena L, et al. Update and review: state-of-the-art management of cytomegalovirus infection and disease following thoracic organ transplantation. Transplant Proc 2011;43:S1–17.

24. Khalifah AP, Hachem RR, Chakinala MM, et al. Respiratory viral infections are a distinct risk for bronchiolitis obliterans syndrome and death. Am J Respir Crit Care Med 2004;170:181–7.

25. Chakinala MM, Walter MJ. Community acquired respiratory viral infections after lung transplantation: clinical features and long-term consequences. Semin Thorac Cardiovasc Surg 2004;16:342–9.

26. Shah JN, Chemaly RF. Management of RSV infections in adult recipients of hematopoietic stem cell transplantation. Blood 2011;117:2756–63.

27. Harris NL, Ferry JA, Swerdlow SH. Posttransplant lymphoproliferative disorders: summary of society for hematopathology workshop. Semin Diagn Pathol 1997;14:8–14.

28. Armitage JM, Kormos RL, Stuart RS, et al. Posttransplant lymphoproliferative disease in thoracic organ transplant patients: ten years of cyclosporine-based immunosuppression. J Heart Lung Transplant 1991;10:877–86.

29. Nalesnik MA. Posttransplantation lymphoproliferative disorders (PTLD): current perspectives. Semin Thorac Cardiovasc Surg 1996;8:139–48.

30. Loren AW, Tsai DE. Post-transplant lymphoproliferative disorder. Clin Chest Med 2005;26:631–45.

31. Kremer BE, Reshef R, Misleh JG, et al. Post-transplant lymphoproliferative disorder after lung transplantation: a review of 35 cases. J Heart Lung Transplant 2012;31(3):296–304.

32. Paranjothi S, Yusen R, Kraus M, et al. Lymphoproliferative disease after lung transplantation: comparison of presentation and outcome of early and late cases. J Heart Lung Transplant 2001;20:1054–63.

33. Hachem RR, Chakinala MM, Yusen RD, et al. Abdominal-pelvic lymphoproliferative disease after lung transplantation: presentation and outcome. Transplantation 2004;77:431–7.

34. Tsai DE, Nearey M, Hardy CL, et al. Use of EBV PCR for the diagnosis and monitoring of post-transplant lymphoproliferative disorder in adult solid organ transplant patients. Am J Transplant 2002;2:946–54.

35. Jagadeesh D, Woda BA, Draper J, et al. Post transplant lymphoproliferative disorders: risk, classification, and therapeutic recommendations. Curr Treat Options Oncol 2012;13(1):122–36.

36. Evens AM, David KA, Helenowski I, et al. Multicenter analysis of 80 solid organ transplantation recipients with post-transplantation lymphoproliferative disease: outcomes and prognostic factors in the modern era. J Clin Oncol 2010;28:1038–46.

37. Trappe R, Choquet S, Oertel SH, et al. Sequential treatment with rituximab followed by CHOP chemotherapy in adult B-cell post-transplant lymphoproliferative disorder (PTLD): the prospective international multicentre phase 2 PTLD-1 trial. Lancet Oncol 2012;13(2):196–206.

38. Husain S, Zaldonis D, Kusne S, et al. Variation in antifungal prophylaxis strategies in lung transplantation. Transpl Infect Dis 2006;8:213–8.

39. Husain S, Paterson DL, Studer S. Voriconazole prophylaxis in lung transplant recipients. Am J Transplant 2006;6:3008–16.

40. Caston JJ, Linares MJ, Gallego C, et al. Risk factors for pulmonary Aspergillus terreus infection in patients with positive culture for filamentous fungi. Chest 2007;131:230–8.

41. Silveira PF, Husain S. Fungal infections in lung transplant recipients. Curr Opin Pulm Med 2008; 14:211–8.

42. Kramer MR, Denning DW, Marshall SE, et al. Ulcerative tracheobronchitis after lung transplantation: a new form of invasive aspergillosis. Am Rev Respir Dis 1991;144:552–6.

43. Singh N, Husain S. Aspergillus infections after lung transplantation: clinical differences in type of transplant and implications for management. J Heart Lung Transplant 2003;22:258–66.

44. Paterson DL, Singh N. Invasive aspergillosis in transplant recipients. Medicine 1999;78:123–38.

45. Husain S, Kwak EJ, Obman A, et al. Prospective assessment of Platelia Aspergillus galactomannan antigen for the diagnosis of invasive aspergillosis in

lung transplant recipients. Am J Transplant 2004;4: 796–802.

46. Husain S, Paterson DL, Studer SM, et al. Aspergillus galactomannan antigen in the bronchoalveolar lavage fluid for the diagnosis of invasive aspergillosis in lung transplant recipients. Transplantation 2007;83:1330–6.

47. Groetzner J, Kaczmarek I, Wittwer T, et al. Caspofungin as first-line therapy for the treatment of invasive aspergillosis after thoracic organ transplantation. J Heart Lung Transplant 2008;27:1–6.

48. Singh N, Limaye AP, Forrest G, et al. Combination of voriconazole and caspofungin as primary therapy for invasive aspergillosis in solid organ transplant recipients: a prospective, multicenter, observational study. Transplantation 2006;81:320–6.

49. Mora-Duarte J, Betts R, Rotstein C, et al. Comparison of caspofungin and amphotericin B for invasive candidiasis. N Engl J Med 2002;347:2020–9.

50. Kuse ER, Chetchotisakd P, da Cunha CA, et al. Micafungin versus liposomal amphotericin B for candidaemia and invasive candidosis: a phase II randomized double-blind trial. Lancet 2007;369: 1519–27.

51. Reboli AC, Rotstein C, Pappas PG, et al. Anidulafungin versus fluconazole for invasive candidiasis. N Engl J Med 2007;356:2472–82.

52. Green H, Paul M, Vidal L, et al. Prophylaxis of Pneumocystis pneumonia in immunocompromised non-HIV-infected patients: systematic review and meta-analysis of randomized controlled trials. Mayo Clin Proc 2008;82:1052–9.

53. Briel M, Bucher HC, Boscacci R, et al. Adjunctive corticosteroids for Pneumocystis jiroveci pneumonia

in patients with HIV-infection. Cochrane Database Syst Rev 2006;3:CD006150.

54. Husain S, Alexander B, Munoz P, et al. Opportunistic mycelia fungal infections in organ transplant recipients: emerging importance of non-Aspergillus mycelia fungi. Clin Infect Dis 2003;37:221–9.

55. Fowler SJ, French J, Screaton NJ, et al. Nontuberculous mycobacteria in bronchiectasis: prevalence and patient characteristics. Eur Respir J 2006;28: 1204–10.

56. Lipuma JJ. The changing microbial epidemiology in cystic fibrosis. Clin Microbiol Rev 2010;(23):299–323.

57. Chalermskulrat W, Sood N, Neuringer IP, et al. Nontuberculous mycobacteria in end stage cystic fibrosis: implications for lung transplantation. Thorax 2006;61:507–13.

58. Chernenko SM, Humar A, Hutcheon M, et al. Mycobacterium abscessus infections in lung transplant recipients: the international experience. J Heart Lung Transplant 2006;25:1447–55.

59. Griffith DE, Aksamit T, Brown-Elliot BA, et al. An official ATS/IDSA statement: diagnosis, treatment, and prevention of nontuberculous mycobacterial disease. Am J Respir Crit Care Med 2007;175:367–416.

60. Aguado JM, Torre-Cisneros J, Fortun J, et al. Tuberculosis in solid-organ transplant recipients: consensus statement of the group for the study of infection in transplant recipients (GESITRA) of the Spanish Society of Infectious Diseases and Clinical Microbiology. Clin Infect Dis 2009;48:1276–84.

61. Centers for Disease Control, Prevention. Treatment of tuberculosis. American Thoracic Society, CDC, and Infectious Diseases Society of America. MMWR 2003;52(RR-11):1–72.

Alternatives to Resectional Surgery for Infectious Disease of the Lung
From Embolization to Thoracoplasty

Marco Alifano, MD, PhD[a], Sonia Gaucher, MD, PhD[b],
Antoine Rabbat, MD[c], Jury Brandolini, MD[a],
Claude Guinet, MD, PhD[d], Diane Damotte, MD, PhD[e],
Jean-François Regnard, MD[a],*

KEYWORDS

- Necrotizing pneumonia • Lung abscess • Aspergilloma • Cavernostomy • Thoracoplasty
- Flap transposition • Bronchoscopy • Embolization

KEY POINTS

- Surgical treatment of lung diseases is generally based on removal of the affected lung tissue, whereas infectious lung diseases are generally treated by exclusive medical therapy. There are cases of lung infection, however, in which alternatives to resectional surgery are indicated.
- Lung abscess, necrotizing pneumonia, and fungal infections, including aspergilloma, may require nonresective surgery, especially when resection is not indicated or associated with an excessively high risk.
- Nonresective surgery of the lung is generally performed in a multimodality management setting to maximize possibility of success in severely ill patients.
- Chest wall surgery, including open window thoracostomy, cavernostomy, and thoracoplasty, may represent am effective tool in the surgical management of severe infectious pleuropulmonary diseases.
- A multistep surgical management is often necessary.

Surgical treatment of lung diseases currently is based on removal of the affected lung tissue. This is achieved by atypical or anatomic lung resection, depending on etiology, topography, results of lung function tests, and coexisting comorbidities.

Infectious lung diseases are generally treated by medical therapy, including medications, chest physiotherapy, bronchoscopic toilet, and respiratory rehabilitation. Such types of multimodal management are possible thanks to progresses in medical management and pharmacology, which have been became increasingly available over the past 6 decades. Before these advances, infectious diseases of the lung often required surgical treatment, which was based on lung resection and, at least as frequently, on nonresectional surgery.

Although indications for surgery for infectious lung diseases have dramatically decreased,

[a] Department of Thoracic Surgery, Hôtel-Dieu Hospital, Paris Descartes University, 1 Place du Parvis Notre Dame, 75181 Paris, France; [b] Department of Plastic Surgery, Hôtel-Dieu Hospital, Paris Descartes University, 1 Place du Parvis Notre Dame, 75181 Paris, France; [c] Department of Pneumology and Intensive Care, Hôtel-Dieu Hospital, Paris Descartes University, 1 Place du Parvis Notre Dame, 75181 Paris, France; [d] Department of Radiology, Hôtel-Dieu Hospital, Paris Descartes University, 1 Place du Parvis Notre Dame, 75181 Paris, France; [e] Department of Pathology, Hôtel-Dieu Hospital, Paris Descartes University, 1 Place du Parvis Notre Dame, 75181 Paris, France
* Corresponding author.
E-mail address: jean-francois.regnard@htd.aphp.fr

Thorac Surg Clin 22 (2012) 413–429
doi:10.1016/j.thorsurg.2012.05.001
1547-4127/12/$ – see front matter © 2012 Elsevier Inc. All rights reserved.

a significant percentage of surgical techniques proposed in the early decades of the past century have maintained some indications in cases of failure of nonsurgical treatment or contraindication to resectional surgery. Most of these techniques have been revisited according to progress in surgery, anesthesiology, and, more generally, perioperative care. Thus, surgical management for infectious disease of lung is integrated in multispecialty care.

Surgical treatment based on lung resection is described in details in articles elsewhere this issue. Thus, this article focuses exclusively on nonresectional surgery and other alternatives to lung resection. This article addresses bacterial infection of lung (including lung abscess and necrotizing pneumonia) as well as fungal disease of lung.

BACTERIAL INFECTIONS OF LUNG

Bacterial infections of lung may occur in a previously healthy lung in an otherwise healthy individual as well as in a previously diseased lung in an otherwise healthy or sick individual.[1,2]

Characteristics of the offending bacteria and host immune response determine the clinical presentation and course of infection as well as susceptibility to administered treatments. Community-acquired pneumonia in otherwise healthy individuals is medically treated in an outpatient, hospital, or ICU setting and almost never requires surgical management.

Uniloculated pleural complications (parapneumonic effusion or empyema) are managed by needle thoracocentesis and/or chest drainage, whereas symptomatic multiloculated pleural effusion requires fibrinolysis or video-assisted thoracic surgery (VATS) débridement. In rare instances,

open lung decortication may be necessary, in cases of late referral to surgery or unsuccessful mini-invasive approach.[1,2] These issues are discussed elsewhere in other articles in this issue.

For severely ill patients with thoracic empyema, in whom VATS débridement fails to control the disease, open window thoracostomy (marsupialization of the cavity via rib[s] resection and open drainage), which is a well-established method of low risk, should be proposed if lung decortication is contraindicated because of operative risk and poor quality of lung parenchyma preventing satisfactory re-expansion.[1,2] Muscle transposition can be proposed as the space becomes sterile-cleansed to fill the residual space if spontaneous closure does not occur. Alternatively, or if myoplasty is not feasible, limited tailored thoracoplasty may be indicated (**Fig. 1**).

The indication of thoracoplasty for primary empyema is accepted but uncommon. If infection is controlled but the lung does not expand and decortication is not feasible or has failed, thoracoplasty can be indicated if sufficient drainage of the pleural space may be achieved by tube thoracostomy.

Pneumonia may be complicated by necrosis and destruction of lung tissue because of factors related to pathogens or host and interaction between the two.[1,2] These changes in lung parenchyma are reflected by two main clinical entities that have some common features but several clinical and pathologic differences: lung abscesses and necrotizing pneumonia (**Figs. 2 and 3**).[1,2] Lung abscess is characterized by focal character, fibrous perilesional reaction (see **Fig. 2**), and a clinical course that is acute or subacute but rarely associated with signs of acute severe sepsis. Necrotizing pneumonias are characterized by

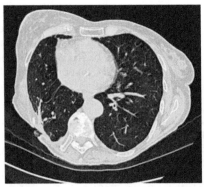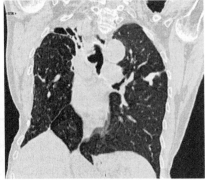

Fig. 1. A 70-year-old woman with history of chronic immunosuppressive therapy for rheumatoid arthritis presented with spontaneous empyema. When VATS débridement failed, open window thoracostomy was indicated, because of contraindication to open decortication. After local control of infection, limited tailored thoracoplasty was necessary to obliterate residual space because of unavailability of muscle for flap transposition. (*Left*) CT scan, axial view. (*Right*) CT scan, coronal view.

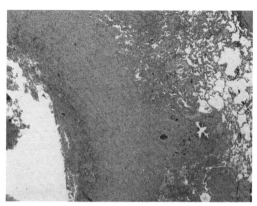

Fig. 2. Pathologic examination of a specimen of lung abscess showing an acute inflammatory reaction surrounding the cavity. Adjacent lung parenchymal is normal. Hematoxylin–Eosin–Safran staining.

diffuse, possibly bilateral, hepatization of the lung parenchyma with multiple cavitations and necrosis area (see **Fig. 3**).[1] Lack of perfusion of the area of necrosis is often shown on injected CT scan of the lungs. In adult patients, necrotizing pneumonia is a rare entity. Lung gangrene is a variant of necrotizing pneumonia whose main feature is loss of perfusion by a central vascular occlusion, frequently by a septic thrombus.[2,3] Anaerobic bacteria are particularly implicated in this latter condition.[4] An intermediate form between necrotizing pneumonia and lung abscess is represented by a third entity, observed only in the chronic phase, the destroyed lung (see **Fig. 3**), which is thought to have originated from progressive confluent piecemeal necrosis. The destroyed lung is characterized by progressive loss of architecture, the net decrease of perfusion, and chronic course marked by recurrent episodes of hemoptysis and bronchopulmonary infection.[5,6]

All 3 entities often require a surgical treatment that is based on resectional or nonresectional surgery, depending considerations about clinical and radiologic presentation, lung function, and comorbidities.

Lung Abscess

Lung abscess is a not infrequent complication of pneumonia in children. In adult patients, primary abscess most frequently results from aspiration of oropharyngeal secretions or gastric contents. Thus, altered levels of consciousness, gastroesophageal dysmotility, and poor dental hygiene represent frequent predisposing comorbidities. Diabetes mellitus, HIV infection, and alcohol abuse are frequently observed in these patients. Less common comorbidities are represented by cystic

fibrosis and α_1-antitrypsin deficiency. Lung abscesses are not infrequently seen after dental surgery and have also been described as a complication of septic thrombosis of a neck vein secondary to dental or pharyngeal infections (Lemierre syndrome).[7,8] Lung abscesses are generally seen on chest radiography or CT performed because of fever and persistent pulmonary symptoms: a cavitary lung mass is seen and differential diagnosis should include tuberculosis, vasculitis, cavitary tumors, and necrotizing pneumonia, among other diseases. In this setting, fiberoptic bronchoscopy is usually performed for sampling purposes as well as to exclude obstructive lesions.[7]

Treatment of pyogenic lung abscesses is based on prolonged antibiotherapy, postural drainage, and optimal management of predisposing illness. This approach allows satisfactorily dealing with the condition in at least 80% to 90% of cases.[9,10] Failure of conservative management is generally a consequence of impossibility to achieve an adequate concentration of antibiotics within the abscess cavity, if the causative germs have been correctly identified by adequate sample collection.[9,11] The question of reliability of diagnosis, however, should be systematically risen; in particular, abscessed bronchogenic carcinoma should be ruled out.

Bronchoscopy may have a therapeutic role in some cases: relief of possibly associated nontumoral bronchial stenoses may be indicated and topic instillation of antibiotics may have some usefulness. In cases of failure of conservative approach, more invasive procedures, namely drainage or resection, are indicated.[8]

Lung resection (segmentectomy or, more frequently, lobectomy) is the definitive procedure and achieves cure rates of 90% but concomitant mortality rates of 11% to 28% are reported.[12] Thus, less-invasive approaches, whose goal is not resection of the diseases area but evacuation of septic collection, may represent a valid alternative.[12] It has been estimated that drainage is performed in 11% to 21% of patients with lung abscesses in whom medical therapy is unsuccessful; drainage may be obtained by direct tube pneumostomy, percutaneous drainage under CT or US guidance, or bronchoscopic drainage.[7]

Pneumonostomy with direct drainage (Monaldi procedure) was initially described in the treatment of tuberculous cavern (intracavitary aspiration). It can achieve the goal of optimal drainage thanks to a large tube, but it is only possible when the pleural space is obliterated. It is indicated in cases of peripheral lesion in close contact with parietal pleura.[8]

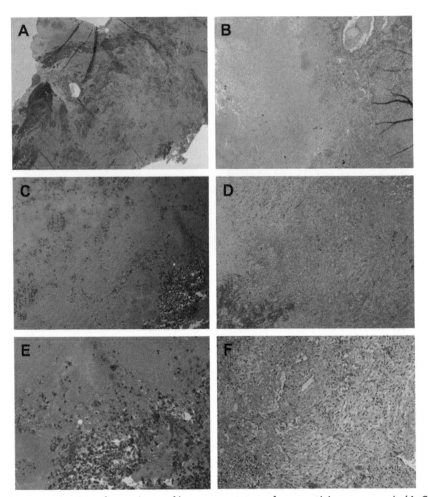

Fig. 3. Pathologic examination of a specimen of lung necrosectomy for necrotizing pneumonia (*A, C, E*) and sur-infected destroyed lung (*B, D, F*). In necrotizing pneumonia specimens, acute extensive lung parenchyma necrosis is evident; the whole-lung specimen is necrotic with hemorrhage and few inflammatory cells. Hematoxylin–Eosin–Safran staining. Original magnification: × (*A*) 40, (*C*) 100, and (*E*) 200. In secondary infection destroyed lung, the lesion is characterized by necrotic area, surrounded by inflammatory cells and fibrotic tissue. Adjacent lung parenchyma is inflamed but still recognizable. Original magnification: (*B*) 40, (*D*) 100, and (*F*) 200. Differences with pathologic examination (shown in **Fig. 2**) are evident.

In the past 2 decades, percutaneous catheter drainage under CT or US guidance has proved effective in appropriately selected adult and pediatric patients and is currently the technique of choice.[7] CT is optimal in determining the wall thickness of an abscess, contents of an abscess, and its relationship to the adjacent lung and pleura. Follow-up CT studies after placement of catheter allow optimal assessment of the efficacy of drainage and help in determining whether an additional catheter is required.[7] Duration of complete obliteration of cavity is variable and has been reported to occur as early as 4 days or as long as 12 weeks but usually takes 4 to 5 weeks.[9]

CT-guided percutaneous catheter positioning may be difficult in cases of centrally located lesions, because of the large amount of lung tissue needed to be traversed and of proximity of vascular structures. In these cases, endoscopic drainage can be proposed.[8]

Bronchoscopic drainage of parenchymal abscess cavities was first reported by Metras and Chapin in 1954.[13] Bronchoscopic drainage does not carry the risk of soiling the pleural space and is less invasive than surgical resection, but endobronchial spillage of abscess contents may be a problem.[10] Endoscopic drainage is possible if an abscess communicates with the bronchial tree (generally at segmental or subsegmentary level). It is performed by flexible bronchoscopy (FOB) through a nasal approach. Selective bronchography may be required first to identify the airway leading into the cavity; this approach has been associated with a success rate of 90%.[8]

Necrotizing Pneumonia

Necrotizing pneumonia is a life-threatening condition whose management is often challenging because of large variability of presentation, impairment of vital function by various mechanisms, and absence of large clinical experience, and as, a consequence, of recommendations, at least in adults. Necrotizing pneumonia is characterized by diffuse, sometimes bilateral, consolidation of lung parenchyma, and presence of necrosis. From a clinical point of view, the disease is rapidly progressive and the main events are represented by respiratory failure and sepsis, which is difficult or impossible to control, in spite of medical treatment.[2,3] An empyema secondary to intrapleural perforation is often associated.[14] Alternatively, parenchymal necrosis often leads to formation of bronchiolar fistula, or, in cases of more proximal process, of bronchial fistula.[15] The latter may be responsible, in patients under mechanical ventilation, for major air leaks with subsequent ventilatory difficulties. Exceptionally, necrotizing pneumonia may have a tumor-like presentation and be responsible for compression of neighboring structures, including the vena cava and right heart cavities, with severe hemodynamic repercussions (**Fig. 4**).

Little is known about the exact epidemiology of necrotizing pneumonia: it is seen more often in children, whereas in adulthood, associated comorbidities and, to a greater extent, immunologic impairment are a frequent feature, as confirmed in the authors' recently published experience.[2,3,5] In children, its incidence seems to increase with time.[16]

With respect to initial causative pathogens, *Streptococcus sp* are often cultured.[14,16,17] Other organisms that cause necrotizing pneumonia with rapid cavitations, microabscess formation, blood vessel invasion, and hemorrhage are also described: *Pseudomonas aeruginosa*[18] and *Clostridium perfringens*.[19] *Staphylococcus aureus* strains producing Panton-Valentine leukocidin seem particularly associated with necrotizing pneumonia.[20,21] Community-associated methicillin-resistant *Staphylococcus aureus* (MRSA) are also increasingly reported in otherwise healthy individuals.[22] Necrotizing pneumonia should be recognized as a distinct element of complicated pneumonia and, in particular, its presence should be considered as a separate complicating feature

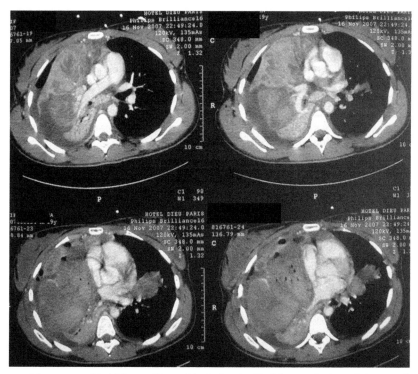

Fig. 4. A 19-year-old women with history of bronchiectasis admitted for respiratory distress and cardiac shock. Necrotizing pneumonia complicating a community-acquired pneumonia was diagnosed. CT scan showing compression of cardiac cavities by parenchymal necrosis.

from the often accompanying pleural effusion.[2,3,14] Diagnosis of necrotizing pneumonia requires CT imaging in patients with complicated pneumonia and continued symptoms despite appropriate medical therapy. Conservative management, including adequate prolonged antibiotics, mechanical ventilation, and pleural drainage, is always necessary for a favorable outcome.[2,3,14] Nevertheless, as previously reported in children,[23] a significant percentage of adult cases requires surgical management.[24]

In almost all the instances, the disease is rapidly progressive and the main events are represented by respiratory failure and sepsis. Because a majority of patients are seriously ill with rapid-onset respiratory failure and or septic shock with multiple organ failure, patient admission in ICU is mandatory.[24]

Medical treatment must include supportive care and adequate antibiotic treatment. Supportive care includes pain management, nutritional support, psychological support, and early physiotherapy to allow recovery with as much minimal functional sequel as possible. The two key points are adequate treatment of septic shock and of respiratory failure.[24]

Severe sepsis and septic shock treatment

Treatment of severe sepsis and septic shock includes fluid resuscitation, vasopressive drugs, and adequate oxygenation. Fluid resuscitation must be carefully adapted to left ventricular loading pressure either indirectly assessed by means of cardiac echography or more-invasive monitoring tools, such as right heart catheterization.[25] Fluid overload may worsen oxygenation. Alternatively, hypovolemia may precipitate other organ failure, such as renal failure.

In these patients, septic shock is usually a hyperkinetic shock. In some patients, a hypokinetic state of septic shock is possible and is well recognized by echocardiography showing a significant decrease in left ventricular systolic function and such patients may benefit from inotropic drugs, such as dobutamine.[26]

As discussed previously, some patients may present a right heart failure mimicking an acute pericardial tamponade with severe hemodynamic disturbances related to compression of the vena cava and/or right heart cavities by tumor-like forms. In these latter cases, relief of the compression by drainage and/or surgery is crucial to reverse a patient's shock (see **Fig. 4**).

Ventilatory support

Treatment of respiratory failure is aimed at insuring correct oxygenation and allowing CO_2 elimination. A key point is to lower, as much as possible, deleterious effect of mechanical ventilation. As discussed previously, parenchymal necrosis often leads to formation of bronchiolar fistula, or, in cases of more proximal process, of bronchial fistula. The latter may be responsible, in patients under mechanical ventilation, of major air leaks with subsequent ventilatory difficulties. Due to the severity of the disease and associated septic shock, or even multiple organ failure, noninvasive ventilation is contraindicated in such patients.

Tracheal intubation with mechanical ventilation is necessary in the large majority of the patients. In all mechanically ventilated patients, a lung protective ventilation strategy should be applied, including low tidal volume (5–8 mL/kg ideal body weight), positive end-expiratory pressure, and avoiding plateau pressure above 30 cm of water. Bronchopleural fistula (BPF) with large air leaks is a major problem because adequate alveolar ventilation may be unachievable with uncontrolled hypercarbia.[27–29]

In such cases, if endoscopic treatment fails (discussed later), extracorporeal lung assist may be useful.[30] Classical extracorporeal membrane oxygenation (ECMO) is able to insure adequate oxygenation and CO_2 removal but requires continuous anticoagulation with a high risk of bleeding. Surgical procedures often necessary in these patients are also difficult to insure while the patients are under ECMO. In patients hemodynamically stable and without major hypoxemia, extracorporeal CO_2 removal with simplest technique, such as with Novalung assist, must be considered.[31] This simplest technique may allow weaning the patients from the ventilator more rapidly in cases of major bronchial fistula.

Bronchoscopic management of bronchopleural fistula

FOB can be used as therapeutic modality in the management of BPF. Because most of the endoscopic techniques require sedation alone, they may be more suited for critically ill patients than surgical procedures that require general anesthesia. BPF may be useful for repair of small leaks as well as for bridging to surgical repair in debilitated patients with large leaks. A BPF greater than 8 mm and large central BPFs are usually unsuitable for bronchoscopic management. FOB can directly visualize the fistula and demonstrate that occlusion of a segmental or lobar bronchus with a balloon catheter decreases or stops the air leak. Although the proximal fistulae are easy to visualize, a peripheral BPF presents a significant challenge even to a skilled bronchoscopist.[27,32]

Once the site is located and the fistula deemed amenable to repair, application of various sealants into the fistula or the bronchial segment leading up to the fistula has been tried. The potential success of this approach seems limited to smaller, low-flow peripheral fistulae. A wide range of synthetic and biologically derived substances has been used with variable success in the management of BPF.[33–38] Alternatively, direct mechanical obstruction of the bronchial segment may be achieved with balloon catheter occlusion,[34] collagen screw plugs, endobronchial coils, and endobronchial valves.[37] One-way endobronchial valves may be placed in the segmental bronchus, allowing unidirectional airflow from the parenchyma to the airway and redirecting the inflowing air away from the affected segment. Unlike other modalities used for mechanical obstruction, these valves allow drainage of distal secretions reducing infectious complications and are easily removable once adequate healing of the fistula has been achieved. There are no controlled studies available to demonstrate the superiority of one modality over the other, and clear guidelines for patient selection for endoscopic management do not exist.

Mechanical obstruction of the airway by the mean of FOB is rarely a definite treatment in large BPF but may be useful as a bridge to surgery.

Antibiotic treatment

All patients should benefit from multiple microbiologic samplings, including arterial blood culture, trachobronchial aspirates culture, FOB-directed bronchial sampling by the mean of protected distal catheter or brush or bronchoalveolar lavage. Pleural fluid culture and lung abscess fluid culture are essential samplings when present. According to the severity of this lung infection, early empiric antibiotic treatment is necessary.[39] Usual guidelines for severe community-acquired pneumonia may be applied but taking account risk factors for potentially resistant pathogen is crucial.[40,41] In cases of previous antibiotic treatment or severe chronic respiratory disease or bronchiectasis, *Pseudomonas aeruginosa* coverage should be considered.[41] In cases of MRSA suspicion, initial antibiotic regiment should include glycopeptides or linezolide. In some regions of high level of multiresistant enterobacteria, initial empiric treatment with carbapenem could be considered. In all cases, antibiotic adjustment according to the antibiotic susceptibility of isolated germs should be achieved. High initial dosages of antibiotics are necessary to achieve high parenchyma and pleural antibiotic concentrations. Prolonged antibiotic treatment (4–6 weeks) is also necessary. Local (pleural or tracheobronchial) antibiotic instillation is not validated. A high level of suspicion of ventilator-assisted pneumonia must be the rule for these patients and requires adequate

diagnostic procedure, including FOB distal microbiologic samplings. In cases of fungal etiology, adequate antifungal treatment is mandatory. Details on antifungal treatments are discussed later.

Surgery

With respect to surgical management, in the authors' practice, the indications are represented by[24]

1. Uncontrolled sepsis in spite of medical therapy and, possibly, chest drainage
2. Major air leaks responsible for ventilatory difficulties with serious hypoxemia/hypercapnia
3. Hemodynamic disturbances by compression of the vena cava and/or right heart cavities by tumor-like forms.

The role of surgical interventions has been rarely evaluated and the subject is difficult to study, mainly because necrotizing pneumonia is a rare complication of community-acquired pneumonia, and the type of surgical treatment should be tailored to each case. In the authors' opinion,[24] the anatomic resection (lobectomy) should be proposed in the acute phase, only in the rare case of necrotic lesions confined to a lobe, and if operative risk is considered acceptable on the basis of general and respiratory conditions. In rare cases, as discussed previously,[24] lobectomy can be proposed as a salvage operation if a bronchial fistula responsible of an air-leak noncompatible with ventilation is present or if arterial erosion is a concern (**Fig. 5**). Lobectomy in a septic context also exposes to specific risks: difficult expansion of residual lung parenchyma with possible occurrence of spaces and persistent infection as well as problems of bronchial sutures healing with occurrence of bronchial or bronchovascular fistula. Thus,[42] the authors prefer the atypical resection of necrotic tissue (necrosectomy) to anatomic resection (**Fig. 6**). This is achieved by 2 different approaches, according to presentation, either standard thoracotomy or elective cavernostomy. In the standard thoracotomy approach, section of adhesions, resection of necrotic tissues by atypical mechanical stapling based on a viable lung parenchyma, and pleural drainage are performed. In the authors' experience, this approach is chosen if a satisfactory re-expansion of lung parenchyma is anticipated and if the lesions are peripheral. The elective cavernostomy approach is chosen when a pleuroparenchymal complete symphysis is already present and if there is extensive and central symptomatic necrosis, provided that the majority of the remaining lung parenchyma is non-necrotic. Furthermore, it is possible that after a necrosectomy by standard thoracotomy,

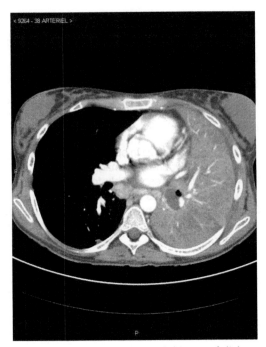

Fig. 5. A 24-year-old woman with history of diabetes mellitus admitted for hemoptysis and respiratory distress revealing pulmonary mucormycosis. CT scan showed the necrosis in close contact with interlobar pulmonary artery. Salvage pneumonectomy was performed and pathology confirmed the ulceration of pulmonary artery.

necrotizing pneumonia continues to evolve and requires elective necrosectomy by cavernostomy (**Fig. 7**).

Once cavernostomy performed, drainage is assured by dressing. Dressing is also efficient in obtaining, by mechanical compression of the fistula, sufficient air seal in patients with major air leaks preventing effective mechanical ventilation. As outlined in sporadic reports,[43] this kind of open drainage may be tolerated by severely ill patients.

All the described operations are regarded as steps in a multimodal treatment. After the control of the acute phase, successive steps of the surgical management are often necessary (see **Figs. 6** and **7**). In the chronic phase, a residual space may require a thoracoplasty, whereas a cavernostomy needs flap transposition to be obliterated (see **Figs. 6** and **7**).[44,45]

The management of necrotizing pneumonia is typically multidisciplinary. Adequate antibiotherapy, mechanical ventilation, and prolonged supportive care are warranted. Surgery must be considered in selected cases and may improve the outcome. Despite the serious morbidity, massive parenchymal damage, and prolonged hospitalizations, long-term outcome after necrotizing pneumonia seems good when multidisciplinary management care is applied to patients with this unusual but severe respiratory infectious disease.[24]

Destroyed Lung

Destroyed lung is thought to have originated from progressive confluent piecemeal necrosis. The destroyed lung is characterized by progressive loss of parenchymal architecture, a net decrease of perfusion, formation of larges cavities, and a chronic course. Initial causative pathogens are represented by bacterial or mycobacterial species and predisposing factors are bronchiectasis, chronic obstructive pulmonary disease (COPD), diabetes mellitus, or other causes of impaired immune response. Destruction may be limited to a lobe or interest an entire lung; in some instances, different lobes on both sides may be affected.[5,6]

Destroyed lung may be asymptomatic, but recurrent episodes of hemoptysis and bronchopulmonary infection are the rule. Responsible pathogens are bacterial or mycotic species, and association of both is possible. In particular, infection of cavities with *Aspergillus* sp[46,47] leads to formation of large tangled fungus balls called aspergillomas or mycetomas. Alternatively, aspergilloma may complicate pre-existing lung cavities present in otherwise healthy or not severely ill lung parenchyma (ie, not inside a destroyed lobe) caused by tuberculosis, lung neoplasms, or granulomatous diseases.

In the absence of effective medical treatment, surgery has been regarded as the treatment of choice of destroyed lung in operable patients with symptoms, with the goal of achieving controls of actual symptoms, preventing their recurrences, some of which (ie, hemoptysis) being possibly life threatening, with possible prolongation of life expectancy. Patient selection for resective surgery depends on the balance between the risk of disease and the risk of surgery: anatomic resection is more morbid than in cases of other indications, with mortality ranging 5% to 44%.[46] Thus, alternatives to resectional surgery have to be considered in patients with important comorbidities, poor lung function, or both. In patients without aspergilloma, association of arteriography with embolization, optimal medical treatment, research, and treatment of a tuberculous reactivation may be sufficient in satisfactorily dealing with the conditions. In some cases, associated renutrition and prolonged physiotherapy may achieve sufficient improvement in general and respiratory conditions to allow resection. Management of destroyed lung complicated with aspergilloma is discussed in detail.

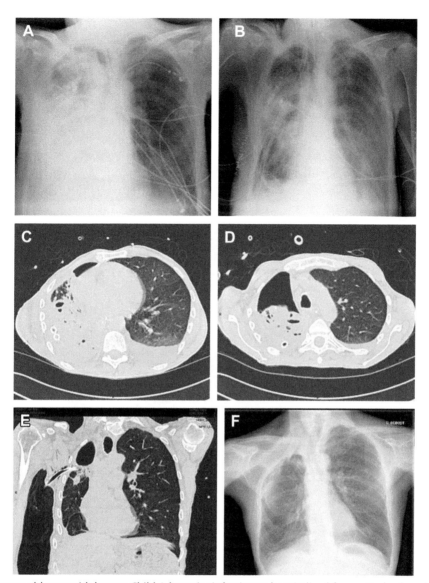

Fig. 6. A 54-year-old man with known Child A hepatic cirrhosis was hospitalized for septic shock and respiratory distress complicated community-acquired pneumonia. In spite of medical treatment and pleural drainage (*A*), sepsis was refractory, justifying open lung necrosectomy (*B*). Hepatization of residual lung (*C*) regressed slowly but persistent pleural space required prolonged drainage (*D*). Some weeks postoperatively, respiratory conditions had dramatically improved but fever secondary to persistent infection of apical space (*E*) required on drain thoracoplasty with fully satisfactory radiologic (*F*) and clinical outcome.

FUNGAL INFECTION OF THE LUNG

A wide range of clinical, radiologic, and anatomo-pathologic entities has been described with a variety of names (eg, simple aspergilloma, semi-invasive/chronic invasive aspergillosis, and chronic necrotizing pulmonary aspergillosis).[48]

Aspergillus sp are ubiquitous but have a low pathogenicity for humans, and invasive infection does not occur unless without immunosuppression from debilitating illness or treatments.[46,47] As discussed previously, pulmonary aspergilloma occurs in pre-existing cavities, which are colonized by the fungus. Complex pulmonary aspergilloma is defined as a thick wall cavity surrounded by diseased lung and containing a fungus ball. Aspergilloma often leads to massive hemoptysis or severe weight loss. Medical therapy has been classically considered poorly effective in pulmonary aspergilloma and resection of diseased lung

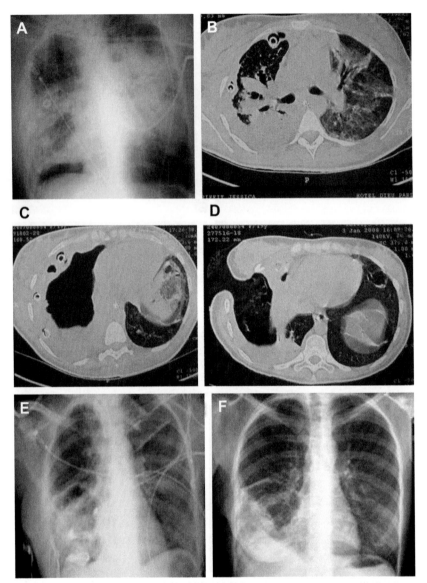

Fig. 7. Same patient as in **Fig. 4**. Initial treatment of necrotizing pneumonia involved right open necrosectomy and pleural drainage (*A*). After an initial improvement, recurrence of sepsis and major air leak, preventing adequate mechanical ventilation (*B, C*) were managed by open necrosectomy and dressing (*D, E*) allowing, together with medical treatment, rapid improvement of clinical condition and weaning from mechanical ventilation. The open window was secondarily closed by serratus anterior transposition (*F*).

parenchyma, by atypical resection, segmentectomy, lobectomy, and even pneumonectomy are often proposed.[49] As discussed previously, however, resection carries a high morbidity and mortality rate, raising the question of alternative treatments in high-risk patients as well as of indication for surgery in asymptomatic patients. Some series reported mortality rates up of 43% and morbidity (including hemorrhage, residual pleural space, BPF, and empyema) rates up to 60%.[46] Also, among patients with normal lung function,

resective surgery for aspergilloma carries a high morbidity: Babatasi and colleagues[49] observed 68% complication rate in their series of 84 patients with normal vital capacity (VC) and forced expiratory volume (FEV)/VC ratio, in most instances.

Thus, resective surgery can be indicated in low-risk symptomatic or asymptomatic patients or in intermediate-risk symptomatic patients, whereas alternatives to resectional surgery should be considered in high-risk patients. Medical treatment has improved because of availability of more efficient antifungal drugs and may be recommended alone or, more frequently, associated with resective surgery or alternative procedures.

Medical Treatment

Fungal lung infection in nonimmunocompromised patients is usually related to aspergillosis, more rarely to other fungi, such as mucorales.[50] There are no codified treatment guidelines for CPA.[51] Antifungal treatment is recommended but only a few drugs are available for long-term treatment. Intravenous amphotericin B and liposomal amphotericin B may be useful as initial therapy in cases of severe fungal pneumonia. Nevertheless the drug-related toxicity may not allow long-term treatment. Local amphotericin B instillation has been proposed in cases of nonresecable aspergilloma, with conflicting results. Caspofungin, an echinocandin, is active against aspergillus but has not been evaluated in this indication; although this drug is well tolerated, it is only available for intravenous route; long-term use is, therefore, difficult. Oral triazoles (ie, itraconazole, voriconazole, and posaconazole) seem to provide suitable treatment for CPA[52]; however, unlike itraconazole, voriconazole has an in vitro fungicidal activity against *Aspergillus*. Moreover, its efficacy was demonstrated in immunocompromised patients with invasive pulmonary aspergillosis.[53] Voriconazole seems the drug of choice and its prolonged oral administration seems possible with an acceptable tolerability. Camuset and colleagues'[54] study showed that useful results were obtained with voriconazole in patients with chronic cavitary pulmonary aspergillosis (CCPA) and patients with CPA who were receiving voriconazole as first-line therapy or after a lack of response to one or several antifungal treatments. A recent study confirmed that voriconazole provides effective treatment of CPA with an acceptable level of toxicity.

In cases of mucormycosis, antifungal treatment is associated with surgical resctions. Amphotericin B is the drug of choice against mucorales. High doses and prolonged administration are necessary. Fluconazole, itraconazole, and voriconazole are poorly effective but pozaconazole shows in vitro activity against mucormycosis. Association of liposomal amphotericin B and posaconazole could be the best regimen.[55] Medical treatment, however, is limited by costs, limited effectiveness when used alone, and possibly important side effects.[46]

Alternative local procedures are represented by bronchial artery embolization, intracavitary amphotericin B instillation, and nonresective surgical procedures, such as cavernostomy or plombage thoracoplasty.[49] Embolization of bronchial arteries has been performed preoperatively, either to reduce perioperative bleeding or to stop massive bleeding in inoperable cases with low side effects but a success rate of approximately only 40%.[45]

Percutaneous instillation of amphotericin B has been suggested for treating aspergilloma and controlling bleeding in patients with compromised lung function or bilateral disease. Giron and colleagues[56] treated 40 patients with amphotericin B paste and achieved the cessation of bleeding in all cases and negative aspergillus serum tests in 26 cases (follow-up time 6 to 28 months). Rumbak and colleagues[57] used potassium iodide in patients with FEV in the first second of expiration (FEV_1) less than 50% and hemoptysis; they achieved cessation of bleeding in 72 hours in all patients. In spite of initial enthusiasm, however, lack of possibility of reproducing these results has prevented generalization of this approach.

Surgical Treatment: Cavernostomy

Cavernostomy is indicated in severely ill patients whose clinical condition does not permit resection.[58] It is a sample procedure, which is generally well tolerated also by patients with poor cardiorespiratory reserve. It achieves immediate mechanical removal of mycetoma with rapid local control of infection and its consequences, especially hemoptysis.

Feasibility of cavernostomy is based on the presence of complete pleuropulmonary symphysis secondary to infection; the tick wall of the caverna should be in close contact with anterior, lateral, or posteroinferior chest wall (the presence of scapula precludes possibility of performing the cavernostomy in some instances). From a technical point of view, resection of 2 or 3 rib arcs and intercostal spaces is followed by incision of pachypleuritis and the tick wall of the caverna (**Figs. 8** and **9**). The fungus ball is mechanically removed and an attempt to closure of bronchial fistula by monofilament stitches is performed. The skin is sutured to the wall of the caverna with some robust stitches (cavernostomy), and dressings are applied and changed each day.[49]

Several surgical teams reported favorably on this approach: Henderson and Pearson,[59] Sagawa and colleagues,[60] and Grima and colleagues.[61] Alternatively, some investigators reported less-favorable results: Oakley and colleagues[58] reported on 24 procedures for treatment of aspegilloma: among the 17 resections and 7 cavernostomies, 30-day mortality rates were 5% and 28.6%, respectively. Patients in the cavernostomy group, however, were probably more severely ill, making comparisons difficult.

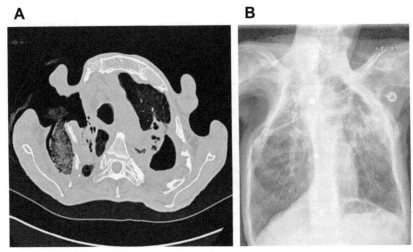

Fig. 8. A 75-year-old man with history of pulmonary tuberculosis treated by extrapleural plombage and severe COPD (FEV$_1$ = 22% of predicted). Severe weight loss led to diagnosis of bilateral aspergilloma. Treatment involved 2-step bilateral cavernostomy, antifungal therapy, and parenteral renutrition. On the right side, cavernostomy (A) was followed by extramuscoloperiosteal thoracoplasty (B) to deal with the infected extrapleural space secondary to the old plombage.

Cavernostomy, closure of bronchial fistulae, and irrigation with amphotericin B, and myoplasty provide good initial therapy and prevent recurrence of the disease in most but not all patients. Ono and colleagues[62] performed 8 cavernostomies and muscle transposition with thoracoplasty in 3 cases but experienced 2 recurrences, 19 and 29 months after the operation.

THORACOPLASTY: NONRESECTIVE SURGERY IN FUNGAL AND NONFUNGAL INFECTION OF THE LUNG

The other nonresective surgical option for treatment of aspergilloma is represented by thoracoplasty, a surgical procedure that allows the reduction of the thoracic cavity by removing the ribs. Thoracoplasty

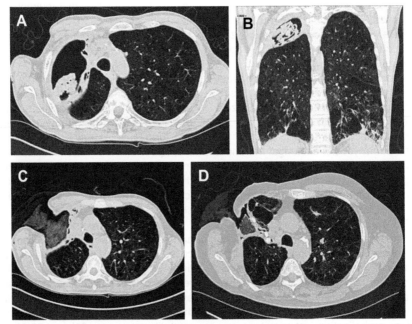

Fig. 9. A 68-year-old man with history of pulmonary tuberculosis, severe COPD (FEV$_1$ = 24% of predicted), and chronic hepatitis C infection. Hemoptysis and weight loss led to discovery of pulmonary aspergilloma (A, B). Treatment involved cavernostomy (C) and subsequent bronchoscopic spigots (D) placement to deal with major airleak. This allowed rapid retraction of cavity, which is suitable for flap transposition.

was originally conceived to collapse cavities of lungs affected by tuberculosis and gained worldwide acceptance in that setting. Subsequently, indications rapidly extended to thoracic empyema. Currently, treatment of postpneumonectomy empyema represents the more frequent, albeit rare, indication for thoracoplasty. The purpose of thoracoplasty is to achieve pleural space obliteration. At present, persistent pleural space in postresectional empyema and unresolving primary empyema with trapped lung are the more common indications for thoracoplasty. Available studies in the last 25 years have shown that thoracoplasty can be an excellent therapeutic option in selected patients,[63–66] used alone or in combination with flap transposition to fill the residual space.[67] An adequate drainage of the space for the control of infection is mandatory for successful thoracoplasty.[64–68]

Since the nineteenth century, various techniques have been developed[69–72]: today only Alexander thoracoplasty[71] (based on extramusculoperiosteal rib resection, without opening of the pachypleuritis) and Andrews thoracoplasty[72] (based on extraperiosteal rib resection and opening of pachypleuritis, which is invaginated and used to close bronchial fistulas and fill the cavity) continues to be used.[44,63,64]

Thoracoplasty is often considered a mutilating operation, leading to undesirable anatomic, functional, and cosmetic sequelae. For these reasons, an almost complete abandon of the technique was observed. Despite the bad reputation, there remain some cases of chronic pleural or pulmonary infection in which thoracoplasty is indicated. In particular, some patients with postresectional empyema or primary empyema or lung infections nonresponsive to other treatments are potential candidates for this operation, which can be performed alone[63–66] or in combination with other procedures.[67] In particular, in the setting of lung infections, thoracoplasty can be used as a primary surgical treatment (almost exclusively in cases of limited aspergilloma in patients not tolerating resection) or as a step in a complex management of lung infection to obliterate a pulmonary (after cavernostomy) or pleural (after thoracostomy) cavity.

The authors perform all thoracoplasties in one stage, especially in the treatment of infectious disease of the lung, where thoracoplasty is limited to some ribs (tailored thoracoplasty). In the setting of aspergilloma, primary Andrews thoracoplasty[72] may be indicated in the treatment of patients with small posterosuperior lesions, whose topography constitutes a contraindication to cavernostomy and whose small volume allows almost complete filling (after removal of the fungus ball) with pachypleuritis and intercostal muscles during the same

operative time. Few patients, however, with small aspergilloma do not tolerate resectional surgery, which remains the treatment of choice. Alternatively, the majority of patients with aspergilloma nonsusceptible to treatment by resectional surgery have large or bilateral lesions and require cavernostomy. In these patients, thoracoplasty may represent an intermediate step to facilitate obliteration of pulmonary space, if it is large enough to prevent filling with available muscular flaps.

The other indication of thoracoplasty is the treatment of a persistent infected pleural space in the setting of an infection of the lung treated by necrosectomy by either thoracotomy or direct open window thoracostomy. Thoracoplasty may be used to obliterate the residual space after cavernostomy or, more frequently, open window thoracostomy, although intrathoracic flap transposition or Clagett procedure may also be indicated.

The Clagett method is simple and safe, but the results can vary and it is unsuitable when bronchial fistulas are present.[73–75] Muscular flap transposition was reported as safe and effective,[45,67,76,77] but there are cases in which the cavity is too large to be filled with muscles or in which there are no muscles available. Thus, thoracoplasty may be used, especially in such case (too large space to be filled with a flap) as an intermediate step to reduce the residual cavity. In this setting, the extramusculoperiosteal thoracoplasty, as originally described by Alexander, is the authors' technique of choice. To achieve satisfactory collapse of the cavity, a sufficient number of ribs (which are selected on the basis of topography of lesions) are resected in a subperiosteal extrapleural manner. The operation is performed in patients who have their infected space already drained by either chest tube (thoracoplasty on drain) or open window thoracostomy. When performed in a patient with an open window thoracostomy, which was usually located in the lateral chest wall, incision extends backward and upward from the posterior limit of the thoracostomy. Special care is taken to avoid entering the thoracostomy cavity. The first rib is removed in all patients with apical space and apicolysis, as described by Semb,[78] is performed: it consists of extrapleural division of adhesions between the pleural dome at the apex and the soft tissues to achieve vertical collapse and to approximate the soft tissues to the mediastinum. The transverse processes are never resected. For posteriorly located spaces, however, special care is taken to remove the back ends of the ribs, and in cases of large posterior spaces, ribs are disarticulated from the costovertebral joint.

When thoracoplasty is performed (on drain), drainage of residual cavity (whose volume has been reduced by thoracoplasty) by chest tube is maintained for several days before progressive withdrawal of the drainage.[44] In cases of thoracoplasty performed in patients with open window thoracostomy, daily change of dressing of cavity remains necessary, but rapid obliteration of cavity is seen in most patients. Residual cavity may completely obliterate spontaneously or require flap transposition possibly associated with skin graft.[44,45]

FLAP TRANSPOSITION

Filling of the residual cavity may be achieved by myoplasty or omentum flap transposition, depending on anatomic considerations, muscle availability, topography and volume of the cavity, topography of the initial thoracotomy incision, and entity of damage caused by previous operations. For all these reasons, it is essential, at the time of the first surgical procedure, to preserve chest wall skin and muscles and respect their pedicles, because they are always likely to be used in subsequent procedure.

Intrathoracic transposition of an extrathoracic muscle was first described in 1911 by Abrashanoff.[79] Techniques of harvesting flaps have been extensively described in the plastic and reconstructive literature.[80] This article highlights specificities of thoracic surgery.

Muscles that are most frequently used for intrathoracic transposition are chest wall muscles, including latissimus dorsi, serratus anterior, and pectoralis major; other flaps may be involved, such as pectoralis minor, subscapularis, trapezius, rectus abdominis, and anterolateral thigh.[81–91] Otherwise, if most of them are pedicled, free flaps have been also reported.[92–95] Achievement of myocutaneous flaps is attractive when possible.[96] It seems that indications and surgical choices are based on surgical team habits more than on immutable decisional algorithm.

In the authors' practice, the edges of the toracostomy are first dissected from the underlying pachypleuritis. Initial incision sometimes requires extension to allow harvesting of the flap through itself. It can be also completed by rib removal through the same incision to reduce the residual cavity. In cases of initial lateral or anterolateral incisions, the authors' first choice is the myoplasty by latissimus dorsi (which is normally spared) due to its ability to fill large residual spaces. Alternatively, in cases of initial posterolateral incisions, the authors' preference is to harvest serratus anterior flap, because the muscle is usually preserved,

allowing its transposition into the cavity trough the thoracotomy itself or through a more cranial intercostal space, ideally the third one.

Filling of residual cavity can be also provided by omentum transposition.[97] In the authors' practice, this procedure is performed when myoplasty is not able to fill all the residual space or muscle flaps are not available. In cases of large spaces, however, myoplasty and omentum transposition could be associated to completely obliterate the cavity. Harvest of omentum is done through a short susombilical incision. A large omental pedicle is created by dividing the left or right gastroepiploïc vessels and detaching the gastroepiploic arch from the greater curvature of the stomach. For transposition, the authors' use the gastroepiploic pedicle of the homolateral cavity, whereas the other pedicle is transected to allow maximal rotation to the flap. Transposition is done through a substernal tunnel or an opening in the diaphragm. The omentum is sutured to possible persistent bronchial fistulas and fixed to the edges of the thoracostomy. Care is used to prevent compression omentum vessels and intestinal herniation.

After transposition, in some instances, direct closure may be not feasible despite thoracoplasty. In these cases, transposition should be associated with an overlay split-thickness skin graft. In the authors' practice, the donor site is chosen according to the installation of the patient and graft is most often harvested on the thigh.

An alternative to the thoracoplasty (described previously) in cases of a small thoracostomy or cavernostomy cavities is represented by thoracomyoplasty, a limited intrapleural thoracoplasty associated with an intrathoracic muscular transposition to totally obliterate the cavity in one stage. In this operation, thoracoplasty consists of the resection of the costal bony extremities of the thoracostomy borders and resection of the 2 ribs above and below the thoracostomy, together with the intercostal muscles, neurovascular bundles, and parietal pleura.

REFERENCES

1. Mansharamani NG, Koziel H. Chronic lung sepsis: lung abscess, bronchiectasis, and empyema. Curr Opin Pulm Med 2003;9(3):181–5.
2. Li HT, Zhang TT, Huang J, et al. Factors associated with the outcome of life-threatening necrotizing pneumonia due to community-acquired staphylococcus aureus in adult and adolescent patients. Respiration 2011;81:448–60.
3. Yangco BG, Deresinski SC. Necrotizing or cavitating pneumonia due to *Streptococcus Pneumoniae*: report of four cases and review of the literature. Medicine (Baltimore) 1980;59(6):449–57.

4. Hammond JM, Lyddell C, Potgieter PD, et al. Severe pneumococcal pneumonia complicated by massive pulmonary gangrene. Chest 1993;104(5):1610–2.

5. Kosar A, Orki A, Kiral H, et al. Pneumonectomy in children for destroyed lung: evaluation of 18 cases. Ann Thorac Surg 2010;89(1):226–31.

6. Ryu YJ, Lee JH, Chun EM, et al. Clinical outcomes and prognostic factors in patients with tuberculous destroyed lung. Int J Tuberc Lung Dis 2011;15(2): 246–50.

7. Kelogrigoris M, Tsagouli P, Stathopoulos K, et al. CT-guided percutaneous drainage of lung abscess: review of 40 cases. JBR-BTR 2011;94(4):191–5.

8. Herth F, Ernst A, Becker HD. Endoscopic drainage of lung abscesses: technique and outcome. Chest 2005;127(4):1378–81.

9. Wali SO, Shugaeri A, Samman YS, et al. Percutaneous drainage of pyogenic lung abscess. Scand J Infect Dis 2002;34(9):673–9.

10. Shlomi D, Kramer MR, Fuks L, et al. Endobronchial drainage of lung abscess: the use of laser. Scand J Infect Dis 2010;42(1):65–8.

11. Mwandumba HC, Beeching NJ. Pyogenic lung infections: factors for predicting clinical outcome of lung abscess and thoracic empyema. Curr Opin Pulm Med 2000;6(3):234–9.

12. Mueller PR, Berlin L. Complications of lung abscess aspiration and drainage. AJR Am J Roentgenol 2002;178(5):1083–6.

13. Metras H, Chapin J. Lung abscess and bronchial catheterisation. J Thorac Surg 1954;27:157–9.

14. Kalaskar AS, Heresi GP, Wanger A, et al. Severe necrotizing pneumonia in children, Houston, Texas, USA. Emerg Infect Dis 2009;15(10):1696–8.

15. Hasan RA, Al-Neyadi S, Abuhasna S, et al. High-frequency oscillatory ventilation in an infant with necrotizing pneumonia and bronchopleural fistula. Respir Care 2011;56(3):351–4.

16. Sawicki GS, Lu FL, Valim C, et al. Necrotizing pneumonia is increasingly detected complication of pneumonia in children. Eur Respir J 2008;31(6): 1285–91.

17. Kerem E, Bar Ziv Y, Rudenski B, et al. Bacteremic necrotizing pneumococcal pneumonia in children. Am J Respir Crit Care Med 1994;149(1):242–4.

18. Crnich CJ, Gordon B, Andes D. Hot tub-associated necrotizing pneumonia due to pseudomonas aeruginosa. Clin Infect Dis 2003;36(3):e55–7.

19. Palmacci C, Antocicco M, Bonomo L, et al. Necrotizing pneumonia and sepsis due to *Clostridium perfringens* a case report. Cases J 2009;2(1):50.

20. Gillet Y, Vanhems P, Lina G, et al. Factors predicting mortality in community acquired pneumonia caused by *Staphylococcus aureus* containing Panton-Valentine leukocidin. Clin Infect Dis 2007;45(3):315–21.

21. Noah MA, Dawrant M, Faulkner GM, et al. Panton-Valentine leukocidin expressing *Staphylococcus aureus* pneumonia managed with extracorporeal membrane oxygenation: Experience and outcome. Crit Care Med 2010;38(1):2250–3.

22. Kohli N, Kochie M, Harber P. Necrotizing community-acquired methicillin-resistant *Staphylococcus aureus* pneumonia: an emerging problem in correctional facilities. AAOHN J 2011;59(3):135–40.

23. Ayed AK, Al-Rowayeh A. Lung resection in children for infectious pulmonary diseases. Pediatr Surg Int 2005;21(8):604–8.

24. Evans B, MacKenzie I, Malata C, et al. Successful salvage right upper lobectomy and flap repair of trachea-esophageal fistula due to severe necrotizing pneumonia. Interact Cardiovasc Thorac Surg 2009;9(5):896–8.

25. Levy MM, Dellinger RP, Townsend SR, et al. The surviving sepsis campaign: results of an international guideline-based performance improvement program targeting severe sepsis. Crit Care Med 2010;38:367–74.

26. Charron C, Caille V, Jardin F, et al. Echocardiographic measurement of fluid responsiveness. Curr Opin Crit Care 2006;12:249–54.

27. Shekar K, Foot C, Fraser J, et al. Bronchopleural fistula: an update for intensivists. J Crit Care 2010; 25:47–55.

28. Bishop MJ, Benson MS, Pierson DJ. Carbon dioxide excretion via bronchopleural fistulas in adult respiratory distress syndrome. Chest 1987;91:400–2.

29. Litmanovitch M, Joynt GM, Cooper PJ, et al. Persistent bronchopleural fistula in a patient with adult respiratory distress syndrome. Treatment with pressure controlled ventilation. Chest 1993;104:1901–2.

30. Hommel M, Deja M, von Dossow V, et al. Bronchial fistulae in ARDS patients: management with an extracorporeal lung assist device. Eur Respir J 2008;32:1652–5.

31. Khan NU, Al-Aloul M, Khasati N, et al. Extracorporeal membrane oxygenator as a bridge to successful surgical repair of bronchopleural fistula following bilateral sequential lung transplantation; a case report and review of literature. J Cardiothorac Surg 2007;2:28.

32. Lois M, Noppen M. Bronchopleural fistulas: an overview of the problem with special focus on endoscopic management. Chest 2005;128:3955–65.

33. Lan RS, Lee CH, Tsai YH, et al. Fibreoptic bronchial blockade in a small bronchial fistula. Chest 1987;92:944–6.

34. Ellis JH, Sequeira FW, Weber TR, et al. Balloon catheter occlusion of bronchopleural fistulae. Am J Roentgenol 1982;138:157–9.

35. Lin J, Iannettoni MD. Closure of bronchopleural fistulas using albumin-glutaraldehyde tissue adhesive. Ann Thorac Surg 2004;77:326–8.

36. Ratliff JL, Hill JD, Tucker H, et al. Endobronchial control of bronchopleural fistulae. Chest 1977;71: 98–9.

37. Ferguson JS, Sprenger K, Van Natta T. Closure of a bronchopleural fistula using bronchoscopic placement of an endobronchial valve designed for the treatment of emphysema. Chest 2006;129:479–81.

38. Hartmann W, Rausch V. New therapeutic application of the fiberoptic bronchoscope. Chest 1977;71:237.

39. Kumar A, Zarychanski R, Light B, et al. Early combination antibiotic therapy yields improved survival compared with monotherapy in septic shock: A propensity-matched analysis. Crit Care Med 2010; 38:1773–85.

40. Niederman MS, Mandell LA, Anzueto A, et al. Guidelines for the management of adults with community-acquired pneumonia: diagnosis, assessment of severity, antimicrobial therapy, and prevention. Am J Respir Crit Care Med 2001;163:1730–54.

41. Mandell LA, Wunderink RG, Anzueto A, et al. Infectious Diseases Society of America/American Thoracic Society consensus guidelines on the management of community-acquired pneumonia in adults. Clin Infect Dis 2007;44:S27–72.

42. Reimel BA, Krishnadasen B, Cuschieri J, et al. Surgical management of acute necrotizing lung infections. Can Respir J 2006;13(7):369–73.

43. Weissberg D, Refaely Y. Pleural empyema: 24-year experience. Ann Thorac Surg 1996; 62(4):1026–9.

44. Stefani A, Jouni R, Alifano M, et al. Thoracoplasty in the current practice of thoracic surgery: a single-institution 10-year experience. Ann Thorac Surg 2011;91(1):263–8.

45. Regnard JF, Alifano M, Puyo P, et al. Open window thoracostomy followed by intrathoracic flap transposition in the treatment of empyema complicating pulmonary resection. J Thorac Cardiovasc Surg 2000;120(2):270–5.

46. Lee JG, Lee CY, Park IK, et al. Pulmonary aspergilloma: analysis of prognosis in relation to symptoms and treatment. J Thorac Cardiovasc Surg 2009; 138(4):820–5.

47. Zmeili OS, Soubani AO. Pulmonary aspergillosis: a clinical update. QJM 2007;100(6):317–34.

48. Kousha M, Tadi R, Soubani AO. Pulmonary aspergillosis: a clinical review. Eur Respir Rev 2011;20:156–74.

49. Babatasi G, Massetti M, Chapelier A, et al. Surgical treatment of aspergilloma: current outcome. J Thorac Cardiovasc Surg 2000;119:906–12.

50. Petri MG, Konig J, Moecke HP. Epidemiology of invasive mycosis in ICU patients: a prospective multicenter study in 435 non-neutropenic patients. Paul-Ehrlich Society for Chemotherapy, Divisions of Mycology and Pneumonia Research. Intensive Care Med 1997;23:317–25.

51. Saraceno JL, Phelps DT, Ferro TJ, et al. Chronic necrotizing pulmonary aspergillosis. Approach to management. Chest 1997;112:541–8.

52. Kohno S, Izumikawa K, Ogawa K, et al, Japan Chronic Pulmonary Aspergillosis Study Group (JCPASG). Intravenous micafungin versus voriconazole for chronic pulmonary aspergillosis: a multicenter trial in Japan. J Infect 2010;61:410–8.

53. Herbrecht R, Denning DW, Patterson TF. Voriconazole versus amphotericin B for primary therapy of invasive aspergillosis. N Engl J Med 2002;347: 408–15.

54. Camuset J, Nunes H, Dombret MC, et al. Treatment of chronic pulmonary aspergillosis by voriconazole in non-immunocompromised patients. Chest 2007; 131:1435–41.

55. Spellberg B, Ibrahim A, Roilides E, et al. Combination therapy for mucormycosis: why, what, and how? Clin Infect Dis 2012;54(Suppl 1):S73–8.

56. Giron J, Poey C, Fajadet P. CT-guided percutaneous treatment of inoperable pulmonary aspergillomas: a study of 40 cases. Eur J Radiol 1998;28:235–42.

57. Rumbak M, Kohler G, Eastridge C. Topical treatment of life threatening haemoptysis from aspergillomas. Thorax 1996;51:253–5.

58. Oakley RE, Mario P, Goldstraw P. Indications and outcome of surgery for pulmonary aspergilloma. Thorax 1997;52:813–5.

59. Henderson AH, Pearson JE. Treatment of bronchopulmonary aspergillosis with observations on the use of natamycin. Thorax 1968;23:519–23.

60. Sagawa M, Sakuma T, Isobe T. Cavernoscopy removal of a fungus ball for pulmonary complex aspergilloma. Ann Thorac Surg 2004;78:1846–8.

61. Grima R, Krassas A, Bagan P, et al. Treatment of complicated pulmonary aspergillomas with cavernostomy and muscle flap: interest of concomitant limited thoracoplasty. Eur J Cardiothorac Surg 2009;36:910–3.

62. Ono N, Sato K, Yokomise H, et al. Surgical menagement of pulmonary aspergilloma. Role of single-stage cavernostomy with muscle flap trasposition. Jpn J Thorac Cardiovasc Surg 2000;48(1):56–9.

63. Icard P, Le Rochais JP, Rabut B, et al. Andrews thoracoplasty as a treatment of post- pneumonectomy empyema: experience in 23 cases. Ann Thorac Surg 1999;68:1159–64.

64. Peppas G, Molnar TF, Jeyasingham K, et al. Thoraco- plasty in the context of current surgical practice. Ann Thorac Surg 1993;56:903–9.

65. Hopkins RA, Ungerleider RM, Staub EW, et al. The modern use of thoracoplasty. Ann Thorac Surg 1985;40:181–7.

66. Horrigan TP, Snow NJ. Thoracoplasty: current application to the infected pleural space. Ann Thorac Surg 1990;50:695–9.

67. Garcia-Yuste M, Ramos G, Duque JL. Open-window thoracostomy and thoracomyoplasty to manage chronic pleural empyema. Ann Thorac Surg 1998; 65:818–22.

68. Deslauriers J, Grégoire J. Thoracoplasty. In: Patterson GA, Pearson FG, Cooper JD, et al, editors. Pearson's thoracic and esophageal surgery. 3rd edition. Philadelphia: Churchill Livingstone Elsevier; 2008. p. 1159–69.

69. Schede M. Diebehandlungderempyeme. Verh Cong Innere Med Wiesbaden 1890;9:41–141.

70. Sauerbruch F. Die chirurgie der brustograne, vol. 11. Berlin: Springer; 1925.

71. Alexander J. The collapse therapy of pulmonary tuberculosis. Springfield (IL): Charles C Thomas; 1937.

72. Andrews NC. Thoraco-mediastinal placation (a surgical tecnique for chronic empyema). J Thorac Surg 1961;41:809–16.

73. Pairolero PC, Arnold PG, Trastek VF, et al. Postpneumonectomy empyema: the role of intrathoracic muscle transposition. J Thorac Cardiovasc Surg 1990;99:958–68.

74. Goldstraw P. Treatment of postpneumonectomy empyema: the case for fenestration. Thorax 1979; 72:319–22.

75. Gharagozloo F, Trachiotis G, Wolfe A, et al. Pleural space irrigation and modified clagett procedure for the treatment of early postpneumonectomy empyema. J Thorac Cardiovasc Surg 1998;116:943–8.

76. Miller JI, Mansour KA, Nahai F, et al. Single-stage complete muscle flap closure of the post- pneumonectomy empyema space: a new method and possible solution to a disturbing complication. Ann Thorac Surg 1984;38:227–31.

77. Zimmermann T, Muhrer KH, Padberg W, et al. Closure of acute bronchial stump insufficiency with a musculus latissimus dorsi flap. Thorac Cardiovasc Surg 1993;41:196–8.

78. Semb C. Thoracoplasty with apicolysis. Oslo (Norway): Nationaltryk- keriet; 1935.

79. Abrashanoff: plastiche methode der Schlessung von Fistelgangen, welche von inneren organen kommen. Zentralbl Chir 1911;38:186.

80. Binder JP, Revol M. Lambeaux musculocutanés, techniques chirurgicales—chirurgie plastique reconstructrice et esthétique. Paris: EMC (Elsevier Masson SAS); 2012. p. 45–85.

81. Pairolero PC, Arnold PG, Piehler JM. Intrathoracic transposition of extrathoracic skeletal muscle. J Thorac Cardiovasc Surg 1983;86:809–17.

82. Arnold PG, Pairolero PC. Intrathoracic muscle flaps: a 10-year experience in the management of life-threatening infectious. Plast Reconstr Surg 1989; 84:92–8.

83. Arnold PG, Pairolero PC. Intrathoracic muscle flaps. An account of their use in the management of 100 consecutive patients. Ann Surg 1990;211:656–60.

84. Michaels BM, Orgill DP, Decamp MM, et al. Flap closure of postpneumonectomy empyema. Plast Reconstr Surg 1997;99:437–42.

85. Widmer MK, Krueger T, Lardinois D, et al. A comparative evaluation of intrathoracic latissimus dorsi and serratus anterior muscle transposition. Eur J Cardiothorac Surg 2000;18:435–9.

86. Li EN, Goldberg NH, Slezak S, et al. Split pectoralis major flaps for mediastinal wound coverage: a 12-year experience. Ann Plast Surg 2004;53:334–7.

87. Seify H, Mansour K, Miller J, et al. Single-stage muscle flap reconstruction of the postpneumonectomy empyema space: the Emory experience. Plast Reconstr Surg 2007;120:1886–91.

88. Okuda M, Yokomise H, Muneuchi G, et al. Obliteration of empyema space by vascularized anterolateral thigh flaps. Ann Thorac Surg 2009;87:1615–6.

89. Botianu PV, Dobrica AC, Butiurca A, et al. Complex space-filling procedures for intrathoracic infections – personal experience with 76 consecutive cases. Eur J Cardiothorac Surg 2010;37:478–81.

90. Botianu PV, Botianu AM, Bacarea V, et al. Thoraco-dorsal versus reversed mobilization of the latissimus dorsi muscle for intrathoracic transposition. Eur J Cardiothoracic Surg 2010;38:461–5.

91. Botianu PV, Botianu AM, Dobrica AC, et al. Intrathoracic transposition of the serratus anterior muscle flap—personal experience with 65 consecutive patients. Eur J Cardiothoracic Surg 2010;38:669–73.

92. Perkins DJ, Lee KK, Pennington D, et al. Free flaps in the management of intrathoracic sepsis. Br J Plast Surg 1995;48:546–50.

93. Jiang L, Jiang G, He W, et al. Free rectus abdominis musculacutaneous flap for chronic postoperative empyema. Ann Thorac Surg 2008;85:2147–9.

94. Takanari K, Kamei Y, Toriyama K, et al. Management of postpneumonectomy empyema using free flap and pedicled flap. Ann Thorac Surg 2010;89:321–3.

95. Walsh MD, Bruno AD, Onaitis MW, et al. The role of intrathoracic free flaps for chronic empyema. Ann Thorac Surg 2011;91:865–8.

96. Tosson R, Peter FW, Steinau HU, et al. Muscle and myocutaneous flaps in reconstructive surgery of thoracic defects. Heart Lung Circ 2004;13:399–402.

97. Mathisen DJ, Grillo HC, Vlahakes GJ, et al. The omentum in the management of complicated cardiothoracic problems. J Thorac Cardiovascular Surg 1988;95:677–84.

Surgical Spectrum in the Management of Empyemas

Matthew D. Taylor, MD[a],
Benjamin D. Kozower, MD, MPH[b],*

KEYWORDS

- Empyema • Decortication • Open thoracostomy • Bronchopleural fistula

KEY POINTS

- Early intervention of pleural space infections is key to prevention of chronic empyemas and the need for surgical intervention.
- Video-assisted thoracoscopic surgery has made it possible to treat stage I and stage II empyemas with significantly less morbidity.
- Decortication or open thoracostomy is largely successful in patients with stage III empyemas.

Empyema thoracis, pleural space infection, represents both a disease of historical importance as well as a common problem faced by the practicing thoracic surgeon. The incidence of empyema continues to grow in both the adult and pediatric populations with an estimated 65,000 patients affected each year with an annual cost of 500 million dollars per year.[1]

Empyema was first described by Hippocrates approximately 2400 years ago when he made the distinction between an empyema and hydrothorax based on its clinical presentation.[2] He is also credited with the first drainage operation creating a burr hole into the infected pleural space and using daily irrigation.[3] Although closed-tube thoracostomy tube placement was first described by Playfair[4] and Hewitt[5] in 1875 and 1876, respectively, it was not until 1925 when Graham[6] first described the role of thoracostomy for management of acute empyema. This discovery was revolutionary to the management of empyema because the previous management, including rib resection and open drainage, resulted in mortality rates of 30% compared with 5% to 10% with closed-tube thoracostomy. Open drainage with

a tissue flap for empyema fibrosis was first described by Eloesser[7] in 1935. More recently, Wakabayashi[8] described video-assisted thoracoscopic surgery (VATS) as a method for both the diagnosis and treatment of acute empyema.

The purpose of this article is to describe the current surgical treatment of the various stages of empyema.

STAGES OF EMPYEMA

Empyema is categorized into three distinct stages as defined by the American Thoracic Society. These include the exudative phase, fibrinopurulent phase, and the organization phase. Transition through the three phases occurs over a 3 to 6 week period. **Table 1** demonstrates the characteristics of each stage of empyema.

DIAGNOSIS

The diagnosis of empyema is entertained by the completion of a thorough clinical evaluation. A clinical history of pneumonia or thoracic intervention is critical to ascertain because greater than

The authors have no disclosures to report.
[a] Department of Surgery, University of Virginia, Box 800300, Charlottesville, VA 22908-0679, USA; [b] Department of Surgery, University of Virginia, Box 800679, Charlottesville, VA 22908-0679, USA
* Corresponding author.
E-mail address: bdk8g@virginia.edu

Thorac Surg Clin 22 (2012) 431–440
doi:10.1016/j.thorsurg.2012.04.007

Table 1
Stages of empyema

Stage	Phase	Characteristics	Status of Lung Parenchyma	Treatment
I	Exudative (Acute)	Pleural membrane thickening Fibrin deposition Presence of exudative fluid	Compliant Reexpansion possible with evacuation of fluid	Thoracentesis Closed-tube thoracostomy
II	Fibrinopurulent	Extensive fibrin deposition Pleural fluid becomes turbid or purulent Presence of loculated empyema	Partial compliance Lung entrapment due to fibrin deposition	Closed-tube thoracostomy with fibrinolytics Thoracoscopy Thoracotomy
III	Organized (Chronic)	Fibroblast in growth Thickened pus Granulation tissue replacement of the pleural space	No compliance Lung completely entrapped by fibrous peel	Thoracotomy (decortication) Open drainage (Eloesser) Open thoracostomy

90% of patients with an empyema have one of these two components in their clinical history. The history is also crucial for establishing the duration of illness, which guides therapy. The presence of leukocytosis, radiographic evidence of a pleural effusion, and the presence of purulent fluid on thoracentesis or thoracostomy are classic findings of empyema. Further characterization of the phase of empyema is accomplished by CT scanning with intravenous contrast to evaluate for the presence of loculated empyemas, the thickness and enhancement of the pleura or rind, presence of trapped lung, and other causes, including malignancy. **Fig. 1** illustrates the classic finding of the posteriorly located inverted D-shaped density.

SURGICAL MANAGEMENT OF ACUTE EMPYEMA

In the presence of an acute empyema, the primary treatments are antibiotic therapy and drainage. Drainage can be accomplished by multiple means, including closed-tube thoracostomy, VATS, or thoracotomy with decortication. Small-bore pigtail catheters have been used in patients with early disease with successes reported to be between 70% and 90%. However, this only works if empyemas are within the early exudative phase. Pigtail catheter placement is not recommended for more advanced infections because the pus and fibrin deposition will clog the tube and ultimately delay definitive treatment.

Closed-tube thoracostomy with a large bore (28–36 F) chest tube remains the gold standard

for treatment of acute empyema. Following insertion into the pleural space, a pleural suction system is used with negative pressure for a few days to facilitate pleural apposition. Huang and colleagues[9] performed a retrospective review of 100 patients with empyema managed by tube thoracostomy to elucidate factors predicting chest tube failure and ultimate surgical decortication. Of the 100 patients managed by chest tube insertion, 53% had resolution without further intervention. Independent predictors of thoracostomy tube failure included the presence of loculated

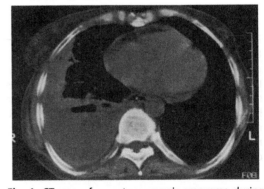

Fig. 1. CT scan of a postpneumonic empyema during the fibrinopurulent stage. A posteriorly located inverted D-shaped density (pregnant lady sign). (*From* Miller DL. Empyema and bronchopleural fistula. In: Patterson GA, Pearson FG, Cooper JD, et al, editors. Pearson's thoracic and esophageal surgery. 3rd edition. Philadelphia: Churchill Livingstone; 2008. p. 1055–71; with permission.)

empyemas on initial imaging and pleural fluid leukocyte count of $\leq$6400/μL.

If tube thoracostomy fails to provide resolution of the empyema, some thoracic surgeons advocate instillation of intrapleural fibrinolytic agents. To date, there have been six randomized controlled trials investigating intrapleural streptokinase or urokinase for empyema. The results of these studies are shown in **Table 2**.[10–15] A recent Cochrane review including these studies found that fibrinolytic therapy reduced the need for subsequent surgical intervention when compared with chest tube insertion alone (risk ratio 0.63; 95% CI 0.46–0.85).[16] The authors occasionally use thrombolytics when there is one loculated collection to drain or to avoid an operative intervention in a patient whose medical comorbidities preclude surgery.

In patients who are of acceptable surgical risk with stage I and II empyema and who have failed conservative management with closed-tube drainage, minimally invasive VATS debridement can facilitate clearing of the intrapleural infection and result in pleural apposition. To perform VATS debridement, the location of the associated pleural effusion can be found by intrapleural aspiration. A thoracoscopic camera port may be placed at the location of fluid aspiration to minimize lung injury. Once the intrathoracic cavity is visualized, 1 to 2 additional thoracoscopic ports may be placed under direct visualization allowing for debridement. Successful debridement is achieved when the lung is fully opposed to the parietal pleura. VATS debridement of empyema was first described by Wakabayashi[8] in 1991. The series achieved lung re-expansion in 18 of 20 patients. Subsequent investigation by Angelillo Mackinlay and colleagues[17]

compared the outcomes of VATS versus open thoracotomy for stage II empyemas in 64 patients. VATS debridement was successful in 90% of cases and was associated with decrease in length of stay and number of days with a chest tube. There was no significant difference between treatments with regard to mortality (both 3%). Subsequently, Cassina and colleagues[18] performed a prospective study of 45 patients with stage II and III empyemas who underwent attempted VATS debridement. VATS was successfully completed in 82% of patients. **Table 3** shows a summary of studies investigating the role of VATS for the treatment of empyema.[17–24] In summary, VATS debridement has been shown to be an effective method of treating acute empyema. The authors frequently use a VATS approach for stage I and II empyemas. The exposure facilitates the breaking up of loculated empyemas and the removal of fibrinous debris. However, we have not found the VATS approach suitable for stage III (organized) empyemas when a true peel needs to be decorticated and has a low threshold for conversion to thoracotomy.

Although drainage and antibiotics are the first-line treatment of acute empyemas, there is evidence that delays associated with ineffective treatment strategies result in increased morbidity and mortality. Wozniak and colleagues[25] investigated the choice of the first intervention for stage II or greater empyemas and its relationship to patient outcomes. In this retrospective study evaluating 104 patients with empyema, tube thoracostomy was successful in 38%, VATS in 81%, and thoracotomy in 89% of patients. Failure of the first attempted procedure was an independent predictor of death.

Table 2
Randomized clinical trials investigating intrapleural fibrinolytic therapy for empyema

Author	Number of Patients	Success (%)	Complications (%)
Bouros et al[10]	Streptokinase group = 25 Urokinase group = 25	Streptokinase group = 92 Urokinase group = 92	28 developed elevation in temperature
Davies et al[11]	Streptokinase group = 12 Control = 12	Streptokinase group = 100 Control = 83	None
Tuncozgur et al[12]	Urokinase group = 25 Control = 24	Urokinase group = 71 Control = 40	None
Diacon et al[13]	Streptokinase group = 22 Control = 22	Streptokinase group = 82 Control = 48	None
Maskell et al[14]	Streptokinase group = 208 Control = 222	Streptokinase group = 69 Control = 73	7 (chest pain, fever)
Misthos et al[15]	Streptokinase group = 57 Control = 70	Streptokinase group = 88 Control = 67	None

Table 3
Thoracoscopic treatment of empyema

Author	Number of Patients	Empyema Stage	Success (%)	Complications (%)	Mortality
Angelillo Mackinlay et al[17]	31	2	90	16	19
Landreneau et al[19]	76	2 & 3	83	3	0
Striffeler et al[20]	67	2	72	4	6
Cassina et al[18]	45	2 & 3	82	11	0
Luh et al[21]	210	2 & 3	86	25	3
Wurnig et al[22]	130	2 & 3	97	9	0
Solaini et al[23]	80	2	97	9	0
Chan et al[24]	41	2 & 3	100	22	0

Adapted from Miller DL. Empyema. In: Selke F, del Nido PJ, Swanson SJ, editors. Sabiston and Spencer's Surgery of the Chest. 8th edition. Philadelphia: Saunders Elsevier; 2010. p. 413–27.

SURGICAL MANAGEMENT OF CHRONIC EMPYEMA

Causes of a chronic empyema are multiple and include delay in diagnosis, ineffective drainage in the acute phase, continued infection such as a bronchopleural fistula (BPF) or lung abscess, as well as the presence of a foreign body. The lung at this stage is incompletely reexpanded and obliteration of the pleural space has not been achieved. Surgical interventions for this phase of empyema include decortication, rib resection with open window thoracostomy, or placement of a long-term empyema tube.

Once an empyema organizes into the fibrinopurulent phase, closed-chest drainage will not be effective in relieving the pleural space infection. In cases in which the empyema has reached an organized phase with significant lung entrapment and the patient is an acceptable surgical candidate, decortication of the affected lung remains an effective procedure for the treatment of their empyema. This procedure is generally approached through a posterior-lateral thoracotomy. In a series of 40 patients, Melloni and colleagues[26] reported 100% resolution of the empyemas and with no mortality. Five patients (12.5%) experienced complications, including two with prolonged febrile syndrome and three with sepsis requiring mechanical ventilation. Multivariable analysis found that symptom duration greater than 60 days and duration of conservative management with drainage alone were associated with increased morbidity. Thoracotomy with decortication remains the mainstay for the treatment of organized empyema. Complete decortication with reexpansion of the lung is essential for success. The authors have found it useful to reexpand the lung after partially decorticating it to ensure that we are in the correct plane. There is frequently a very thin peel that remains on the lung, preventing reexpansion, and it is imperative to complete the decortication in the correct plane. Importantly, this requires adequate exposure. The thoracotomy should be centered over the infection and a counterincision may be required between different ribs to facilitate a safe and complete procedure.

In patients that are poor surgical candidates with sufficient fibrous adhesions between the parietal pleura and visceral pleura, chronic empyemas may be managed with large drainage chest tubes or open-window thoracostomy. In the case of chronic empyema with significant adhesions between pleura, a chest tube may be slowly retracted over the course of weeks to months while the infected space heals behind it. This is an effective means of managing patients with chronic empyemas as outpatients with close surveillance. This is also a useful management strategy for post–lung resection empyemas that result from a prolonged air leak and residual pleural space, provided that most of the lung is expanded.

Open-window thoracostomy was first described by Robinson,[27] in 1916, for nontuberculous empyema and Eloesser,[7] in 1935, for tuberculous empyema. This procedure is indicated when long-term drainage is expected. Some advantages of this procedure include the ease with which the cavity can be cleaned and dressings changed. Symbas and colleagues[28] described a modified Eloesser flap procedure using an inverted "U" skin and subcutaneous flap. This modification has become the preferred choice of open-window thoracostomy used by thoracic surgeons. **Figs. 2–4** illustrate the procedure for

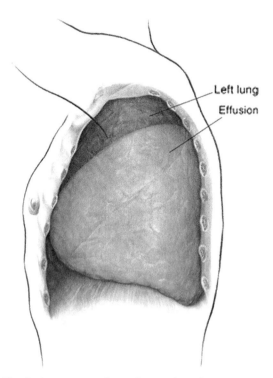

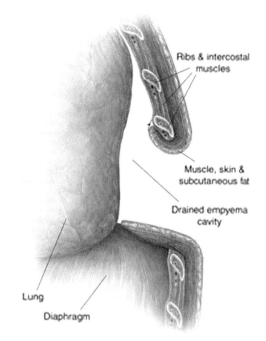

Fig. 2. An empyema shown fromc a lateral perspective. (*From* Denlinger CE. Eloesser flap thoracostomy window. Operat Tech Thorac Cardiovasc Surg 2010;15:61–9; with permission.)

Fig. 4. Coronal view of the Eloesser flap window demonstrating the apposition of the skin surface of the inferiorly based soft tissue flap to the diaphragmatic surface. (*From* Denlinger CE. Eloesser flap thoracostomy window. Operat Tech Thorac Cardiovasc Surg 2010;15:61–9; with permission.)

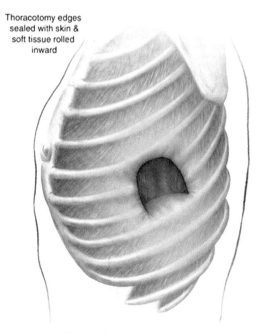

Fig. 3. The inferiorly based soft tissue flap is folded inward against the diaphragm and the skin edges of the flap are secured to the pleural surface using absorbable sutures. (*From* Denlinger CE. Eloesser flap thoracostomy window. Operat Tech Thorac Cardiovasc Surg 2010;15:61–9; with permission.)

creation of a modified Eloesser flap.[29] Thourani and colleagues[30] published their experience with 78 patients undergoing a modified Eloesser flap for empyema. Interventions before open thoracostomy in this group included antibiotics alone (88%), image-directed catheters (14%), tube thoracostomy (77%), and decortication or VATS (29%). In this group, no intraoperative complications occurred, adequate drainage was achieved in all patients, and mortality was 5%. Open drainage is the treatment of choice for debilitated patients with chronic empyemas when a large pleural space exists and prolonged drainage is anticipated. It is imperative to place the window at the inferior aspect of the cavity and to make the chest wall opening large enough to accommodate one's fist. The hole closes faster than expected and needs to be large enough to facilitate healing over several months.

In conjunction with open thoracostomy for chronic empyemas, muscle transposition has been used to obliterate an infected pleural space. Most commonly, rotational muscle flaps using the latissimus dorsi, pectoralis major, or serratus anterior are harvested to eliminate the infected pleural space. The latissimus dorsi flap is the largest of these three

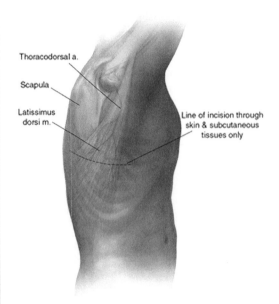

Fig. 5. The latissimus dorsi is the largest chest wall muscle and is a versatile flap that is easily harvested through a standard incision. (*From* Babu AN, Mitchell JD. Technique for muscle flap harvest for intrathoracic use. Operat Tech Thorac Cardiovasc Surg 2010;15: 41–52; with permission.)

flaps and is able to fill approximately 20% to 30% of the thoracic cavity. Its blood supply is based on the thoracodorsal bundle. **Figs. 5** and **6** illustrate the procedure for latissimus dorsi flap creation.[31] Pectoralis major is the second largest muscle and is well-suited for placement in the apical thoracic space. Its blood supply is through the thoracoacromial bundle. **Fig. 7** illustrates the procedure for pectoralis flap creation.[31] Serratus anterior is another option used by thoracic surgeons to fill the infected pleural space. This flap has a long vascular pedicle (thoracodorsal) and relatively low flap complication rate. **Figs. 8** and **9** illustrate the procedure for creation of a serratus anterior flap.[32] Botianu and colleagues[32] reported on 76 consecutive patients who underwent muscle flap creation for chronic empyemas. In their series, 148 flaps were constructed with 60 serratus anterior, 55 latissimus dorsi, 27 pectoralis, and 6 subscapularis. Mortality in the series was 5%, hospital stay averaged 40 days, and all patients were discharged with healed wounds. The authors have found it difficult to obliterate an infected pleural space with muscle flaps. However, they can be very useful in buttressing repairs, such as BPF (see later discussion), and helping to decrease the size of the infected pleural

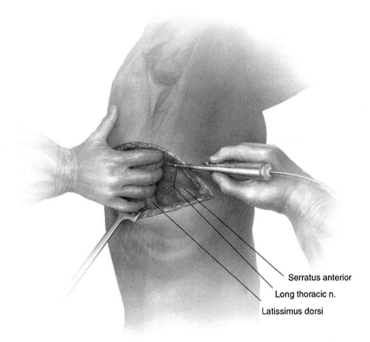

Fig. 6. The anterior border of the latissimus dorsi is identified and retracted outward. The undersurface of the latissimus dorsi is separated from the underlying serratus muscle using electrocautery. (*From* Babu AN, Mitchell JD. Technique for muscle flap harvest for intrathoracic use. Operat Tech Thorac Cardiovasc Surg 2010:15;41–52; with permission.)

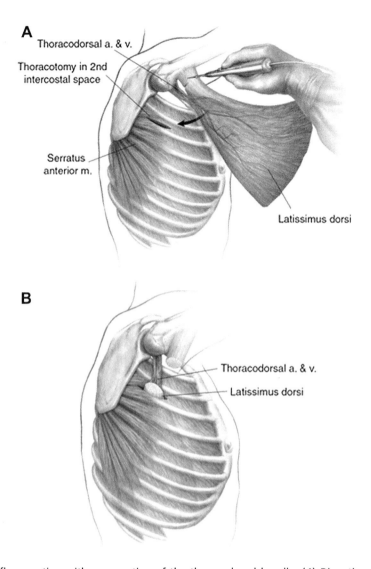

Fig. 7. Pectoralis flap creation with preservation of the thoracodorsal bundle. (*A*) Dissection of the latissimus dorsi muscle flap. (*B*) Intrathoracic transposition of the muscle flap. (*From* Babu AN, Mitchell JD. Technique for muscle flap harvest for intrathoracic use. Operat Tech Thorac Cardiovasc Surg 2010;15;41–52; with permission.)

space. The other flap that may be of significant value is an omental flap brought through the diaphragm and used in the hilum or at the base of the thoracic cavity.

BPF

BPF is a complex form of empyema and represents a major challenge to thoracic surgeons. This is most commonly a complication of pulmonary resection. The overall incidence of BPF following pulmonary resection is estimated to be between 1.6% and 2.7% and two-thirds

of these patients have received neoadjuvant therapy.[33,34]

Following lobectomy or sublobar resection, the diagnosis of a BPF is suggested by a continuous air-leak through the chest tube or failure to maintain lung expansion. After pneumonectomy, the pleural space fills with fluid and the presence of a new air-fluid level or a new productive cough of rust colored liquid suggest a BPF. Diagnosis is confirmed by bronchoscopy.

The treatment of BPF depends on the cause of its formation: bronchial stump leak or peripheral alveolar leak. In the case of a peripheral alveolar leak,

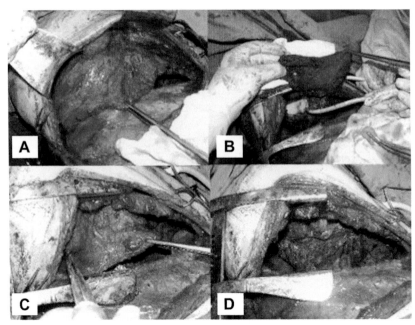

Fig. 8. Creation of a serratus anterior flap. (*A, B*) The serratus flap raised from the chest wall and scapula. (*B*) An unresectable pulmonary abscess with a drain and hemostatic sponge inside. (*C*) Intrathoracic transposition of the serratus flap. (*D*) The pulmonary cavity is completely filled with the muscle, which is secured inside the abscess with a few separate stitches. (*From* Botianu PV, Botianu AM, Dobrica AC, et al. Intrathoracic transposition of the serratus anterior muscle flap–personal experience with 65 consecutive patients. Eur J Cardiothorac Surg 2010;38:669–73; with permission.)

conservative management with suction drainage of the pleural cavity is performed. If the lung reexpands and there is good pleural apposition, these leaks will typically heal. If there is a large residual

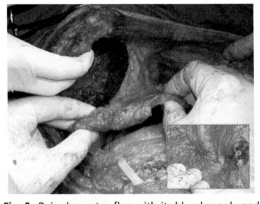

Fig. 9. Raised serratus flap with its blood supply and details with the origin of the main blood supply from the thoracodorsal vessels. (*From* Botianu PV, Botianu AM, Dobrica AC, et al. Intrathoracic transposition of the serratus anterior muscle flap–personal experience with 65 consecutive patients. Eur J Cardiothorac Surg 2010;38:669–73; with permission.)

space, the space may become infected and require intervention with prolonged closed drainage or the creation of open drainage after the remainder of the lung has scarred to the parietal pleura. If a bronchial stump leak is present, surgical intervention with a Clagett procedure, as described by Clagett and Geraci,[35] may be beneficial. This procedure consists of closure of the bronchial stump, reinforcement of the stump with a muscle flap, and pleural space drainage. **Fig. 10** illustrates bronchial stump reinforcement with the latissimus dorsi following a BPF repair. Once the space is clean, pleural sterilization is performed using intrapleural instillation of antibiotics followed by chest closure.

Zaheer and colleagues[36] reported on 84 patients with postpneumonectomy empyema of whom 55% had associated BPF all treated with the Clagett procedure. All BPFs remained closed in patients and 81% had a healed chest without evidence of infection. Massera and colleagues[37] have demonstrated that both late presentation of BPF and performing immediate open window thoracostomy are independent predictors of successful closure of open window thoracostomy. The authors advocate early open window thoracostomy for BPF presentation.

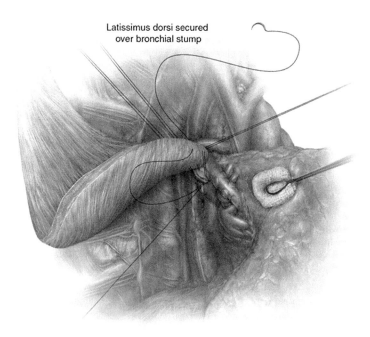

Latissimus dorsi secured
over bronchial stump

Fig. 10. Reinforcement of a bronchial stump leak with a latissimus dorsi flap for a BPF. (*From* Babu AN, Mitchell JD. Technique for muscle flap harvest for intrathoracic use. Operat Tech Thorac Cardiovasc Surg 2010; 15;41–52; with permission.)

SUMMARY

Empyema remains a major source of morbidity and health care expenditure in the thoracic surgery community. Early intervention of pleural space infections is key to prevention of chronic empyemas and the need for surgical intervention. The advent of VATS has made it possible to treat stage I and stage II empyemas with significantly less morbidity. Although management of chronic empyema remains a significant challenge, current surgical interventions are largely successful in clearing the pleural space infection.

REFERENCES

1. Colice GL, Curtis A, Deslauriers J, et al. Medical and surgical treatment of parapneumonic effusions: an evidence-based guideline. Chest 2000;118: 1158–71.
2. Chadwick J. The medical works of Hippocrates. Springfield (IL): Charles Thomas; 1950.
3. Paget S. Empyema. In: Paget S, editor. The surgery of the chest. New York: EB Treat; 1897. p. 204–9.
4. Playfair GE. Case of empyema treated with aspiration and subsequent drainage: recovery. Br Med J 1875;1:45.
5. Hewitt LF. Thoracentesis: the place of continuous aspiration. Br Med J 1876;1:317.
6. Graham EA. Some fundamental considerations in the treatment of empyema thoracis. St Louis (MO): CV Mosby; 1925.
7. Eloesser L. An operation for tuberculous empyema. Surg Gynecol Obstet 1935;60:1096.
8. Wakabayashi A. Extended application of diagnostic and therapeutic thoracoscopy. J Thorac Cardiovasc Surg 1991;102:721.
9. Huang HC, Chang HY, Chen CW, et al. Predicting factors for outcome of tube thoracostomy in complicated parapneumonic effusion or empyema. Chest 1999;115(3):751–6.
10. Bouros D, Schiza S, Tzanakis N, et al. Intrapleural urokinase versus normal saline in the treatment of complicated parapneumonic effusions and empyema. Am J Respir Crit Care Med 1999; 159(1):37–42.
11. Davies RJO, Traill ZC, Gleeson FV. Randomised controlled trial of intrapleural streptokinase in community acquired pleural infection. Thorax 1997; 52:416–21.
12. Tuncozgur B, Ustunsoy H, Dikensoy O, et al. Intrapleuravel urokinase in the management of parapneumonic empyema: a randomised controlled trial. Int J Clin Pract 2001;55(10):658–60.
13. Diacon AH, Theron J, Schuurmans MM, et al. Intrapleural streptokinase for empyema and complicated parapneumonic effusions. Am J Respir Crit Care Med 2004;170(1):49–53.

14. Maskell NA, Davies CW, Nunn AJ, et al. First Multi-center Intrapleural Sepsis Trial (MIST1) Group. U.K. Controlled trial of intrapleural streptokinase for pleural infection. N Engl J Med 2005;352(9): 865–74.

15. Misthos P, Sepsas E, Konstantinou M, et al. Early use of intrapleural fibrinolytics in the management of postpneumonic empyema. A prospective study. Eur J Cardiothorac Surg 2005;28(4):599–603.

16. Cameron R, Davies HR. Intra-pleural fibrinolytic therapy versus conservative management in the treatment of adult parapneumonic effusions and empyema. Cochrane Database Syst Rev 2008;2:CD002312.

17. Angelillo Mackinlay TA, Lyons GA, Chimondeguy DJ, et al. VATS debridement versus thoracotomy in the treatment of loculated postpneumonia empyema. Ann Thorac Surg 1996;61:1626–30.

18. Cassina PC, Hauser M, Hillejan L, et al. Video-assisted thoracoscopy in the treatment of pleural empyema: stage-based management and outcome. J Thorac Cardiovasc Surg 1999;117(2):234–8.

19. Landreneau RJ, Keenan RJ, Hazelrigg SR, et al. Thoracoscopy for empyema and hemothorax. Chest 1996;109(1):18–24.

20. Striffeler H, Gugger M, Im Hof V, et al. Video-assisted thoracoscopic surgery for fibrinopurulent pleural empyema in 67 patients. Ann Thorac Surg 1998; 65(2):319–23.

21. Luh SP, Chou MC, Wang LS, et al. Video-assisted thoracoscopic surgery in the treatment of complicated parapneumonic effusions or empyemas: outcome of 234 patients. Chest 2005;127(4): 1427–32.

22. Wurnig PN, Wittmer V, Pridun NS, et al. Video-assisted thoracic surgery for pleural empyema. Ann Thorac Surg 2006;81(1):309–13.

23. Solaini L, Prusciano F, Bagioni P. Video-assisted thoracic surgery in the treatment of pleural empyema. Surg Endosc 2007;21(2):28.

24. Chan DT, Sihoe AD, Chan S, et al. Surgical treatment for empyema thoracis: is video-assisted thoracic surgery "better" than thoracotomy? Ann Thorac Surg 2007;84(1):225–31.

25. Wozniak CJ, Paull DE, Moezzi JE, et al. Choice of first intervention is related to outcomes in the management of empyema. Ann Thorac Surg 2009; 87(5):1525–30.

26. Melloni G, Carretta A, Ciriaco P, et al. Decortication for chronic parapneumonic empyema: results of a prospective study. World J Surg 2004;28(5):488–93.

27. Robinson S. The treatment of chronic non-tuberculous empyema. Surg Gynecol Obstet 1916;22:557.

28. Symbas PN, Nugent JT, Abbott OA, et al. Non-tuberculous empyema in adults. Ann Thorac Surg 1971; 12:69.

29. Denlinger CE. Eloesser flap thoracostomy window. Operat Tech Thorac Cardiovasc Surg 2010;15:61–9.

30. Thourani VH, Lancaster RT, Mansour KA, et al. Twenty-six years of experience with the modified eloesser flap. Ann Thorac Surg 2003;76:401–5.

31. Babu AN, Mitchell JD. Technique for muscle flap harvest for intrathoracic use. Operat Tech Thorac Cardiovasc Surg 2010;15:41–52.

32. Botianu PV, Botianu AM, Dobrica AC, et al. Intrathoracic transposition of the serratus anterior muscle flap–personal experience with 65 consecutive patients. Eur J Cardiothorac Surg 2010;38:669–73.

33. Malave G, Foster ED, Wilson JA, et al. Bronchopleural fistula: present day study of an old problem. Ann Thorac Surg 1971;11:1.

34. Vester SR, Faber LP, Kittle F, et al. Bronchopleural fistula after stapled closure of bronchus. Ann Thorac Surg 1991;52:1253.

35. Clagett OT, Geraci JE. A procedure for the management of post-pneumonectomy empyema. J Thorac Cardiovasc Surg 1963;45:141.

36. Zaheer S, Allen MS, Cassivi SD, et al. Postpneumonectomy empyema: results after the Clagett procedure. Ann Thorac Surg 2006;82:279.

37. Massera F, Robustellini M, Pona CD, et al. Predictors of successful closure of open window thoracostomy for postpneumonectomy empyema. Ann Thorac Surg 2006;82:288–92.

Index

Note: Page numbers of article titles are in **boldface** type.

Thorac Surg Clin 22 (2012) 441–448
http://dx.doi.org/10.1016/S1547-4127(12)00040-0
1547-4127/12/$ – see front matter © 2012 Elsevier Inc. All rights reserved.

Moving?

Make sure your subscription moves with you!

To notify us of your new address, find your **Clinics Account Number** (located on your mailing label above your name), and contact customer service at:

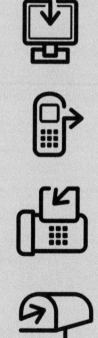

Email: journalscustomerservice-usa@elsevier.com

800-654-2452 (subscribers in the U.S. & Canada)
314-447-8871 (subscribers outside of the U.S. & Canada)

Fax number: 314-447-8029

Elsevier Health Sciences Division
Subscription Customer Service
3251 Riverport Lane
Maryland Heights, MO 63043

Printed and bound by CPI Group (UK) Ltd, Croydon, CR0 4YY

03/10/2024

01040359-0011